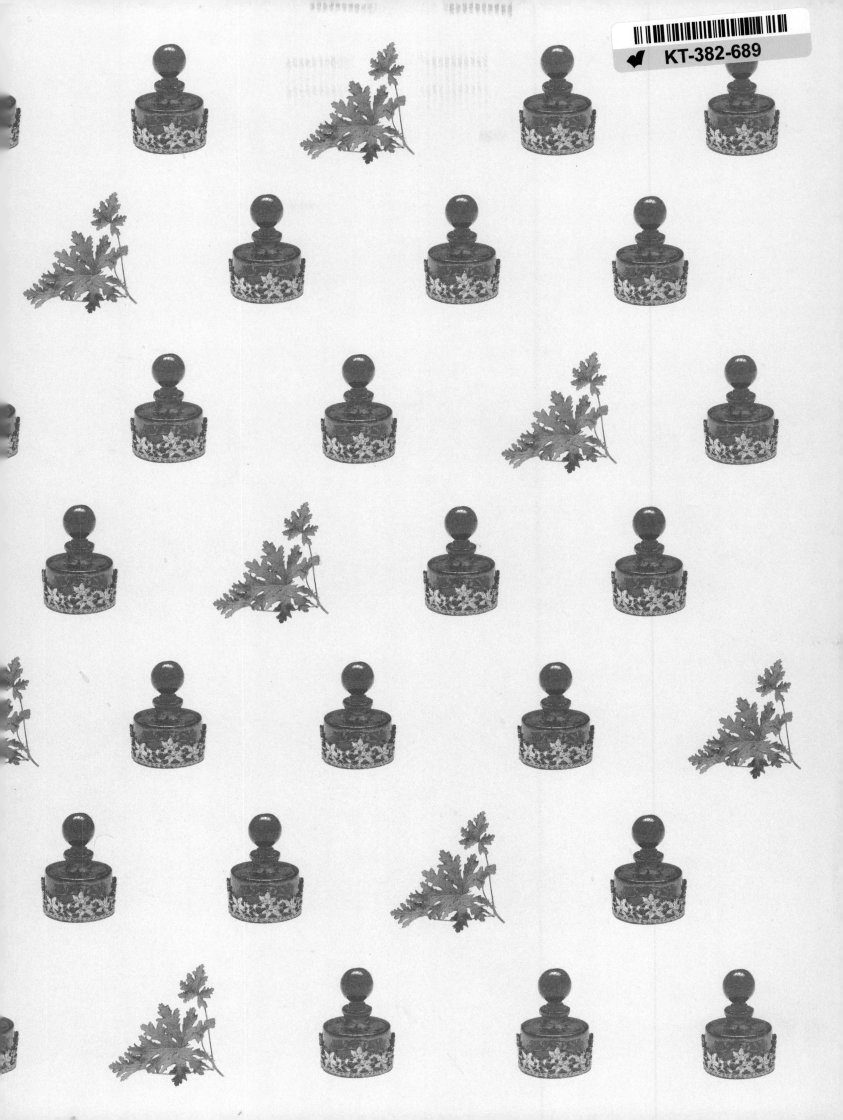

THE BOOK OF
MASSAGE &
AROMATHERAPY

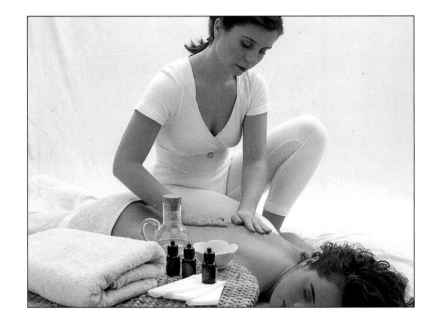

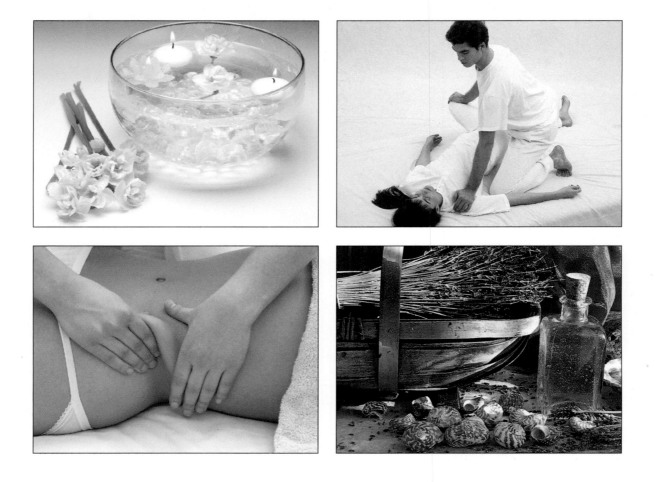

THE BOOK OF
MASSAGE &
AROMATHERAPY

Nitya Lacroix & Sharon Seager

Special Photography by Alistair Hughes

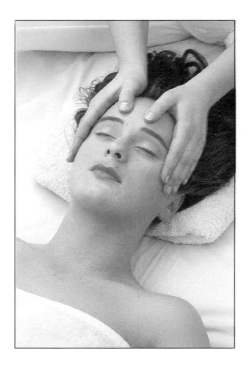

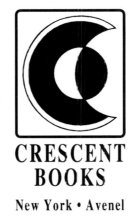

CRESCENT
BOOKS

New York • Avenel

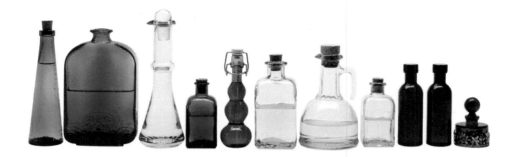

This 1997 edition published by Crescent Books, a division of
Random House Value Publishing, Inc., 201 East 50th Street, New York, NY 10022

Crescent Books and colophon are trademarks of Random House Value Publishing, Inc.

Random House
New York · Toronto · London · Sydney · Auckland
Http://www.randomhouse.com/

© Anness Publishing Limited 1994

Produced by
Anness Publishing Limited
Hermes House
88-89 Blackfriars Road
London SE1 8HA

ISBN 0-517-10256-0

A CIP catalogue record for this book is available from the British Library

Printed and bound in Singapore by Star Standard Industries Pte. Ltd.

3 5 7 9 10 8 6 4 2

PUBLISHER'S NOTE

The reader should not regard the recommendations, ideas, and techniques expressed and described in
this book as substitutes for the advice of a qualified medical practitioner. Any use to which the
recommendations, ideas, and techniques are put is at the reader's sole discretion and risk.

Contents

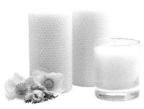

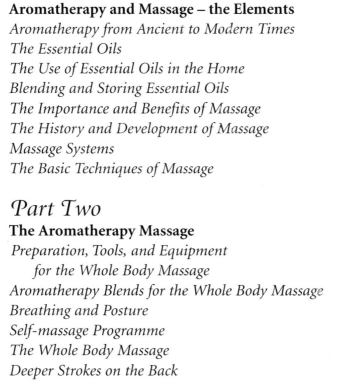

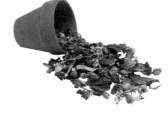

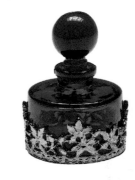

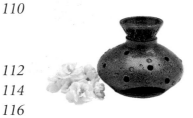

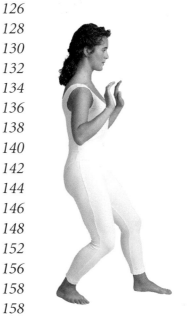

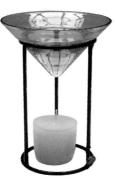

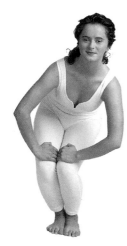

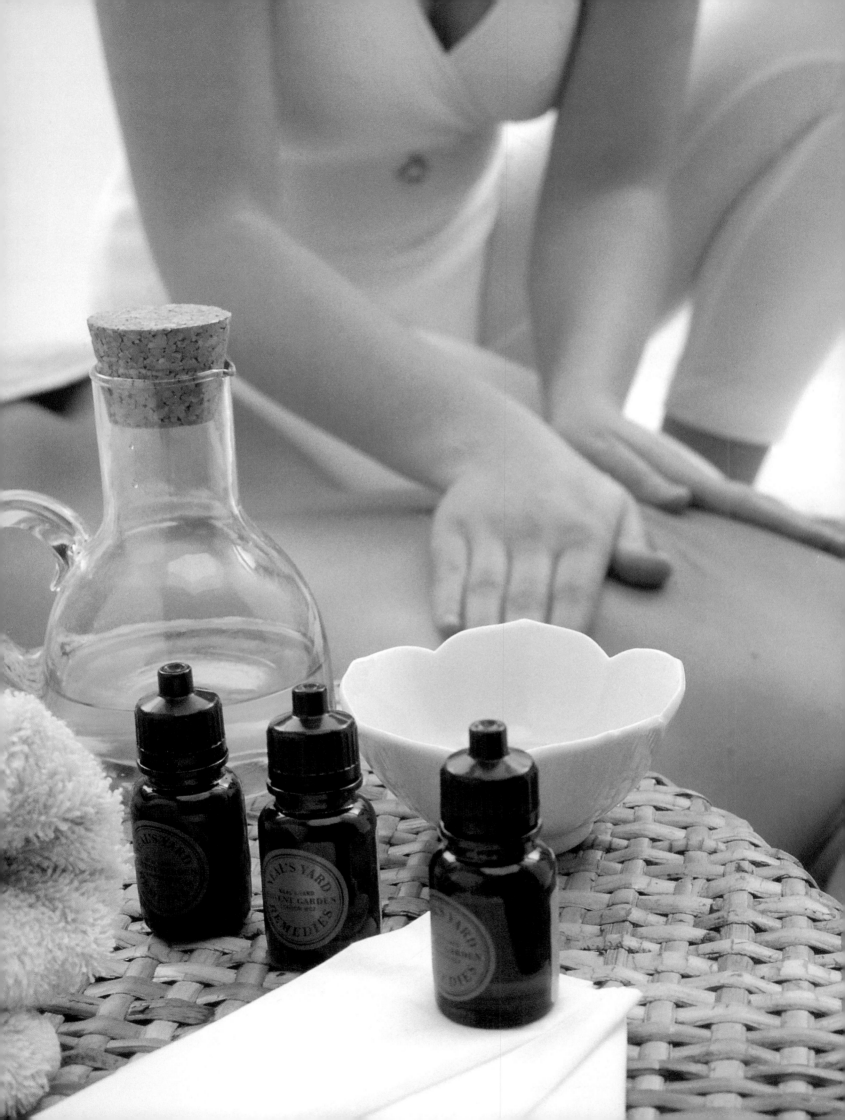

Preface

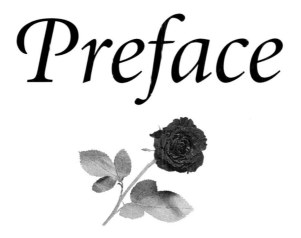

Writing about aromatherapy massage has given us the opportunity to pool our knowledge about two of the main sources of natural healing – the power of touch, which evokes changes in body, mind, and spirit, and aromatic plants, which bring remedial benefits to the whole person.

Together, the skills of massage through which touch is applied in the caring application of strokes and techniques, and a knowledge of the therapeutic properties of essential oils, form a potent healing art. Our hope is that the reader can learn from this book, not only to gain new skills, but to be able to bring comfort and pleasure, relaxation and invigoration, to friends and family. There is something tremendously satisfying about being able to respond positively to another's need, whether it is in the physical or emotional dimension. We hope the reader will discover that it is just as rewarding to give an aromatherapy massage as it is to receive one. Of course, there are few experiences more luxurious, relaxing, and nourishing than to receive a whole body massage with the added benefits of essential oils, which have been carefully selected and blended according to your needs. While the hands relax and soothe the body and mind, the oils work their intrinsic aromatic magic, to uplift the spirits, and balance the whole system.

Finally, we hope the reader will use this book to embark on a joyful journey of discovery that demonstrates how to use and then share some of nature's finest gifts.

Part One
Aromatherapy & Massage — the Elements

The association of aromatherapy with massage is not a new one. Indeed the beneficial effects of both were known to the ancients, who in their healing arts combined the use of essential oils from herbs and other plants with therapeutic strokes. In Part One the basic elements of aromatherapy and massage are examined separately in preparation for the demonstrations and discussions of how they work together that are detailed in Parts Two and Three.

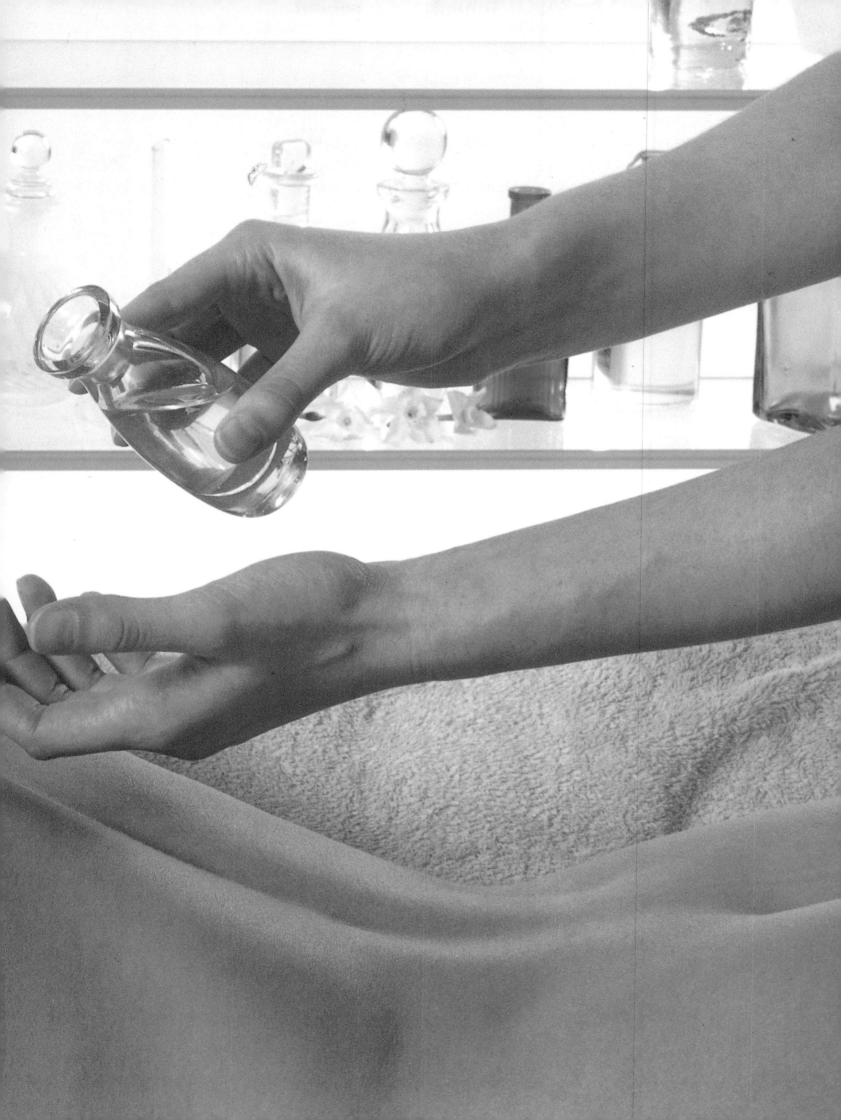

Aromatherapy – from Ancient to Modern Times

There is well-documented evidence from the great civilizations of the past to indicate that the use of herbs and aromatics in ancient times was commonplace, and that a large body of knowledge existed concerning the properties of these plants. During the intervening millennia much of this knowledge was lost or ignored, and the importance of herbs and aromatics in holistic healing was devalued. It is only relatively recently that the wisdom of ancient healers in the application of essential oils has been rediscovered.

The Ancient Egyptians applied their knowledge of aromatic plants to almost all aspects of life. They used them for healing, as ingredients in cosmetics, and in burial rituals such as mummification. A papyrus dating from 1550 BC, unearthed in 1875, details the recipes for treating a variety of ailments, which are very similar to the remedies we might use today.

The Chinese, too, used aromatics for religious practices as well as for health, and applied them during massage as an additional means of maintaining a healthy body. The Chinese knowledge of herbs some 2500 years BC is documented in *The Yellow Emperor's Classic of Internal Medicine*, written by the Emperor Kiwang-Ti. More than 4000 years later, after 26 years of study, Li Shih-Chên published the *Pên T'sao* (1579), an enormous and valuable volume in which he recorded the use of 2000 herbs and 20 essential oils. This book documents the greatest range of herbs studied in any tradition.

In India the traditional Ayervedic medical practice was developed from 2000-year-old texts, which list 700 useful aromatics, all valued for their spiritual and health-giving properties. There, as in China, the principal aspect of this form of medicine was the aromatic massage.

Aromatic substances were one of the earliest traded goods, rare and highly prized. Phoenician merchants spread the trade of aromatic material into the Arabian peninsula and across the Mediterranean to Greece and Rome. The Greek physician Marestheus first recorded the stimulating and sedative qualities of different aromatic flowers, and in the 1st century AD Dioscorides compiled the *Herbarius,* a five-volume study of the sources and uses of plants and aromatics. This became the standard medical treatise for the following thousand years.

Distilling

Revolutionary developments in science that began during the Renaissance led to the analysis and study of an increasing number of essential oils and other aromatic substances. The famous perfume industry in Grasse, France, developed, and by the end of the 17th century the distinction between apothecaries, who dealt with herbs for medicinal purposes, and the perfume manufacturers, was quite pronounced. The advent of mechanized printing meant that the publication of popular herbals became possible, making texts such as *Banckes' Herbal* (1527) available to a wider public.

Such changes gave a background against which modern aromatherapy could develop. In 17th-century England, Nicholas Culpeper, John Parkinson, and John Gerarde, among others, led the way in what was the Golden Age of English herbalism. At the same time natural philosophy that had been such an important part of the alchemists work was left behind to be developed in isolation by artists and thinkers. This development marked the beginning of the separation of body and spirit that is so evident in medical practice today.

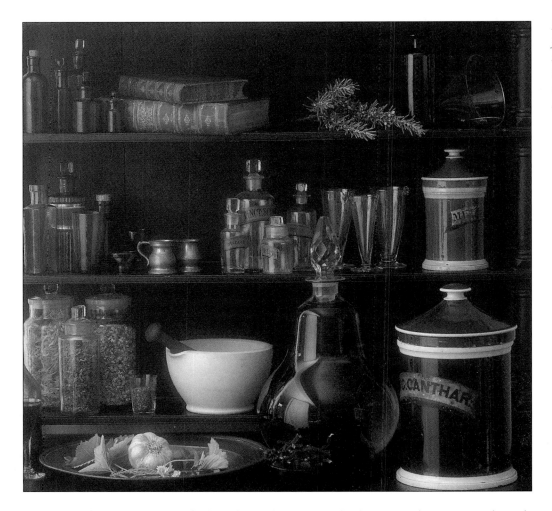

Practitioners of the healing arts have for thousands of years relied on herbs and other aromatic plants to treat illness. Many of the common herbs they used are plants from which essential oils are extracted.

During this time, as scientific knowledge about essential oils grew, their use in medicine became less important, and the concept of holism was lost, albeit temporarily. In the mid 17th century the separation between the traditional herbalists and the physicians who favoured chemical drug therapy began. However, at the same time philosophers exploring alchemy further refined the art of distillation, allowing more and more aromatic essences to be created for a wide range of uses.

The Modern Art and Practice

The French doctor and scientist René-Maurice Gattefossé is the 20th-century father of modern aromatherapy. Gattefossé is credited with coining the name "aromatherapy" to describe treatments with essential oils. His main achievement was to discover the powerfully antiseptic nature of many essential oils. He also discovered that the essential oils are more powerful in their natural state than when their active chemicals are used in isolation. Gattefossé published the results of his findings in his book *Aromathérapie*, published in 1937.

Many of those who came after Gattefossé helped to rediscover the link between the mind and spirit and healthy bodies. The Frenchman Jean Valnet, also a doctor and scientist, used essential oils to treat wounds during the Second World War, as well as to treat specific illnesses. Today in France there are many medical doctors prescribing essential oils for internal use to heal ailments.

Valnet's work was taken up and developed by Madame Marguerite Maury, a beauty therapist who was interested in incorporating essential oils into her treatments. Her principle was to revitalize each client by using a personal aromatic blend, which she based on the individual's temperament and specific health disorders. Madame Maury was dissatisfied with the oral administration of essential oils, and rediscovered the method of applying them in diluted form during massage, as had been practised by the ancient healers.

Today, widespread use is made of aromatherapy in many fields of conventional medicine. Aromatherapy has been found to be useful in the care of patients suffering long-term illnesses such as cancer and AIDS. Most imaginatively, it has recently been used by volunteers working with orphaned children in Romania, and one enterprising South African teacher uses essential oils to create a calm atmosphere of learning and concentration in her township nursery school.

The Essential Oils

An essential oil is the essence of a plant, or its personality, the plant's life force distilled for use. The fragrance and character of each oil are as individual and unique as a finger print, as are its therapeutic properties and the effects they have on the individuals.

Essential oils are natural, volatile substances that evaporate readily, quickly releasing their aroma into the air, as happens, for example, when someone brushes against an aromatic plant in a garden. The Germans refer to essential oils as "ethereal oils", which is a much more accurate and a more evocative name. Approximately 300 essential oils are commercially available, but of these only 50 to 100 have health giving properties and are suitable for home use and for the aromatherapist.

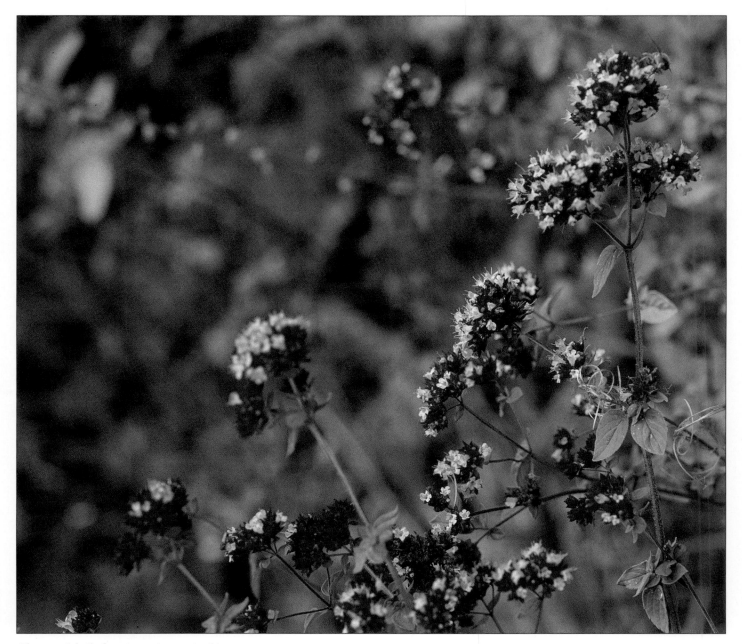

The essential oil of marjoram is contained in tiny hairs on the surface of the leaves.

A fragrance may conjure up a vivid image from the past – perhaps of a secluded garden visited in childhood. Both memory and emotion are linked to our sense of smell; all three are governed by the same area of the brain, the limbic system.

Sources and Properties of Essential Oils

Not all plants contain essential oils. In those that do the oil, or essence, is contained in highly specialized glands that are present in the foliage, flower, or other plant material. The purpose of the oil is to help prevent water loss in the plant. As the oils evaporate they create a barrier around the leaf or other plant part, and so reduce water loss through evaporation in the plant itself. Essential oils may also provide some defence against infection, and attract insects that are vital to pollination.

The plants that contain essential oils are found mainly in hot, dry habitats. In some plants, such as marjoram, the essential oil glands are present in the minute hairs on the leaves, but in woody plants such as rosewood they are embedded in the fibrous bark or wood. In others the oil glands can be seen clearly as shiny, coloured discs on the surface of the leaf or flower.

At certain times of the day, and particular times of the year, the essential oils are present at optimum levels, and this is the best time for harvest and distillation. The amount of oil produced by a

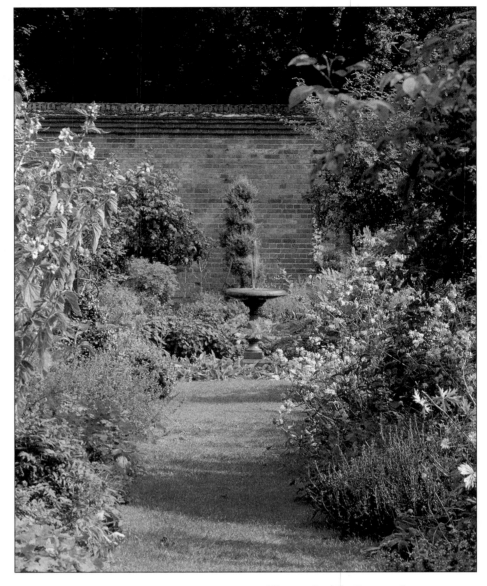

plant is also affected by the growing conditions, including the type of soil, the amount of sunlight it receives, and rainfall.

Essential oils have a consistency similar to that of water and most are lighter than water, although benzoin is an example of an essence that is heavier. All of them differ from vegetable oils in that they are not greasy. Most are colourless; those that are coloured include bergamot, which is green, lemon oil, which is yellow, and chamomile, blue.

Chemical Constituents

The chemicals present in essential oils are acids, alcohols, aldehydes, ketones, esters, phenols, oxides, and terpenes. Each of these chemicals has its own properties, and these are imparted to the essential oil when the chemical is present in large quantities. The chemical complexity of essential oils is responsible for their various characteristics and the actions they produce in the body.

A particular oil may contain between 50-500 different chemicals. Rose oil contains the greatest number, some of which are found in such minute quantities that they have not yet been identified. This has made it impossible to reproduce accurately the most exquisite of the essential oils.

The chemicals in essential oils unlock the body's ability to heal. They enter the body through the skin and are carried to all parts in the blood, after which they are

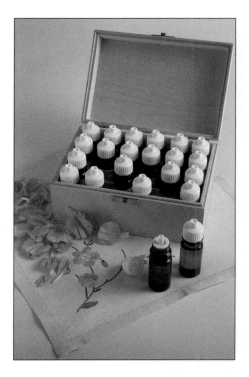

In the distillation process the plant is placed in a sealed container. Water in a second container is heated to produce steam, which is passed under pressure through the plant material. The steam causes the glands containing the essence to burst, allowing the volatile chemicals to dissolve in the steam. This rises and is taken into a condensing chamber, where it is cooled. As it cools the oil is separated from the water. Floral water is a by-product of distilling, and like essential oil has therapeutic and commercial uses.

A different process, solvent extraction, is favoured for releasing essential oil from more delicate material, such as jasmine flowers. The plant material is washed with a solvent such as alcohol until the essence dissolves. The resulting material is then distilled at a precise temperature to separate the solvent and the aromatic oil. Oil made by this process is known as an absolute.

Buying the Finest Oils

For the best results use only the finest oils. In general, price is an excellent guide to quality, and it is wise to compare various suppliers' prices so that you can recognize an extremely expensive oil and

excreted through the lungs and in urine. Diluting the oils delays their passage through the body but does not detract from the efficacy of the essential oils. After a treatment the essential oil remains in the body for three to four hours, activating the healing process, which can continue for two to three weeks.

Essential oils are able to influence all aspects of the body's functions, from tissues to organs, to body fluids and cells, as well as the emotional state and the spiritual aspects of the person.

Extracting Essential Oils

Most essential oils are produced by distillation or expression. Generally, because of the fragile nature of the raw material, the processing takes place in the country of origin. More robust materials, such as wood, bark, and seeds, are sometimes exported for distillation elsewhere. Herbs and flowers can be distilled fresh or dried, and hardier material such as wood needs to be chipped or even powdered before processing can begin The citrus oils, which contain their essence in the peel of the fruit, are all expressed (squeezed), often by hand. Other essential oils are produced by dry, water, or steam distillation.

The commonest method of production is steam distillation. By this method the volatile and water soluble parts are separated from the rest of the plant. The resulting mixture may need to be distilled a second time to remove non-volatile matter.

The Mechanics of Smelling

When the scent of something is inhaled, the odour molecules float to the back of the nasal cavity. Here they dissolve in the moist environment, and in this form unite with receptor, or olfactory cells. The olfactory cells then trigger off electrical signals via the nerve pathways to the olfactory bulb in the brain. Most of the essential oil molecules that have triggered the system are breathed out, although some will enter the blood stream via the lungs. Only eight molecules of an odoriferous substance are needed to trigger the smell mechanism.

The areas of the brain to which messages concerning smell are sent are the cerebral cortex and limbic system. The limbic system controls many vital activities, such as sleep, sexual drive, hunger, and thirst, as well as smell. This is also

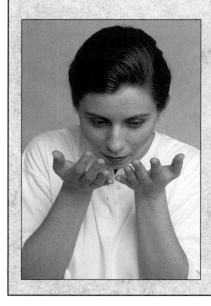

the area of the brain that relates to emotion and memory, and thereby gives the clue to the link between smell, emotion, and memory. Odours also connect with the part of the brain called the hypothalamus, which controls the endocrine system and nervous system. Through this mechanism the brain comes into direct contact with the outside world.

The fading of a scent occurs when all the receptor cells are full, but after ten minutes or so they are vacated and can be reoccupied, causing the scent to "come back". This explains why we may fail to notice a scent after a while, while a person just entering the same area may comment on it.

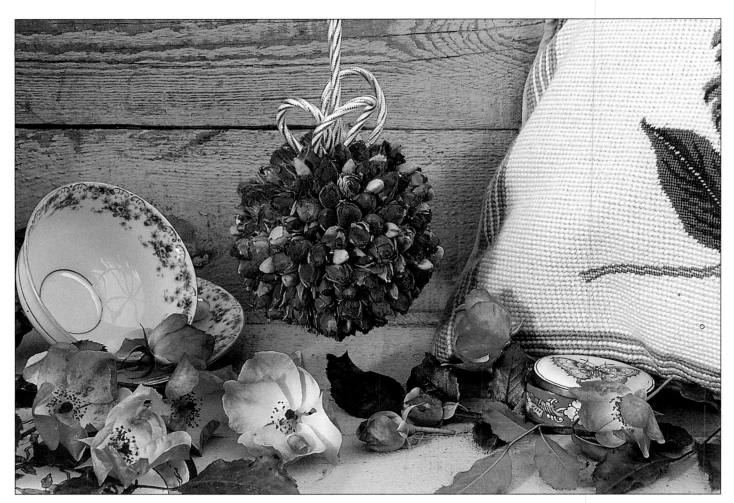

an unbelievably cheap one. Be aware that essential oils are easily adulterated, and do not be misled by unscrupulous marketing practices. For example, there is no such thing as cheap rose oil; cheap rose oil is probably a similar-smelling product to which geranium or palmarosa oil has been added. Rosemary is another oil that may be adulterated by the addition of camphor or eucalyptus.

If you buy from a reputable source you will also avoid those unscrupulous manufacturers who, although offering a pure essential oil, market oils from a second or third distillation. These will contain only a few active ingredients; the majority will have been removed during the first processing.

When purchasing essential oils it is best to know the Latin, or scientific name, of each oil, which is in fact the name of the plant from which it comes. Most reputable suppliers put this name on the label of the bottle. The bottle containing the oil should be of dark glass and have a stopper incorporating a drop dispenser. If you are in any doubt about where to purchase oils, seek the advice of a qualified practitioner, who will recommend a reputable retail supplier.

Oil Profiles

Twenty-eight essential oils are profiled in the following pages. They constitute the main oils that are suitable for use in the home and that play a large part in the aromatherapist's practice. The oils are arranged alphabetically by their Latin names.

Essential oils are used to produce a variety of fragrant objects, such as scented candles (below), pot pourri and pomanders (above).

ANTHEMIS NOBILIS
Roman Chamomile

There is a long tradition of use for this gentle yet strengthening herb. The Moors and Egyptians recognized its calming qualities and the Saxons used it as part of their mixture of nine sacred herbs in an incense known as "maythen". There are several varieties of chamomile from which essential oils are obtained, but the most commonly used are Roman chamomile and German chamomile (Matricaria chamomilla). They have similar properties, although they differ in appearance. Roman chamomile is a creeping perennial with tiny, needle-like leaves; German chamomile is a taller, upright annual with fragile, feathery leaves. Both have small white, daisy-like flowers. The essential oil of German chamomile has a larger proportion of the anti-inflammatory chemical azulene, which is useful for treating skin conditions.

Applications and Effects

Calming. Particularly effective for teething pain, headaches.

Skin and teeth: Acne, allergies, boils, burns, chilblains, earache, inflammations, insect bites, toothache.

Circulatory, muscular systems: Arthritis, muscular pain, rheumatism, sprains.

Digestive system: Colic, indigestion, nausea.

Reproductive and excretory systems: Painful periods, menopause, premenstrual syndrome (PMS), cystitis.

Immune system: Thrush, fever.

Nervous system: Insomnia, nervous tension, bed wetting.

Mental/emotional effects: A gently sedative oil for the highly strung and overenthusiastic. Useful where symptoms are related to anger, irritability, or unexpressed emotions.

Precautions
Some people may find it causes dermatitis.

BOSWELLIA THURIFERA
Frankincense

Frankincense (also known as olibanum) is an inspiring and contemplative oil that comes from the gum of a small tree or shrub grown mainly in the Middle East, with most of the oil produced in Iran and Lebanon. The gum is extracted by incising the trunk and peeling away the bark. The oozing juice slowly hardens on contact with the air and is then collected for distillation. The gum was highly prized in ancient times and was known simply by the old French name franc encens, "frank" meaning luxuriant. Frankincense is known primarily in its biblical connection as one of the three gifts to the infant Jesus; at that time its value was almost as great as the value of gold. In Ancient Egypt it was used as an incense in religious ceremonies and in cosmetics, where it was valued for its rejuvenating properties.

Applications and Effects

Particularly effective for mature skin, bronchitis, and anxiety.

Skin: Dry skin, scars, wounds, sores, ulcers.

Respiratory system: Catarrh, coughs, laryngitis, rheumatic conditions.

Reproductive and excretory systems: Cystitis, painful periods, heavy periods.

Immune system: Colds, 'flu.

Nervous system: Nervous tension, fear, nightmares.

Mental/emotional effects: Regulating oil, yet stimulating. This makes it useful in cases of exhaustion and mental fatigue. Useful for those who lack confidence and are weary of spirit. An excellent aid to meditation, as it deepens and slows the breath.

Precautions
Generally completely safe to use.

CANANGA ODORATA
Ylang Ylang

The name ylang ylang means "flower of flowers", and the very fragrant plant is sometimes called "poor man's jasmine". The source of this essential oil is a beautiful evergreen tree native to Madagascar and the Philippines. It is now cultivated in several parts of the world, including Sumatra, Java, and the Comores. The oil comes from the tree's delicate yellow flowers, which have a very sweet scent reminiscent of almonds and jasmine. Many different qualities of oil are available; the finest are said to come from the flowers of trees grown in Réunion and picked in early morning at the beginning of summer. In Indonesia the voluptuously fragrant flowers are ceremonially scattered on the beds of newly married couples. The essential oil is widely used in perfumes and other types of fragrance.

Applications and Effects

Particularly effective for accelerated breathing and palpitations, insomnia, and bowel infections.

Skin: Combination skin.

Circulatory, muscular systems: High blood pressure.

Digestive system: Gastro-enteritis.

Nervous system: Depression, anxiety.

Mental/emotional effects: This exotic, luxurious oil creates a feeling of peace and dispels anger, especially anger born of frustration. Its voluptuous nature is reassuring and builds confidence.

Precautions

Some people may feel headachy or nauseous after using the oil, especially if it is used in concentrated form.

CEDRUS ATLANTICA
Cedarwood

Cedar is a Semitic word meaning "the power of spiritual strength". The tree from which the essential oil is extracted is native to the Atlas mountains of Morocco, but it is now grown more widely, particularly in Lebanon and some parts of the Far East. The majestically tall, pyramid-shaped evergreen gives an oil that embodies the ancient qualities of its name – confidence and firmly rooted spiritual strength. The oil is extracted by steam distillation from the wood of the tree. It was used in ancient times by the Egyptians in the form of a gum, as a main ingredient for the preservation of mummies, and it is thought to be one of the earliest-known oils. The oil is still used today by Tibetans as a temple incense and by natives of North Africa for medicinal purposes.

Applications and Effects

Particularly effective for long-standing complaints rather than acute ones; has aphrodisiac properties.

Skin: Acne, dandruff.

Circulatory, muscular systems: Arthritis, rheumatism, poor circulation.

Respiratory system: Bronchitis, catarrh, coughs, chest infections.

Reproductive and excretory systems: Cystitis.

Mental/emotional effects: This uplifting oil is useful for lack of confidence or fearfulness. It has euphoric properties that help eliminate mental stagnation in depressed states. It is relaxing and soothing and can be a good aid to meditation.

Precautions

Best avoided during pregnancy.

CITRUS AURANTIA
Orange

The essential oil called orange and the preserve, marmalade, come from the small, bitter fruit known as the Seville orange, which differs from the familiar edible, sweet orange Citrus sinensis. C. aurantia has dark, shiny green oval leaves that are pale beneath; the smooth grey-green branches have long blunt spines and the small white flowers are highly fragrant. The plant has become a symbol of both innocence and fertility. The Crusaders brought it back to Europe with them from North Africa and early missionaries introduced it into California. The United States is now one of the main producers of the oil. Because the oil oxidizes very quickly it cannot be kept for very long.

Applications and Effects

Mellow, warming, and soothing. Has similar properties to neroli and can be used in similar conditions.

Skin: Dull and oily complexions, mouth ulcers.

Circulatory, muscular systems: Muscular aches and pains, water retention, detoxifying.

Respiratory system: Bronchitis, chills.

Digestive system: Constipation, colic, indigestion (aids digestion of fats), diarrhoea, stimulates appetite.

Immune system: Colds, 'flu, fevers.

Nervous system: Nervous tension, insomnia due to anxiety.

Mental/emotional effects: Lifts gloomy thoughts and depression and encourages a positive outlook. Useful for replenishing cheerfulness. Revives the spirit when it is lacking in energy and relieves boredom. Quells "butterflies" in the stomach.

Precautions

Generally safe to use, although like other citrus oils it increases the photosensitivity of the skin and can cause irritation under ultraviolet light, particularly from the sun. Occasionally causes dermatitis.

CITRUS AURANTIUM
Neroli

The evergreen tree from which the essential oil is produced is native to China, where it was used by traditional Chinese herbalists. The expressed oil is produced in Israel, Cyprus, Brazil, and North America. It is a less robust and smaller plant than the sour orange variety and without the spiny branches or the heart-shaped leaves. The flowers were traditionally used in wedding bouquets to symbolize innocence and to secure love. Orange flower water features in Eastern European cooking and is an ingredient in eau-de-cologne, which was very popular with those Victorian ladies who would be overcome with the "vapours". Neroli is one of the finest of the floral essences.

Applications and Effects

Simple happiness; nourishing to the soul. Particularly effective for nervous diarrhoea, and stress-related conditions.

Skin: Dull, oily, dry, and sensitive skin, mouth ulcers, broken veins.

Circulatory, muscular systems: Palpitations, poor circulation.

Respiratory system: Bronchitis, chills.

Reproductive and excretory systems: PMS, menopausal symptoms.

Digestive system: Constipation, indigestion, flatulence, nausea.

Immune system: Colds, 'flu.

Nervous system: Nervous tension, headaches, and insomnia.

Mental/emotional effects: Hypnotic and euphoric. Gives a feeling of peace; useful during times of anxiety, panic, hysteria, or shock and fear. Invaluable for soothing when difficulties stem from a relationship. It can help in the development of self-esteem and self-love, comfort the sad, and bring people into contact with their feminine aspect.

Precautions

Distilled oil is phototoxic, but the expressed oil is not. Generally safe to use although some individuals may get dermatitis.

CITRUS BERGAMIA
Bergamot

Bergamot is the name of an ornamental citrus tree that produces a small fruit, which is green at first but later ripens to yellow. The peel of the ripe fruit yields an oil that is mild and gentle. The oil has a sweet, aromatic odour and is one of the main constituents of eau-de-cologne and lavender water, and is also found in some sun tan preparations. It is extracted by expression (squeezing and pressing). The plant is native to tropical Asia and is now cultivated in Italy and on the Ivory Coast. The common name of the plant may have come from the city of Bergamo in northern Italy. Bergamot leaves are used in Earl Grey tea.

Applications and Effects

Particularly effective for boils (to draw out infection), eczema, psoriasis, anxiety, and depression.

Skin: Acne, cold sores, insect bites, insect repellent, oily complexions, especially stress-related, spots, wounds.

Respiratory system: Bad breath, sore throat, tonsillitis, bronchitis.

Digestive system: Flatulence, poor appetite (has a regulating action, which may be useful for anorexia), colic, indigestion.

Reproductive and excretory systems: Cystitis, thrush.

Immune system: Colds, fever, 'flu, cold sores, chicken pox, immune deficiency, herpes.

Nervous system: PMS (mood swings), insomnia, nightmares.

Mental, emotional effects: Its cooling and refreshing action helps soothe anger and frustration. Bergamot is useful for grief; the uplifting nature of this oil makes the bereaved receptive to joy and love, having been blocked to these emotions as a result of their grief.

Precautions

Not to be used before going out into the sun, even when diluted. It can cause discoloration of the skin that results in a rash when oiled skin is exposed to the sun.

CITRUS LIMONUM
Lemon

The lemon tree is native to Asia, although it now grows wild in the Mediterranean, particularly in Spain and Portugal. It is cultivated extensively in many parts of the world, including North and South America, Israel, Guinea, Cyprus, Sicily, and Italy. The tree grows to only 2 m/6½ ft in height; it is evergreen with small serrated oval leaves and highly fragrant pink or white flowers. The fruits ripen from green to yellow. The oil was used by the Ancient Egyptians as an antidote to food poisoning, and to cure epidemics of fever. In most European countries it was regarded as a cure-all, but its main use was as a treatment for infectious diseases.

Applications and Effects

Fresh, strong, and versatile, it harmonizes well and adds character. Particularly effective for arthritis, rheumatism, cellulite, nausea, diarrhoea, and haemorrhoids.

Skin: Acne, brittle nails, boils, chilblains, greasy skin, cold sores, insect bites, mouth ulcers, spots, warts, verrucas, bruises.

Circulatory, muscular systems: Nosebleeds, congestion, poor circulation, muscular aches and pains.

Respiratory system: Throat infections, bronchitis, catarrh, sinusitis.

Digestive system: Indigestion, flatulence, heartburn, constipation.

Nervous system: Headaches, migraine.

Immune system: Colds, 'flu, fever, coughs, infections (chronic and recurrent), candida, allergies.

Mental/emotional effects: Can help refresh and clarify thoughts. Good for feelings of bitterness or resentment about life's injustices, and useful when someone is feeling touchy, or when begrudging others good fortune and success.

Precautions

May sensitize the skin in some individuals. Use with caution if sunbathing as it may cause skin discoloration and rash.

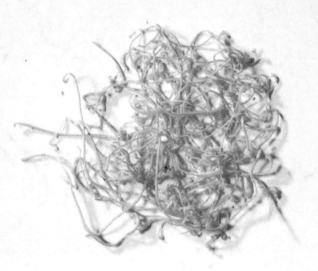

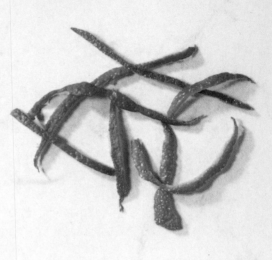

CITRUS PARADISI
Grapefruit

The grapefruit tree is cultivated for its delicious large, yellow fruits. The tree reaches about 10 m/33 ft in height and bears dark glossy leaves and white flowers. It is native to tropical Asia and the West Indies, although it probably originated in Asia as a hybrid of the orange tree. Grapefruit trees are grown as ornamental trees all over the Mediterranean and are also cultivated in Florida, Brazil, and Israel. California is the main producer of the oil. The yield of oil from the fresh peel is small when compared to the yield from the orange and lemon.

Applications and Effects
Cleansing, balancing, brightening, and refreshing. Particularly effective for congested pores and oily skin, cellulite, and the digestion of fatty foods.

Skin: Acne.

Circulatory and muscular systems: Muscle fatigue, exercise preparation, stiffness, water retention, migraine.

Digestive system: Loss of appetite, cleansing the kidneys, liver tonic.

Immune system: Chills, colds, 'flu.

Reproductive and excretory systems: PMS.

Nervous system: Depression, headaches, migraine, performance stress, nervous exhaustion, jet lag, restoration of balance after ear infections.

Mental/emotional effects: Use this uplifting oil when feeling apathetic or indecisive. Its euphoric nature may help with feelings of resentfulness, jealousy, and envy.

Precautions
Presents a very slight risk of producing photosensitivity in the skin. Like other citrus oils it has a relatively short shelf life.

CITRUS RETICULATA
Mandarin

The fruit of the mandarin tree was the ancient and traditional gift to the mandarins of China, where the plant is a native species. It is an evergreen tree with shiny leaves, fragrant white flowers, and the familiar juicy, edible fruit. The tree was introduced to Europe at the beginning of the 19th century, and some 40 years later into the United States. The Americans renamed the tree and fruit the tangerine, but the latter is in fact a larger and rounder fruit with a more yellow skin than the mandarin. The mandarin is grown in Italy, Spain, Algeria, Cyprus, Greece, the Middle East, and Brazil.

Applications and Effects
Refined, soft, cheerful, uplifting, sweet. Particularly effective for congested pores and oily skin, and fluid retention.

Skin: Acne, spots, stretch marks.

Circulatory, muscular systems: Helps to tone and improve the circulation.

Digestive system: Digestive problems, pain, flatulence, heartburn, nausea, hiccups.

Nervous system: Insomnia, restlessness, nervous tension.

Mental/emotional effects: This is a balancing oil that can be relaxing or a tonic, according to the individual's needs. It is good for dejected spirits and feelings of emotional emptiness, or the regretting of the passage of time and losses of the past. It is cheering and uplifting, and brings the message of happiness to children. It also helps adults make contact with their own inner child.

Precautions
Generally safe to use. Other citrus oils are known to cause photosensitivity in the skin, but there have been no conclusive findings for mandarin. However, it should still be used with caution in the sun and under other sources of ultraviolet light.

CUPRESSUS SEMPERVIRENS
Cypress

The cypress tree is a statuesque evergreen that grows wild in southern France, Italy, Spain, Portugal, Corsica, and North Africa. The specific Latin name sempervirens *means "everlasting", and both the Egyptians and Romans dedicated it to their deities of the underworld. The essential oil is yellow and has a rich scent similar to the scent of pine needles. It is extracted from the cones of the plant by steam distillation; the main centres of production are in Europe, in Germany and France.*

Applications and Effects

Useful when there is an excess of fluids in some way. Particularly effective for diarrhoea, water retention, and watery colds.

Skin: Oily and puffy skin, sweaty feet (when blended with peppermint), wounds.

Digestive system: Haemorrhoids.

Circulatory and muscular systems: Cellulite, muscular cramps, poor circulation, rheumatism.

Respiratory system: Bronchitis, spasmodic coughing, 'flu.

Reproductive and excretory systems: Heavy and painful periods, menopausal problems, cystitis.

Nervous system: Nervous tension.

Mental/emotional effects: The solemn nature of cypress makes it useful during periods of transition such as bereavement. It is also helpful at times for feelings of sadness and self-pity. It can be useful for soothing anger and quietening over-talkative people. It is spiritually cleansing and aids the removal of psychic blocks.

Precautions

Should be used with caution during pregnancy.

CYMBOPOGON MARTINI
Palmarosa

This herbaceous plant is native to India and Pakistan but it is now cultivated in parts of Africa, in Indonesia, the Comoro Islands, and Brazil. Palmarosa has fine, elegant stems, and bears flowers on the tip of each stem. The oil is extracted from the leaves. At one time it was exported from the sub-continent and shipped from Bombay to the Red Sea ports. From there it was taken overland to Istanbul (then Constantinople) and to Bulgaria, where it was used to adulterate the highly prized rose oil known as attar of roses, gaining the name "Indian" or "Turkish" oil.

Applications and Effects

Gentle and comforting. Particularly effective for skin inflammations, scars, weak digestion, and headaches.

Skin: Acne, dermatitis, minor skin infections, scars, sores, all skin types.

Circulatory and muscular systems: Rheumatic conditions.

Respiratory system: Palpitations.

Digestive system: Intestinal infections.

Reproductive and excretory systems: Candida, cystitis.

Immune system: Myalgic encephalomyelitis (ME).

Nervous system: Nervous exhaustion.

Mental/emotional effects: This is a refreshing oil that can be an aid to spiritual healing. Its cooling quality is useful for anger, jealousy, irritability, hot headedness, and burning, passionate feelings.

Precautions

Generally safe to use.

EUCALYPTUS GLOBULUS
Eucalyptus

Some 15 species of this tall evergreen tree yield a useful essential oil. They include Eucalyptus citriadoria *and* E. radiata, *as well as* E. globulus. *The leaves and oil of the plant have long been a household remedy in Australia, where the Aborigines, who know it as "kino", use it to dress wounds. The young trees, which have round, bluish leaves, are valued by florists and gardeners. As the plants mature the foliage becomes long, narrow, and yellowish in colour. The flowers are white and the smooth bark is often covered with a white powder.*

Applications and Effects

Useful in congested and toxic states. Particularly effective for muscular aches, bronchitis, colds, coughs, sinusitis, and throat infections.

Skin: Insect bites, insect repellent.

Circulatory and muscular systems: Poor circulation, arthritis.

Reproductive and excretory systems: Cystitis, diarrhoea.

Immune system: 'Flu, fevers.

Nervous system: Headaches.

Mental, emotional effects: This oil has a deeply grounding quality, which can help cool overheated emotions. Its cleansing and harmonizing nature makes it useful for places where there has been emotional or physical conflict, and for places that just feel uncomfortable. It may also aid concentration.

Precautions

Safe for external use, although some people may find it irritates the skin. Not to be taken internally.

JASMINUM OFFICINALE
Jasmine

Described as "the king of flower oils", and "the scent of angels", jasmine is renowned as an aphrodisiac and is often used in love potions. It is a tall evergreen vine with bright green coloured leaves and highly fragrant, white star-shaped flowers. The flowers are harvested at night in order to obtain the most intense aroma. In India guests are often welcomed with garlands of the flowers. Jasmine is popular as a tea in China; and in Europe it is used medicinally. The plant is grown in many parts of the world, including the Middle East, China, North Africa, France, and Italy.

Applications and Effects

It has a strong, masculine scent and produces feelings of optimism, euphoria, and confidence.

Skin: Dry skin, greasy skin, irritated skin, sensitive skin (but see precaution, below).

Circulatory and muscular systems: Muscular spasm, sprains.

Respiratory system: Catarrh, coughs, laryngitis, hoarseness.

Reproductive and excretory systems: PMS, painful periods; promotes labour and lactation.

Nervous system: Depression, nervous exhaustion.

Mental/emotional effects: This emotionally warming oil has the ability to unite the opposing factors within us. It is most useful at times when there is apathy, indifference, and coldness.

Precautions

Generally safe to use, although some individuals may have an allergic reaction to it. It can give some people a headache and its narcotic quality may impede concentration.

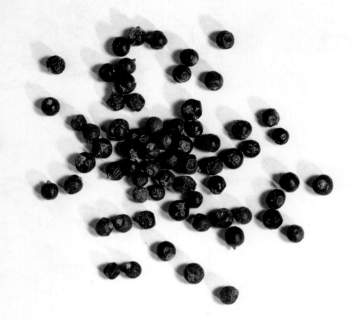

JUNIPERUS COMMUNIS
Juniper

This evergreen tree or shrub has fine, stiff, needle-like leaves of bluish-green and small flowers that are followed by tiny berries. The tree is native to Scandinavia, Siberia, Canada, northern Europe, and Asia. Its medicinal properties are known throughout the world. The Greeks, Romans, and Arabs valued its antiseptic properties, while the Mongolians used it to assist women in labour. More recently, juniper and rosemary were burned to clear the air in French hospitals. In the Bible, Elijah sleeps under a juniper tree (Kings 1:19:4-5) connecting it with the ability to revive the spirits.

Applications and Effects

Its most important use is as a detoxifier. Also particularly effective for cellulite, absence of menstrual periods, cystitis, water retention, and painful periods.

Skin: Acne, dermatitis, eczema, haemorrhoids, toner for oily skin, wounds.

Circulatory and muscular systems: Toxic states generally, gout, arthritis, cramps, rheumatism.

Digestive system: Detoxifying.

Immune system: Colds, 'flu, coughs, purification of the blood, useful following infection.

Nervous system: Anxiety, nervous tension.

Mental/emotional effects: Strengthens the spirit and purifies the atmosphere. Can help in challenging situations and when overcome with feelings of regret for past actions.

Precautions

Some people may find it irritating, and it is best avoided during pregnancy. Not to be used by people with kidney disease.

LAVANDULA ANGUSTIFOLIA/OFFICINALIS
Lavender

Lavender has been the most popular essential oil for centuries. The plant is an easily recognized evergreen shrub with narrow, pale silver-green leaves and spikes of flowers ranging in colour from pink and white to pale or deep blue. It is widely cultivated in France, Bulgaria, and England. Lavender was used by the Romans to bathe in and cleanse wounds. In England it was commonly used to scent linen boxes, as an aid to controlling insects. Lavender water was the favourite perfume of Queen Marie Henrietta, wife of Charles I of England, who was responsible for it becoming popular and fashionable.

Applications and Effects

Mellow, peaceful, and the most versatile of all the essential oils. Particularly useful for burns, stress headaches, and insomnia.

Skin: Sunburn, bruises, earache, insect bites, cuts.

Circulatory and muscular systems: Muscular aches and pains, rheumatism.

Digestive system: Nausea, vomiting, flatulence, indigestion.

Reproductive and excretory systems: Painful and scanty periods.

Immune system: 'Flu, colds, myalgic encephalomyelitis (ME).

Nervous system: Stress headache, insomnia, shock, vertigo.

Mental/emotional effects: Gently sedative, its balancing action makes it useful for panic states, or impatience and anger. Lavender cleanses both physically and spiritually. It aids in breaking bad habits and is soothing during a crisis.

Precautions
None.

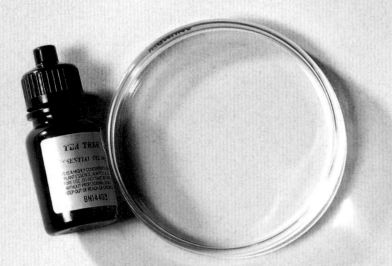

Melaleuca alternifolia
Tea Tree

The tea tree is native to Australia, and is cultivated for its oil along the coasts of New South Wales. It has narrow leaves and bears yellow or purple flowers. The essential oil is one of only a few that have been extensively studied. The results revealed that tea tree oil is active against the three types of infectious organisms: bacteria, fungi, and viruses. It is also a very powerful immune stimulant, increasing the body's ability to respond to these organisms. The oil was a component of tropical first aid kits during the Second World War, but as antibiotics were developed it was dropped from use, only to be rediscovered as aromatherapy has gained in popularity.

Applications and Effects

Particularly effective in fighting infectious organisms.

Skin: Abscess, acne, athlete's foot, blisters, cold sores, dandruff, dry scalp, insect bites, rashes (nappy rash), spots, verrucas, warts, infected wounds.

Respiratory system: Bronchitis, catarrh, coughs, sinusitis, throat infections, ear infections.

Reproductive and excretory systems: Thrush, cystitis.

Immune system: Colds, fevers, 'flu, infectious diseases including chickenpox, systemic candida, mouth ulcers, myalgic encephalomyelitis (ME), post-operative shock, reducing the risk of infection, in convalescence to boost immune system.

Mental/emotional effects: The oil is vigorous and revitalizing, and is particularly useful after shock. It is also very refreshing.

Precautions

Generally safe to use, but some individuals may develop a sensitivity to it.

Mentha piperita
Peppermint

Peppermint is a perennial herb that is cultivated throughout the world. White peppermint has green stems and leaves, the black variety has dark-green, serrated leaves, purplish stems and reddish-violet flowers. Legend relates how Mentha, a nymph pursued by Hades, was trampled into the ground by Hades' jealous wife Persephene. Out of compassion for her treatment, Hades transformed Mentha into the herb. Peppermint's medicinal qualities were widely appreciated by the Ancient Egyptians, Chinese, and Indians. The Romans used to crown themselves with peppermint wreaths during feasts, in order to take advantage of its detoxifying effects.

Applications and Effects

Particularly useful for muscular aches and pains, sore feet, headache, indigestion and flatulence, stomach cramps, nausea, colds, fevers.

Skin and teeth: Acne, dermatitis, toothache.

Circulatory and muscular systems: Palpitations.

Respiratory system: Bronchitis.

Digestive system: Morning and travel sickness, bad breath.

Immune system: 'flu, sinusitis.

Mental/emotional effects: Useful for mental fatigue and as an aid to clear thinking. Helpful for anger or hysteria, nervous trembling, shyness and hypersensitivity. Overcomes feelings of inferiority by dispelling pride. Associated with cleanliness and the wish to live ethically.

Precautions

Can be a slight irritant for sensitive skins. May counteract the effects of homeopathic remedies, and suppress milk flow in breast-feeding mothers. Too much in the evenings may cause disturbed sleep patterns.

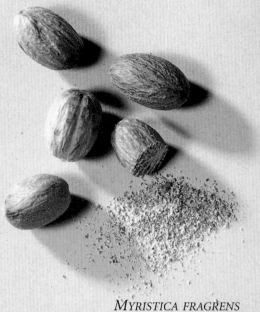

MYRISTICA FRAGRENS
Nutmeg

Nutmeg and mace are most widely used as a culinary spice both in the East and West. The fruit is like a small peach and is contained in a bright red husk. Mace, the husk, is used independently as a milder spice than the actual nut. The tree is cultivated in Indonesia, Sri Lanka, and the West Indies – particularly Granada – and the oil is distilled in Europe and the United States. Nutmeg oil has been used in diverse ways, for example in Malaysia as a tonic for pregnant women, and in the manufacture of candles and soap. The Egyptians used it in embalming and in Italy it was an ingredient in incense, used to give protection against the plague.

Applications and Effects

Particularly effective for muscular aches and pains, poor circulation, sluggish digestion, loss of appetite, and the early stages of a cold.

Circulatory and muscular systems: Arthritis, gout, rheumatism.

Digestive system: Flatulence, indigestion, nausea, constipation.

Immune system: Bacterial infection, convalescence.

Nervous system: Nervous fatigue.

Mental/emotional effects: This oil is warming, stimulating, and a euphoric. It can be comforting to those who find themselves physically and emotionally isolated, such as the elderly.

Precautions

Use in moderation and care during pregnancy.

ORIGANUM MAJORANA
Marjoram

Marjoram is a small perennial plant, with hairy stems and dark-green oval leaves. It is native to the Mediterranean region and North Africa and was often planted in graveyards to bring peace to the departed spirits. The Latin name may be derived from major, meaning "greater", not because there is a lesser variety, but in the sense of conferring longevity. The species name, oreganos, is derived from two Greek words, oros and ganos, which together mean "joy of the mountains". The herb is used extensively in cooking. The essential oil is extracted from the leaves; it has a very bitter taste and a refined fragrance.

Applications and Effects

Gentle, warming, and comforting. Particularly effective for constipation, flatulence, menstrual disorders, anxiety, tension, panic, and insomnia.

Skin: Chilblains, bruises.

Circulatory and muscular systems: Arthritis, muscular aches and stiffness, rheumatism, sprains, strains.

Respiratory system: Bronchitis, coughs.

Digestive system: Colic.

Reproductive and excretory systems: PMS.

Immune system: Colds.

Nervous system: Headaches.

Mental/emotional effects: A sedative oil and aphrodisiac. Helps in highly excitable states and may be useful for hyperactive children. Strengthens the mind and aids in confronting difficult issues such as recent grief.

Precautions

Best avoided during pregnancy.

PELARGONIUM GRAVEOLENS
Geranium

This adaptable oil has been widely used since antiquity, when it was thought to keep evil spirits at bay. The essential oil is strong when pure but when diluted sweetens. It comes from a perennial shrub covered in tiny hairs, which bears small pink flowers and has pointed, serrated leaves from which we obtain the essential oil, though all parts of the plant are scented. The plant is native to Africa but is now cultivated in many parts of the world, as a house plant as well as commercially for its oil. Production of the oil is centred mainly in Réunion; other producers include France, Italy, China, and Egypt.

Applications and Effects

Particularly effective for sluggish, oily complexions and combination skin, irregular menstrual periods, mood swings, and post-natal depression.

Skin: Acne, bruises, burns, chilblains, dermatitis, eczema, herpes, wounds.

Circulatory and muscular systems: Cellulite, poor circulation, fluid retention, detoxifying the body.

Respiratory system: Sore throats, tonsillitis.

Reproductive and excretory systems: PMS, menopause, urinary infections.

Nervous system: Nervous tension, diarrhoea resulting from a nervous condition, anxiety, depression.

Mental/emotional effects: Balancing, harmonizing and cleansing. Can be stimulating and uplifting. A useful alternative to bergamot as an anti-depressant oil.

Precautions
Generally safe to use.

PIPER NIGRUM
Black Pepper

The essential oil of black pepper comes from the fruit of a tropical vine. These fruit are the same peppercorns used for culinary purposes, the familiar spice commonly added to food. The vine, which has heart-shaped leaves and white blooms, is extensively cultivated in South-east Asia. Black pepper comprises one of the three oldest-known spices, the other two being cloves and cinnamon. The oil is warming and comforting and surprisingly sweet; it can often add a mysterious depth to a blend. In ancient times it was very highly valued: it is said of Attila the Hun that he demanded black pepper as part of the ransom for Rome.

Applications and Effects

Particularly effective for muscular aches and pains, fevers, colds, 'flu.

Skin: Chilblains.

Circulatory and muscular systems: Arthritis, neuralgia, poor circulation, rheumatic pain, sprains, stiffness, poor muscle tone.

Respiratory system: Catarrh, chills. Used as a homeopathic remedy, it can relieve fevers.

Digestive system: Colic, constipation, sluggish digestion, diarrhoea, flatulence, heartburn, loss of appetite, nausea.

Immune system: Colds, 'flu, infections caused by bacteria (urinary, respiratory, or digestive), viral infections.

Mental/emotional effects: Gives stamina where there is frustration, and enthusiasm where there is indifference. Can help where there is lack of interest and vitality, such as when recovering from an infection.

Precautions
Care should be taken by those with sensitive skins, as in high concentrations it can occasionally cause irritation. Too frequent use may over-stimulate the kidneys.

ROSA X DAMASCENA TRIGINTIPETALA / R. CENTIFOLIA
Rose

The fresh rose petals used to produce the essential oil are harvested early in the morning just after the dew has settled, and distilled immediately to maximize the yield. The finest oil – the famous and extremely expensive attar of roses – comes from an area in Bulgaria lying halfway between Sofia and the Black Sea, and known as the Valley of Roses. Other roses used in the production of rose oil include Rosa centifolia, or the Provence rose. Many of these are also cultivated in Grasse, the centre of the perfume industry in the South of France.

Applications and Effects

Promotes a feeling of well-being and the development of tolerance. Particularly effective for mature skin and stomach upsets with an emotional origin.

Skin: Broken veins, conjunctivitis, dry skin, eczema, sensitive skin.

Circulatory and muscular systems: Palpitations, poor circulation.

Respiratory system: Coughs, allergies affecting the lungs.

Digestive system: Liver congestion (caused by a surplus of blood), nausea, constipation.

Reproductive and excretory system: Irregular and painful periods.

Nervous system: Depression, insomnia, headache, nervous tension.

Mental/emotional effects: Loneliness, grief, and past emotional trauma, such as repressed anger or problems in relationships, can all be helped by this euphoric oil. Useful for bitter feelings such as jealousy or smouldering anger. Helps people make a fresh start, as it is emotionally healing and cleansing.

Precautions
Generally safe to use.

ROSMARINUS OFFICINALIS
Rosemary

Rosemary is a shrubby evergreen bush cultivated in most parts of the world, but native to the Mediterranean region. It has scented, silver-grey, needle-like leaves and pale lilac or blue flowers, from which the oil is distilled. In Ancient Greece it was burned in shrines, and in Ancient Rome it was regarded as a symbol of regeneration. The Moors planted it around their orchards as an insect repellent and it was used in the Middle Ages as a fumigant to drive away evil spirits. More recently, the French used it as a disinfectant in hospital wards during epidemics.

Applications and Effects

Vigorous, penetrating, and stimulating. Particularly effective as a remedy for fluid retention and muscular pain.

Skin: Acne, dandruff, dermatitis, eczema, greasy hair, insect repellent.

Circulatory and muscular systems: Gout, palpitations, poor circulation, rheumatism.

Respiratory system: Bronchitis.

Digestive system: Flatulence, indigestion.

Reproductive and excretory systems: Painful menstrual periods.

Nervous system: Debility, headaches, high blood pressure, mental fatigue, nervous exhaustion.

Mental/emotional effects: It can also be useful for mental fatigue or lethargy, poor memory, or confusion. Rosemary strengthens the mind where there is weakness and exhaustion, and can be used when feeling apathetic or desiring to escape. It is a psychic protector for both individuals and places.

Precautions
Should be avoided in pregnancy and by epileptics, and used with caution by those with sensitive skins.

SALVIA SCLAREA
Clary Sage

This tall, biennial herb grows in most parts of the world and provides a powerful aromatic, yet benevolent, euphoric oil. Its leaves are rather similar to those of common sage, although they are broader, wrinkled, and hairy. The blue-white flowers are smaller than those of the more familiar herb and are enclosed in greeny-yellow, sometimes purplish, bracts. The Latin name salvia means "good health", and sclerea means "clear". Because of its euphoric properties it was sometimes substituted for hops in the brewing of beer. Today it is more widely used as a culinary herb in soups and stews as well as in the perfume industry.

Applications and Effects
Particularly effective for reproductive and excretory disorders.

Skin: Acne, boils, dandruff.

Circulatory and muscular systems: High blood pressure, muscular aches, pains.

Respiratory system: Throat infections.

Digestive system: Colic, cramp, flatulence.

Immune system: Myalgic encephalomyelitis (ME), convalescence.

Nervous system: Depression, migraine, nervous tension, insomnia, panic.

Mental/emotional effects: Useful for difficulty in adjusting to change. Helps put things into perspective. Encourages dream recall; may help the individual see more clearly.

Precautions
Should be avoided by pre-menopausal women with a history of breast, cervical, ovarian, or uterine cancer. May cause problems in some women on the contraceptive pill or hormone replacement therapy (HRT). Avoid using with alcohol as it may exaggerate the effects or cause nausea. Not to be used before driving.

SANTALUM ALBUM
Sandalwood

Sandalwood has a persistent, sensuous perfume, and is one of the oldest known scented materials, with perhaps as many as 4000 years of uninterrupted use. The essential oil of Santalum album is distilled from the heartwood of 30- to 60-year-old evergreen trees growing in Mysore, India. Because the wood is resistant to ant infestation, it was used in the construction of both furniture and buildings, a use that eventually resulted in near extinction of the species. Export of the wood is now illegal and all trees are owned by the India Government. Oils originating from countries other than India are far inferior in quality.

Applications and Effects
Gentle and sedative. Particularly effective for acne, dry and oily skins, persistent coughs, cystitis, stress and fear.

Skin: Dehydrated, cracked, or chapped skin, barber's rash, itching, inflammation, dry eczema, boils, cuts, and wounds.

Respiratory system: Bronchitis, catarrh, dry coughs, laryngitis, sore throat.

Immune system: Immune system booster for persistent conditions.

Nervous system: Depression, insomnia, diarrhoea caused by nervous conditions, paranoia; a sensual stimulant.

Mental and emotional effects: Can help encourage self-expression and boost lack of confidence. Brings peace and acceptance, and is therefore useful for grieving, helping the individual cut their ties with the past. Creates a balance for possessive and manipulative people who have difficulty in forgiving. Quietens mental chatter while meditating, allowing deeper meditative states to be reached; useful for healing and self-healing.

Precautions
May sometimes cause contact dermatitis.

STYRAX BENZOIN
Benzoin

Benzoin is a warming and comforting oil produced from a tall tree native to tropical Asia. It is extracted from a grey- and red-streaked gum that forms when the trunk is cut. Benzoin is most familiar to people in the West as one of the ingredients in friars balsam, a mixture used to treat respiratory complaints. It was also, together with lavender and ethanol, one of the main ingredients in an old-fashioned toilet water called Virgins Milk, which reputedly left the skin "clear and brilliant". Like sandalwood, it is a traditional ingredient in incense.

Applications and Effects

Calming and soothing. Particularly effective for respiratory conditions and mental and emotional disorders.

Skin: Cracked, dry, and chapped skin, also wrinkled skin, chilblains, rashes, wounds, sores, itching, soothing to irritation resulting from sunburn, rashes and hives.

Circulatory and muscular systems: Arthritis, gout, poor circulation, muscular aches and pains, rheumatism.

Digestive system: Flatulence.

Respiratory system: Bronchitis (very effective on congested mucous membranes), chills, colic, chesty coughs, sore throats, and laryngitis.

Immune system: 'Flu, cystitis, mouth ulcers.

Mental/emotional effects: Calms stress and tension, comforts sad, lonely, and depressed individuals. Helps to let go of worries, gives confidence, and helps in exhausted emotional and psychic states.

Precautions
Can cause drowsiness.

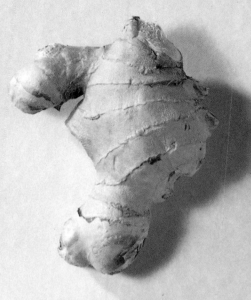

ZINGIBER OFFICINALE
Ginger

Like benzoin, the essential oil of ginger is known for its warm and comforting nature. The oil is extracted from the dried tuberous root of a plant that is native to south Asia. The plant itself has a reed-like stalk with narrow, spear-shaped leaves and yellow or white flowers that are carried on a spike arising straight from the tuber. There is some debate as to the derivation of its name: the Greeks call it ziggiber, and in Sanskrit writings it is listed as srngavera. However, its name may come from the area in India called Gingi, where it was drunk as a tea to cure stomach upsets.

Applications and Effects

Quintessentially balancing; counteracts ailments caused by dampness. Particularly effective for muscular aches and pains, catarrh, coughs, and colds (especially runny colds).

Skin: Clears bruises.

Circulatory and muscular systems: Poor circulation, rheumatism, sprains, strains.

Digestive system: Diarrhoea, colic, cramp, flatulence, indigestion, hangovers, loss of appetite, nausea, travel sickness.

Respiratory system: Congestion, sinusitis, chills.

Reproductive and excretory systems: Regulates menstruation after colds.

Immune system: Fever, 'flu, infectious disease, sore throats.

Nervous system: Debility, nervous exhaustion or fatigue.

Mental/emotional effects: This oil is comforting and grounding at the same time. When emotions are flat and cold it can be used to warm them. Ginger sharpens the senses and may aid memory.

Precautions
May be slightly phototoxic. In high concentrations it may cause skin irritation in some individuals.

The Use of Essential Oils in the Home

Aromatherapy has a wide range of applications in the home, not the least of which is the creation of an aromatic environment that will prove beneficial to the whole household.

A widely used method of employing essential oils in the home is to fragrance the rooms by means of a vaporizer, or oil burner. Vaporizers are widely available, and range from the simple utilitarian version to the highly decorative, hand-crafted piece.

Although they come in many forms, they all work on the same principle. The reservoir, or receptacle, is filled with water, to which is added drops of essential oil. The reservoir is then heated, causing the oil and water to evaporate.

Choosing and Using a Vaporizer

When choosing a vaporizer there are two important points to consider. First, there should be a suitable distance between the source of heat and the reservoir for oil and water. This will reduce the risk of completely evaporating the water and burning the oil. Second, the vaporizer should be easy to clean.

The simplest type of vaporizer makes use of a candle as the heat source; a more efficient, but more expensive, type is the electric vaporizer. Under certain circumstances these are

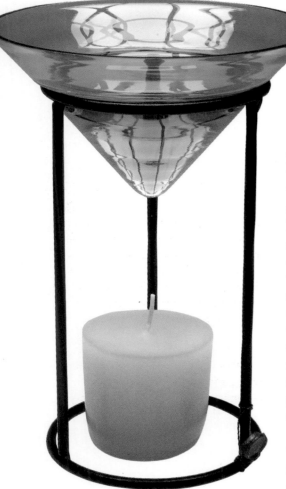

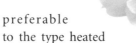

preferable to the type heated by a candle – for example in the reception area of an office, in a hospital ward, or at home, when you want to disperse oils for a long period of time without the necessity of frequent supervision. Some electric vaporizers have a silent fan that disperses the evaporating oils; others employ a heated ceramic dish. Either would be suitable for a child's bedroom, or a room occupied by someone who is bed-ridden. Wherever you use a vaporizer of any kind, do make certain that you place the burner in a safe position, out of the reach of children and pets.

Any of the suggested blends for the Whole Body Massage are suitable for use in a burner. The number of drops of oil depends on the size of the room: two to three drops for a small room, and as many as six to ten for a larger one. It is better to use fewer drops and refresh the burner more frequently, rather than use too many and saturate a room with scent.

The electric vaporizer on the left dispels fragrance by means of a fan; the one on the right by means of a heated ceramic dish.

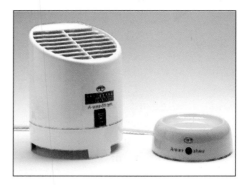

Room Sprays

To fragrance a room without a vaporizer, purchase a commercially-made scented

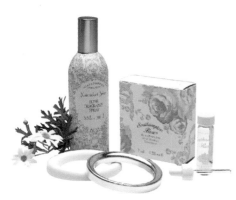

spray, or make your own with water and essential oils. For the latter option, use a plant spray or a smaller plastic spray dispenser of the type available from chemists. Fill it with 300 ml/¹/₂ pt of spring water and add 4 drops of essential oil. Shake the spray vigorously, as the oils will not dissolve completely in water. Then spray into the air as needed throughout the day. Without anything to preserve it the mixture will deteriorate rapidly, so it is best to make up only what you think you will need for one day.

Any of the following essential oils are suitable for a room spray: eucalyptus, fennel, geranium, lavender, lemon, marjoram, orange, peppermint, rosemary, and ylang ylang.

The Scented Bath

Essential oils make a luxurious addition to the bath, whether they are chosen to aid recovery from a particular illness, to lift the spirits, or to promote relaxation after a stressful day. The essential oils that are recommended for the bath affect the body as they are inhaled in the steam, but some will also cling to the skin and penetrate through skin pores that have opened in the warm atmosphere.

In order to add the oils to the bath safely it is important to dilute them. There are a variety of ways to do this, the most common of which is to use a vegetable oil – any one of the carrier oils used for massage will be suitable. For those who do not need or like an oily bath, a commercial dispersing agent (available from many shops specializing in health foods), some ordinary dairy cream, or full-fat milk can be used

instead. These non-slip carriers are especially important when preparing an essential oil bath for the elderly and for young children.

Adults bathing in an average-sized bath in which the water is at a reasonable temperature (neither too hot nor too cold) should dilute 6-10 drops of essential oil in 15 ml/1 tbsp of the carrier substance. For a child's bath, which will contain less water, use only the following dilution: 1-3 drops of essential oil in 15 ml/1 tbsp of the carrier for a child aged 6-12 months, and 3-4 drops for a child aged 1-5 years.

Any of the blends suggested for the specific programmes or the Whole Body Massage would make a lovely and useful bath blend for adults. Essential oils suitable for young children include geranium and mandarin.

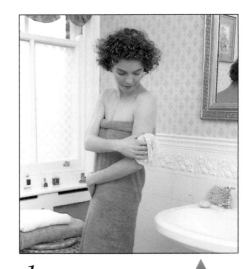

1 Preparation for the aromatherapy bath should include the removal of dead skin cells. Use a massage mitt or a loofah that has been thoroughly dampened with water, and rub it firmly but gently over the whole body.

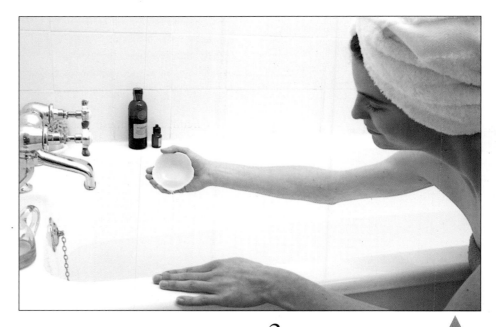

2 Dilute your chosen oil in a vegetable carrier oil, or a carrier of cream or full-fat milk. Add the blend to the water just before the bath has filled to the desired depth, pouring it in slowly under the hot water tap so that the oil is dispersed through the air and the water.

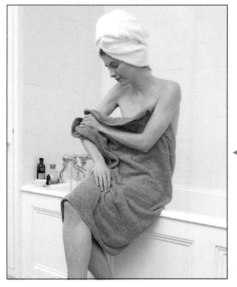

3 After the bath, gently pat the skin dry with a soft towel. This is a time for relaxation, not for a vigorous rub-down.

Foot Baths

A warm, relaxing foot bath is ideal for easing aching feet after long periods of standing. Take a large bowl, such as a clean washing up bowl, and add warm water until the bowl is one-quarter full. To this add five drops of essential oil diluted in one of the recommended carriers – either a vegetable oil, milk, cream, or alcohol such as vodka. The essential oils most useful for a foot bath are rosemary, peppermint, and lavender.

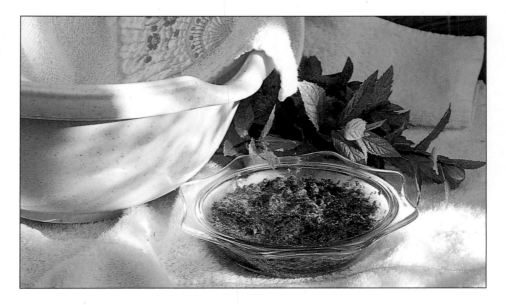

Peppermint is cooling and counteracts tiredness. The essential oil is ideal for using in a refreshing foot bath.

Jacuzzis and Saunas.

In a private jacuzzi, add the oils of your choice directly into the water. For a sauna, the oils can be added to the water that is poured over the hot coals. When sharing either of these with friends it is useful to add one of the anti-bacterial oils to keep everyone free of infections – eucalyptus, bergamot, lavender, or lemon.

Lotions and Creams

The use of essential oils for skin care combines simple pleasure with health benefits. The oils can be used in a number of ways: as a cream or face oil for massage, for daily application as part of your skin care routine, or for treating a specific skin condition such as acne, eczema, or psoriasis. Use the opaque plastic, screw-top jars and bottles available from chemists as containers for your preparations.

The proportion of cream, lotion, or gel to drops of essential oil is 25 drops of oil for every 50 gm/2 oz of the base substance and 25 drops to every 50 ml/10 tsp. In other words, half the number of grams or millilitres will indicate the number of drops needed for a blend. Mix the oils into the base with a teaspoon or a cocktail stick. The lotion or cream bases can be bought from good cosmetic companies. Choose a mild, fragrance-free vegetable-based product and then add the oils suited to your particular skin type or condition. As with all home-made preparations the mixture will be preservative-free, so it is best to mix up small amounts as you need them. It will also help to store them in the fridge.

Recipes for Facial Preparations

Fragrant facial lotions are easily prepared at home using a blend of base carrier oils and essential oils

- Dry skin base: 25 mls/5 tsp avocado, peach, or apricot oil and 5 passion flower oil capsules
- Essential oils for dry skin: Benzoin, frankincense, jasmine, neroli, rosewood, rose, sandalwood, palmarosa
- Oily skin base: 25 mls/5 tsp of jojoba and hazelnut
- Essential oils for oily skin: Bergamot, cypress, orange, fennel, grapefruit, jasmine, sandalwood, rosewood, neroli, lemon, mandarin
- Mature skin base: 25 ml /5 tsp almond and jojoba oils and 5 capsules of Evening Primrose oil
- Essential oils for mature skin: Fennel, frankincense, palmarosa, rose, rosewood
- Eczema base: 50ml/10 tsp of peach or apricot oil and 10 capsules of evening primrose oil
- Essential oils for eczema: Bergamot, chamomile, cedarwood, geranium, juniper, lavender, rosemary
- Acne base: 50 mls/10 tsp of jojoba oil
- Essential oils for acne: Bergamot, chamomile, cedarwood, clary sage, geranium, grapefruit, juniper, lemon, mandarin, peppermint, palmarosa, rosemary, rosewood, sandalwood, tea tree
- Psoriasis base: 25 mls/5 tsp almond, 15 ml grapeseed, 5 ml/1 tsp avocado, 5 capsules borage oil
- Essential oils for psoriasis: Bergamot, lavender

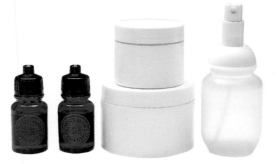

Simple, well-designed plastic jars and bottles for home-made beauty preparations can be found at most chemists. The plastic spray dispensers are particularly useful when making room refresher spray.

Flower Waters

Flower waters are lovely to use as part of your daily skin care routine, or for any common skin problem. The essential oils do not dissolve completely in water, but their scent and their healing properties can be transferred to it. Simply take a sterile, dark-coloured glass bottle that can hold 100 ml/3½ fl. oz of spring water, fill it and add 30 drops of your chosen essential oils. Leave the bottle in a cool, dark place for a few days, then filter the water through a coffee filter-paper into a second, similar bottle, and use as required. As with the room sprays, the water has no preservative in it, so it is best to make small quantities to use within a few days and replenish the supply often. Flower waters can also be kept in the fridge. Any of the oils suggested for your particular skin type would make a lovely flower water to complement your skin care routine.

Scented Clothes and Linen

Wooden acorns, balls, and fruit that have been scented with aromatic oils will add fragrance to drawers used for storing clothes. Alternatively, you can make your own scented paper drawer-liners. Simply add the oil of your choice directly on to pieces of decorated or plain paper. Gift wrap or a light-weight wallpaper are both suitable. Padded coat hangers can also be scented with essential oils, fragrancing your clothes with the perfume of your choice. The oil will need to be replenished regularly.

Essential Oils in Inhalations

Making an inhalation for someone suffering from cold symptoms, a cough, or a chest infection is a comforting and highly effective way to ease their suffering. A facial steam is also an effective and pleasantly relaxing aid to skin care. Recent studies have shown that essential oils not only have a strong emotional effect as they pass to the brain via the nose, they can also penetrate to the cells of the body and effect positive changes when the rising vapours are breathed in. This makes a steam

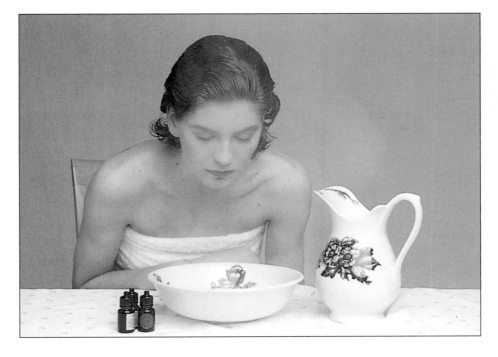

inhalation a valuable and simple way to receive the benefits of essential oils when time or circumstances prevent massage.

To make an inhalation, choose a bowl large enough to take at least 600 ml/1 pt of water. Fill it with boiling water and add 2-3 drops of essential oil. There is no need to dilute the oils as they do not come into direct contact with any part of the body.

Some people like to drape a towel over their heads, as this directs the steam on to the face, but it is not essential. Simply inhale the steam, allowing the vapours to relax you and relieve any symptoms. This procedure can be undertaken up to four times a day. For the last inhalation before bedtime, you may like to choose a sleep-inducing oil such as rose, neroli, or sandalwood. For coughs, colds, and related symptoms use eucalyptus, lemon, or ginger.

Hot and Cold Compress

This is an excellent way to use essential oils on an area of the body that cannot be massaged, for example, a joint that is very red and swollen following an injury, or an area affected by a severe skin infection. Lay a compress, either hot or cold, over the body to receive the beneficial qualities of the essential oils you have chosen to ease the condition.

A compress is simple to make. All that is required is a large bowl filled with water and a soft cloth, such as a baby's cotton nappy or a clean flannel. Fill the bowl with either cold or hot, not boiling, water and float four to five drops of the chosen oil on the surface. Stroke the cloth over the surface of the bowl, allowing the oils to be picked up without soaking the cloth. Squeeze out any excess water and then lay it gently over the affected part of the body. For a hot compress, leave in place until it has cooled, and for a cold one, until it has taken the heat from the body. The treatment can be repeated three to four times during the day.

Hot compresses are good for long standing conditions such as backache, arthritic and rheumatic pain, and menstrual pain. Cold compresses alleviate recent injuries and acute pain such as sprains, bruises, swelling, and headaches.

Mouth Washes

To make a gargle for sore throats, add two drops of geranium or tea tree essential oil

Below: Fresh flowers are one source of essential oils. Bottom: A few drops of geranium oil on a hairbrush add a delightful fragrance to the hair, while chamomile makes an excellent rinse for fair hair.

to $^1/_2$ pt of spring water, which you have placed in a screw-top container. Shake or briskly stir the mixture before using, so that the oil and water blend temporarily. Use as a gargle three to four times a day, or as a mouthwash.

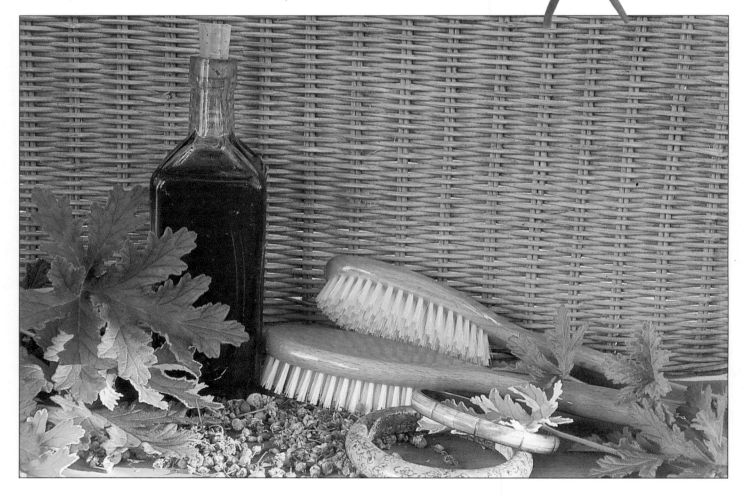

Three drops of oil stirred into a 5 ml/ 1 tsp of vodka or brandy can also be used as a mouth wash for gum diseases or mouth ulcers, or it can be wiped on to the affected area with a clean cottonwool bud.

The Use of Undiluted Essential Oils

Generally speaking you should avoid using essential oils in their undiluted form. There are, however, some useful exceptions to this important rule when treating a few specific conditions.

To treat burns, immediately flush the burned area with cold water to prevent contact with the air and to reduce the heat. When the heat has definitely been reduced apply undiluted lavender oil directly on to the burned area. If there is excessive burning and blistering you should see your family doctor immediately. You can, however, continue the lavender treatment in conjunction with other treatments.

Sports Blends

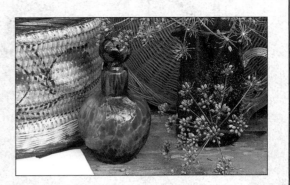

The oils listed below are grouped according to their usefulness before and after sporting activities.

Before

- Juniper, eucalyptus, and rosemary
- For supple, toned muscles: Black pepper, ginger, rosemary, lavender, cypress, juniper, peppermint, grapefruit, orange
- To aid a good strong respiratory system for aerobics: Eucalyptus, peppermint and rosemary, geranium
- To aid mental preparation prior to a competitive event: A blend of rosemary, lemon, lavender, chamomile
- To promote good circulation: Rose and palmarosa

After

- To soothe and prevent aching muscles: Eucalyptus, ginger and peppermint
- To eliminate stress following a competition: Lemon, nutmeg, clary sage, orange

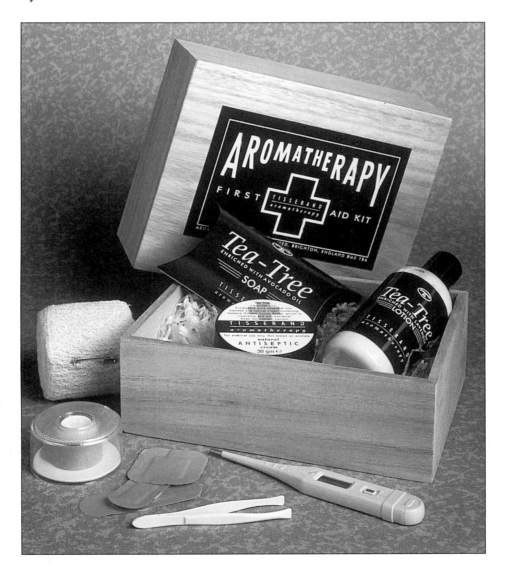

Lavender and tea tree can both be used undiluted on mosquito bites. Tea tree is also good in its undiluted form for those occasional spots that flair up.

Note: Under no circumstance should essential oils be taken internally.

Basic Travel Kit

This is a suggested group of oils covering the common ailments that can spoil holidays. These oils can be used in any of the ways suggested throughout the book, and to save on valuable packing space an extra large container of body moisturizer can be used for its intended purpose, but also as a carrier for essential oils as you require them. This will also be safer to pack than a bottle of vegetable oil. The specially designed boxes that are available for storing and transporting essential oils are highly recommended. They are best carefully packed upright in hand luggage where it is possible to ensure they are not stowed upside down. Add your particular favourites to the following list of suggested oils: lavender, peppermint, geranium, chamomile, ginger, eucalyptus, tea tree, black pepper, and sandalwood.

Aromatherapy first aid kits are available from some suppliers of essential oils.

Blending and Storing Essential Oils

When essential oils are used for aromatherapy massage, different oils are combined to increase their therapeutic effect. As you become more practised in the art of blending you will begin to develop a nose for compatibility, in much the same way as a perfumer blends scents, and you will be able to judge the best blend for your requirement by its aroma. Once you have mixed your oils, store and use them immediately, as they are perishable.

Blending oils for massage enables you to alleviate various physical and emotional symptoms in a single treatment, and while the combination of therapeutic properties is of prime importance, the value of fragrance should also be taken into account – no-one enjoys taking unpleasant medicine, so don't underestimate the beneficial effects of a pleasing and sweet-smelling odour when mixing your oils.

The ratio of essential oil to carrier oil may vary, but as a general rule, 10 drops of essential oil in 20 ml/4 tsp carrier oil is enough for a body massage. This gives a standard 2.5 per cent dilution, the recommended dilution for most purposes.

However, if you are using oils for purely emotional problems, half the number of drops can be equally effective, while physical symptoms often respond better to a higher percentage. If your massage partner has a lot of body hair you will need more carrier oil, but keep the amount of essential oil the same. If you are using bottles or jars bought from the chemist they will usually have their capacity marked on them. To work out how many drops of essential oil you will need in a container, simply divide its capacity by two. For example, if you have a 30 ml bottle of carrier oil you will need to add 15 drops of essential oil, or for a 50 g jar, 25 drops of oil.

Useful Conversion Guide

1 ml	= 20 drops of essential oil
5 ml	= 1 teaspoon
30 ml	= 1 fluid ounce
600 ml	= 1 pint

Synergy

When essential oils are blended, a chemical reaction occurs and the oils combine as a new compound. For example, when lavender is added to bergamot the sedative qualities of bergamot are increased; but if lemon is added to bergamot then its uplifting, refreshing aspect is enhanced. This process is known as synergy. Using this principle, oils can be blended so that they treat a person's emotional and physical needs at the same time. The blend can also be modified from treatment to treatment, depending on the time of day or the person's mood (for example, changing the balance of the blend, or substituting a different oil to the basic blend, can raise someone's spirits if they are low).

Top, Middle, and Base Notes

Essential oils are categorized by what are known as top, middle, and base "notes". This is the way perfumers categorize scents, using different combinations of notes to create a new perfume. A good blend combines an oil from each category, and each oil is classified according to its dominant characteristic. You will eventually develop your own nose for which oils relate to each note, but in general the fresh, herbaceous oils such as lemon, eucalyptus, or tea tree are good top notes. The floral oils and some herb oils make up the majority of the middle notes, while woody, resinous oils form the base notes. There are, however, some exceptions; rose and jasmine are unusually heady fragrances, and although they are floral oils they are usually considered to be base notes.

Because they evaporate quickly, most blends should contain a higher percentage of top-note oil to middle-note and base-note oil. For example, a well-balanced blend would be made up from three drops of orange (top note), two drops each of clary sage and geranium (both middle notes), and two drops of cedarwood (base note).

Top notes: fresh, light and immediately detectable because of their high evaporation rate.

Middle notes: the heart of the mixture, perceptible immediately after the top notes when smelling the blend for the first time.

Base notes: rich, heavy odours that linger and emerge after more prolonged exposure to the blend.

Carrier Oils

Vegetable carrier oils are more than just vehicles for essential oils, as they often have health-giving qualities of their own. Choosing the appropriate carrier oil will add considerably to the dynamic nature of a massage and can have specific benefits, such as helping to guard against heart disease or inflammatory diseases such as arthritis. They can also help to boost the immune system.

Vegetable oils are made up from essential fatty acids and contain the fat-soluble vitamins A, D, and E. Some vegetable oils also contain large amounts of gamma linoleic acid (GLA), useful for the treatment of PMS. The fatty acid compounds help to reduce blood cholesterol levels and strengthen cell membranes, thereby slowing down the formation of fine lines and wrinkles and helping the body to resist attack from free radicals.

Heat-treated oils lose some of their nutritional value, so always use a cold pressed, unrefined vegetable oil as a base oil for the dilution of essential oils. Likewise, use a certified organic vegetable oil as this guarantees that no chemical fertilizers, pesticides, or fungicides have been used in its production. The darker the colour and stronger the odour, the less refined the oil, so it will be richer in health-giving properties. The following oils can be used on their own, or as a carrier oil for essential oils. Once they are opened, keep them in the refrigerator.

Almond oil is a good source of vitamin D. It is suitable for all skin types, but is especially good for dry or irritated skin.

Avocado oil is easily absorbed into the deep tissues and is therefore excellent for mature skin. It can help to relieve the dryness and itching of psoriasis and

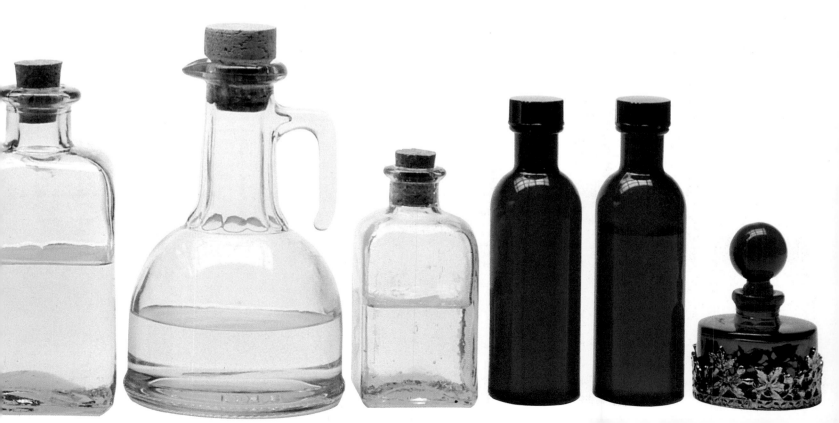

eczema. Although this oil blends well with others, it has a distinctive fruity smell, so choose essential oils with complementary fragrances.

Borage oil is one of the richest sources of GLA. It is useful for the relief of eczema and psoriasis, as well as for the symptoms of PMS.

Carrot oil is a valuable source of beta carotene, and is useful for healing scar tissue and soothing acne and irritated skin.

Evening primrose oil is a rich source of GLA and is useful for the relief of eczema, psoriasis, dry skin, PMS, and tender breasts. It is also suitable for face treatments, but as it is quite a sticky oil it should be mixed with a lighter oil, such as grapeseed, soya, peanut, or peachnut, for this purpose.

Grapeseed oil is non-greasy and suits all skin types. It is most readily available in a refined state, so it is best to mix it with almond oil to enrich the blend.

Hazelnut oil has unusual astringent qualities that are particularly valuable for oily and combination skins.

Jojoba oil is good for all skin types and penetrates more easily than other oils. Because it is rich in vitamin E it is excellent for massaging faces with sensitive or oily complexions. It also contains antibacterial properties, making it a useful oil for the treatment of acne.

Olive oil is too sticky for massage, but makes an excellent addition to a blend for mature or dry skin.

Peachnut oil is a fine oil rich in vitamin E and is good for delicate skin. It encourages elasticity and suppleness, and is particularly suitable for face massage.

Peanut oil is highly nutritious in its unrefined state, but this is rarely available. In its refined form it makes a good carrier oil for massage purposes, but it is best to enrich it with a more nutritious oil if you want it to be more than just a slippage medium.

Safflower oil has a light texture and penetrates the skin well. It is cheap and readily available in an unrefined state, making it a useful oil base for a blend.

Sesame oil made from untoasted seeds is good for skin conditions. It has sun screening properties and is used in many suncare preparations. Use commercial preparations with a stated SPF number except in an emergency.

Sunflower oil is a light oil rich in vitamins and minerals. It can be enriched by the addition of more exotic oils.

Walnut oil contains small amounts of GLA and has a pleasant, nutty aroma.

Wheat germ oil is rich in vitamin E and is useful for dry and mature skin. It is well known for its ability to heal scar tissue, smooth stretch marks, and soothe burns. As it is too sticky to use on its own as a massage oil, add small amounts of it to a lighter oil. This oil should not be used on people with wheat intolerance.

Storage of Essential Oils

Essential oils last for a relatively long time if a few simple precautions are taken. They should always be bought in dark-coloured glass bottles with a stopper that automatically dispenses them a drop at a time. Keep the lid firmly closed to prevent evaporation, and store them in a cool place out of direct sunlight and away from direct heat. The citrus oils tend to go off more quickly than other oils, so it is a good idea to buy them in small quantities as you need them. It is easy to tell if an oil has deteriorated: it will become cloudy and give off a distinctly unpleasant odour.

Blending Essential Oils for Massage

Experiment with different types of vegetable oil to achieve the ideal blend for your massage style. Try adding a teaspoonful of another vegetable oil as well as the essential oils for a highly personal mixture. It is worth remembering that even the weather affects the state of our skin, and in the winter central heating and cold temperatures will cause it to dry out. These variations can be accommodated by changing the exotic vegetable oils used to enrich each blend.

1 Before you begin, wash and dry your hands and make sure that all your utensils are clean and dry. Have your essential oils at the ready, but leave the lids on the bottles until they are required. Carefully measure out approximately 10 ml/2 tsp of your chosen vegetable oil.

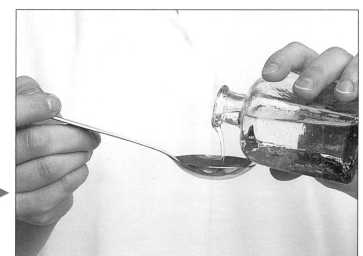

2 Gently pour the vegetable oil into your blending bowl.

3 Bearing in mind the ratio of essential oil to carrier oil (generally 10 drops of essential oil in 10 ml/2 tsp base oil), and the combination of top, middle, and base notes required, add the first essential oil a drop at a time. Add the remaining oils a drop at a time and mix gently with a clean, dry cocktail stick or toothpick, to blend.

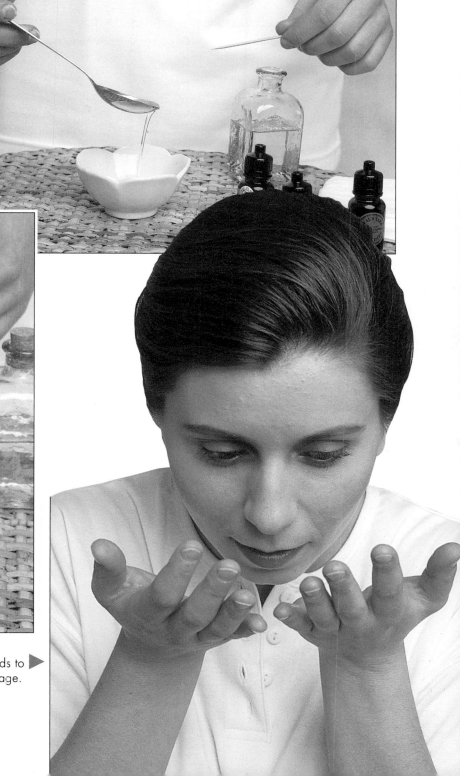

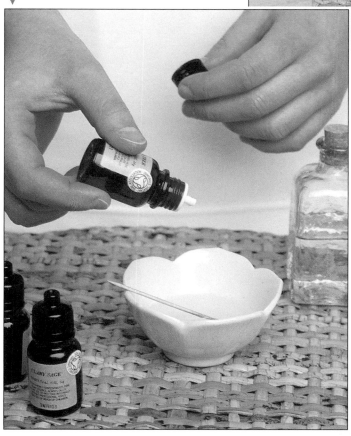

4 Rub a little of the blend between the palms of your hands to warm it, then test the fragrance before beginning the massage. It may require slight adjustment before you are happy with the result.

The Importance and Benefits of Massage

Massage is a complementary therapy that, when applied with skill, love and care, can evoke many beneficial changes within the body, mind, and spirit of the whole person.

Massage is a powerful treatment precisely because it works on both the physical and psychological levels, and because it has the ability to relax and invigorate the person receiving it. While the techniques and strokes of massage can ease pain or tension from stiff and aching muscles, boost a sluggish circulation, or eliminate toxins, the nurturing touch of the hands on the body soothes away mental stress and restores emotional equilibrium at the same time. As tensions dissolve there is an ensuing integration between the physical body and underlying emotions, which breaks the vicious cycle of tension between mind and body.

Massage allows time for the replenishment of innate resources of vital energy. This is particularly relevant in a modern world when stress is known to be the root cause of many serious physical and mental conditions. Stress is a natural factor of life, but if it is not discharged appropriately, or is suffered for a prolonged period of time, it robs the body of health and energy. Stress can also lower the natural defences of the body's immune system and its ability to fight disease. When a person is constantly exposed to the adverse effects of stress, the situation can result in anxiety, depression, lethargy, insomnia, and panic attacks. Increasingly, both the medical profession and the public recognize the benefits of massage as a successful treatment of symptoms arising from stress.

The Importance of Touch

Massage provides a safe and neutral situation in which to receive loving touch and stimulation of the skin senses, which is so important for emotional health and self esteem. Touch is fundamental to the development of a healthy human being, and touch deprivation in the early stages of life is known to inhibit the emotional and physical growth of a child. Yet the need to be touched in a caring way does not stop with the advent of adulthood. Unfortunately, in many societies, physical contact between people has become strictly limited to intimate relationships. The power of a loving touch, and its ability to heal, share empathy, and to comfort, has been largely forgotten. Massage should combine skilful techniques with loving touch, so that as the hands stroke the body, they unlock not only the physical tensions trapped in muscles, but also acknowledge, with

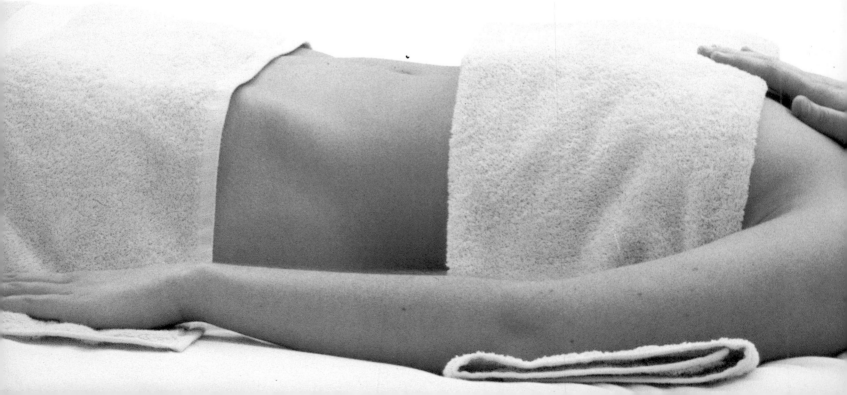

complete acceptance, the essence of the person within. While massage itself is active, the underlying quality of the touch is one of stillness and calm, a sense of being totally present with that person. This is why massage is such a beneficial therapy, because it helps the person receiving it to feel safe enough to relax and unwind from the deepest parts of the mind.

Physiological Benefits

Massage benefits the entire physiological system. Soft, flowing strokes calm and soothe the nervous system, stimulate the sensory nerve-endings in the skin, and warm and loosen the superficial tissue. They integrate the different parts of the body, defining its shapes and contours to bring a renewed sense of body image and self-esteem. Deeper strokes remove tension from the muscles and increase suppleness and mobility. Massage assists the cardiovascular system by boosting blood and lymph circulation, so that vital nutrients reach all the cells and toxins are eliminated from the tissues. Revitalizing strokes invigorate energy levels, and leave the skin with a healthy glow. Breathing deepens as the person becomes more relaxed and energized through massage, increasing the intake of oxygen into the body and the expulsion of carbon dioxide from the lungs. Calm, still holds enable the person to relax deeply and discharge pent-up feelings of stress.

Massage, combined with the healing properties of essential oils, is a truly holistic therapy.

To touch or rub, and to caress and hold as a response to emotional or physical pain, is natural to people. The laying of hands on the body as a means of healing the sick is well described in the Bible, but its practice is found in every culture.

The History and Development of Massage

Over the last 200 years, Western medicine has achieved many remarkable breakthroughs in the treatment of human disease. However, in the pursuit of scientific knowledge, and as a result of an increasing reliance on pharmaceutical drugs for the treatment of disease, many of the traditional wisdoms concerning simple healing remedies tended to be neglected. Under the clinical scientific eye, the human body was seen simply as a mechanism in need of repair, as though it were an organism functioning separately from the mind, emotions, and spirit. The symptoms of disease became the focus of medicine, and the intrinsic wholeness of the patient was overlooked.

In more recent times, there has been a growing willingness among medical practitioners and lay people alike to acknowledge the value of alternative or complementary healing arts in the treatment of physical and psychological conditions, and, more importantly, in the maintenance of health. Most of these disciplines share a common holistic principle – that the well-being of body, mind, and spirit is interlinked and inseparable. In other words, to treat one aspect is to treat the whole person. Many complementary therapies, such as naturopathy, acupuncture, aromatherapy, and, in particular, massage, have re-emerged to the forefront of these holistic treatments.

Holistic Massage

Massage, or body work as it is known in its wider context, is now perceived as a holistic therapy and is enjoyed by many people as a means of achieving psychological as well as physical relaxation. Its function as a bridge between the human psychic and somatic processes was largely endorsed during the growth of the Humanistic Psychology Movement, which gained in popularity in the United States during the 1960s and 70s, and has continued to influence therapeutic practices throughout the world to this day. The humanistic approach to therapy moved away from classic psychoanalysis, perceiving the client basically in terms of health rather than illness, and recognizing the importance of the body, mind, and spirit connection. Techniques of body manipulation and massage, breath work and exercises, were used to help people dissolve muscular tensions that had formed in the body as a result of emotional repression. Hands-on techniques proved invaluable as a means of directly accessing and transforming the client's inner reality, and bringing a healthier integration between the body and the mind.

There are many different schools of body work and massage, but holistic massage, as described in this book, has become one of the most popular. The return to the basic premise that caring touch in itself is a powerful agent for the healing process, combined with skilful techniques drawn from both ancient and more modern approaches to the science of massage, has made it a successful treatment for an increasingly varied clientele.

Massage as an essential aid to medical recovery or as a method of alleviating physical symptoms has been well documented through the ages. Its first known mention is in *The Yellow Emperor's Classic of Internal Medicine*; ancient Sanskrit texts advocate the benefits of massage, and to this day in countries such as India its use is natural and common between family members. Hippocrates, known as the father of medicine, wrote in praise of its benefits in the 5th century BC. He assured his students that rubbing was an excellent remedy for the binding and loosening of joints. The Greeks and Romans enjoyed massage and anointing their bodies with oils, especially after sporting events or to ease their battle-weary bones. Julius Caesar had regular massages in an attempt to cure his epilepsy.

The renowned Roman physician, Galen, wrote 16 manuals on the subject of massage, and introduced a variety of techniques and strokes that are still commonly used in massage today. France's eminent physician of the 14th century, Guy de Chauliac, wrote a classic text book on surgery in which he promoted hands-on techniques of manipulation as being highly complementary to this medical science.

The foundations of modern massage and physiotherapy are drawn from a system of strokes devised by the Swede, Per Henrik Ling, (1776-1839). He combined his method with the use of gymnastics and a thorough knowledge of anatomy and physiology. Many health spas, leisure, and sports facilities throughout Europe and America have continued to this day to offer Swedish massage as a treatment to alleviate muscular aches and pains.

Holistic massage uses the basic strokes of Swedish massage but tends to work in a softer and slower way, with emphasis on relaxing the client psychologically and emotionally as well as physically. The focus on relaxation applies to the practitioner as well, so that the experience has a calm and meditative quality for both people concerned. While the strokes and techniques remain important to the treatment, the caring and loving quality of the touch is fundamental to the holistic principle.

Touch transcends language and personality. It speaks directly to the innermost core of the human heart, soothing away pain and dissolving tension from body and mind.

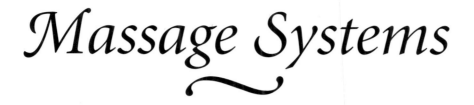

Massage Systems

There are various approaches to the art of healing through touch, massage, and bodywork. Some systems focus directly on the physiology of the body, and others on the release of emotional tension. Others work more subtly on energy levels within the body. These days, many touch therapies combine ancient and modern techniques drawn from both the East and the West. What they all have in common is the aim to bring harmony and well-being to the recipients by removing tension and congestion, thereby allowing the restoration of natural vitality.

Soft tissue massage – the system described in this book – makes use of a variety of techniques to stroke and manipulate the skin and the superficial muscles and tissues in order to alleviate pain and tension. The strokes themselves help to boost the circulatory system and increase the exchange of tissue fluids. Variations such as Swedish massage, sports massage, physiotherapy, and lymphatic massage are particularly beneficial for these purposes, as they work directly with the anatomy and physiology of the body to restore vitality and a state of relaxation.

Holistic massage also works with the body's soft tissue, but is usually more concerned with psychological relaxation. Soporific strokes predominate, lulling the mind, calming the nervous system, and restoring a sense of equilibrium, thereby producing an inner release of tension. A nourishing touch and the delivery of massage in an atmosphere of loving care is seen as the main medium of transformation. A holistic session can also combine the strokes of therapeutic and remedial massage, but its main emphasis always remains on relaxation.

Deep Tissue Massage

Deep tissue massage works mainly on the body's connective tissue, or fascia, which wraps, binds, supports, and separates all the internal structures, including the skeletal muscles, bones, tendons, ligaments, and organs. The aim is to restore structural alignment and balance within the body by removing chronic tensions, formed by deep muscular tension, which inhibit postural ease and movement. This muscular "armour" in the body may be the result of injury, habitual bad posture, or the repression of emotions.

Connective tissue is present throughout the entire internal structure of the body, and is best recognized by its shiny white fibres, which are formed mainly from a type of protein called collagen. When the body is free of trauma (injury) and tension, the fascia is generally elastic, but if the system is sluggish or inactive, or muscular armour has formed in the body, the fascia can become rigid and immobile. Since connective tissue envelops and connects every internal

structure, tension in one area can have a detrimental effect on the whole system.

Deep tissue massage strokes manipulate the fascia by the action of friction and stretching, releasing blocks that impede the flow of energy and vitality throughout the whole body. This is a skill that requires a professional training and a thorough knowledge of anatomy and physiology. While the strokes penetrate the body at a deeper level than in soft tissue massage, the practitioner's hands must work with great sensitivity and patience, and the client must be willing to release tension. Causing undue pain in the attempt to free the body from tension is counter-productive, as the neuromuscular response of the tissues will be to contract in defence.

Deep tissue massage is usually based over a series of at least 10 sessions, so that the whole structure of the body can be balanced and re-aligned. In the process of breaking down chronic tensions, breathing becomes deeper and the body regains its vitality and feeling. Emotions

and memories that have been repressed within the body by the muscular armour may be released. It is important, therefore, for a deep tissue bodyworker to be aware of the psychosomatic link between the emotions and physical tension, and to understand that behind the most defended areas of the body there is a great deal of vulnerability.

A deep tissue practitioner may use the thumbs, fingers, knuckles, and forearms to stretch and manipulate the fascia. Pressure is applied slowly, and in conjunction with the client's awareness and breathing. The tissue is then stretched and moved in specific directions, depending on its location in the body. By ungluing and freeing the fibres, the tissue becomes warm and revitalized, and returns to its natural fluidity. When the whole body is treated systematically in a series of sessions it is able to regain its vitality, structural alignment, and ease of movement.

There are a number of schools of deep tissue bodywork. The most established of these is rolfing, also known as structural integration, which was founded in the United States by Ida Rolf. Rolf pioneered many new techniques in her work with connective tissue, and it is her profound understanding of its role in the body's structural balance that has laid the foundations for the ensuing development of connective tissue massage.

A deep tissue worker may apply pressure from the elbow or forearm to sink into the connective tissue before stretching and manipulating it.

Reflexology

Reflexology is based on the principle that energy flows through the body along specific paths, or meridians. When a person is healthy, energy moves freely along these channels. However, if the energy is impeded through tension, congestion, imbalance, or sluggishness within the system, then all those organs and internal structures that lie in the energy path have the potential to succumb to disease.

Reflexologists maintain that an individual's health can be restored when pressure is applied to certain points on the body. This helps to unblock the energy channel, thereby having a revitalizing effect on all the organs, glands, and other structures that lie within its zone.

Reflexologists divide the body into 10 vertical zones, 5 on each side of the medial line that runs from the top of the head to the tips of the fingers and toes. Although the pressure-point therapy can be applied on the hands, the treatment is more effective when used on the feet.

The technique involves pressing the reflex points on the sole, sides, and top of each foot in turn, for up to three seconds – using the top or side of the thumb or finger – before walking, or inching, the digit to its next position. The foot must be securely held, and leverage applied by the fingers or thumb opposing the movement.

The client should be sitting comfortably so that their legs are relaxed and the soles of the feet are facing the therapist. Passive movements to loosen and warm the foot and ankle provide an excellent way to start the session. A qualified reflexologist will be able to detect or locate a disorder within a corresponding body part, because of tenderness or the accumulation of granular deposits at certain points of the foot. If the spot is particularly sore, the reflexologist may return to it several times but takes care not to overwork it. Several sessions may be needed to erase the sensitivity or complete a full treatment.

The principles of reflexology date back to ancient times. It is known that the Chinese, Indians, Egyptians, and Amer-Indians used pressure therapy on the feet to maintain or restore good health. In Saqqara, Egypt, a wall painting originating from 2330 BC clearly depicts foot reflexology being administered as a treatment. Modern zone therapy in the Western world was developed at the beginning of this century by the American physician William H Fitzgerald, who researched the benefits of Chinese acupuncture, with its inherent belief in the energy meridians. It was Fitzgerald who proposed the theory that the body was divided into 10 zones, and

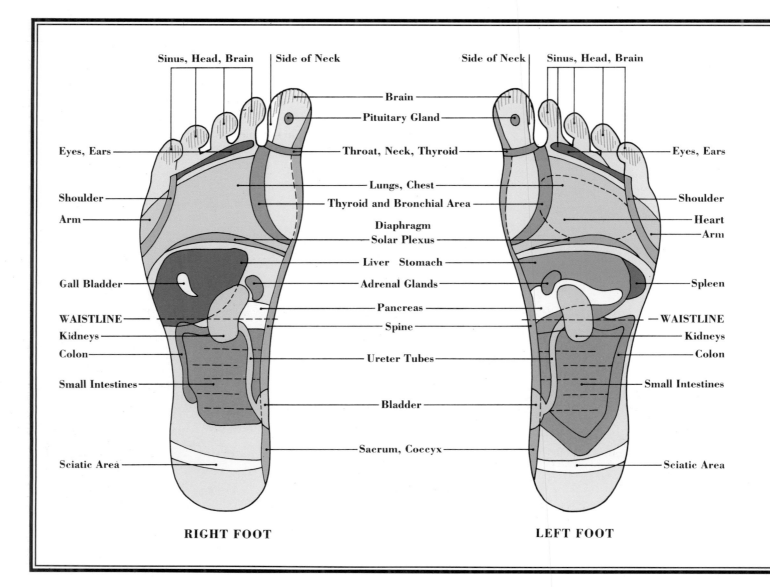

RIGHT FOOT

LEFT FOOT

that by pressing on certain points, an analgesic effect could be achieved in other areas of the related zone.

In the 1930s Eunice Ingham, a hospital physiotherapist, further developed Fitzgerald's work and discovered that the feet were particularly responsive to zone therapy. Ingham introduced a specific pressure technique and began to refine reflexology into the specialized treatment that exists today.

While no scientific explanation, as yet, can be given to explain how reflexology works, it is widely accepted as a successful treatment for many ailments. When applied skilfully it can relax and invigorate the entire physiology of the body, stimulating the nervous system and the blood circulation, and boosting the elimination of toxins, in addition to clearing congestion within the organs. Reflexology has become firmly established as a complementary healing art.

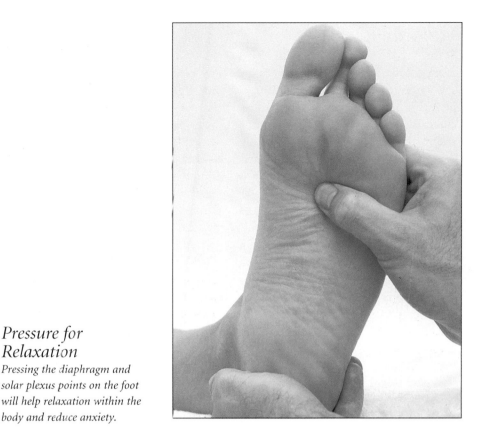

Pressure for Relaxation

Pressing the diaphragm and solar plexus points on the foot will help relaxation within the body and reduce anxiety.

Reflexologists regard the feet as a map of the whole body structure. The big toe represents the head, the arches relate to the spine, and the heel is the pelvic bowl. The organs are then located on the right or left foot, corresponding to their position within the body. For example, the liver point is on the right foot, and the spleen is on the left foot. By superimposing the body map on to the feet as a guide, the reflexologist can directly stimulate an internal organ or gland by pressing the related point on the foot. In some circumstances, when an area of the body is too tense or sore to be massaged directly, reflexology can bring about the desired relief. This works especially well in easing a painful back or neck, relieving the symptoms of migraine, or clearing blocked sinuses.

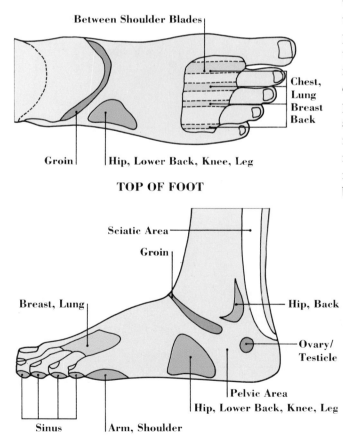

TOP OF FOOT

OUTER FOOT

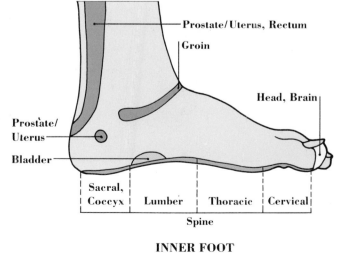

INNER FOOT

Shiatsu

Shiatsu is a relatively modern Japanese body therapy that derives its principles from the ancient wisdom of Chinese medicine. It operates on the belief that health is restored when a balance is reached between the energetic forces of yin and yang within the body, mind, and spirit. Yin and yang are the polar, yet complementary energies of existence: yin is feminine and passive, yang is masculine and active. Shiatsu helps to bring a harmony between the yin and yang energies of the body and its internal organs.

In Shiatsu there are 14 energy meridians, and pressure is applied to key points along those pathways where the energy, or *ki (chi)*, is blocked or overstimulated. The word "shiatsu" translates literally as "finger pressure", although the practitioner can use the hands, elbows, knees, and feet to apply pressure on specific meridian points. Shiatsu can also incorporate the passive movements of Western osteopathy to stretch and manipulate the joints and ease tension from the major segments of the body, thereby helping to clear congestion in the energy pathways. The aim of shiatsu is to restore a balance in the flow of *ki* as it interconnects the vital organs.

The Shiatsu Session

The Shiatsu practitioner assesses the client's state of health through observation of skin colour and muscle tone, or by taking a case history. He then leans a steady weight into the key points of the relevant meridian for up to 10 seconds before slowly releasing the pressure. A whole body session may also be given as a maintenance treatment or as a way of detecting an imbalance between the organs. The session, which can last 45-60 minutes, is always carried out on the floor, with the client, fully but comfortably dressed, lying on a mattress.

Thumb Pressure

The bladder meridian is the largest in the body and runs down each side of the spine to the sacrum (the triangular bone forming the back of the pelvis). A steady thumb pressure applied on the sacral points can relieve sciatica and lower-back pain.

The qualified Shiatsu therapist knows that one of the essential components of the treatment is to focus on his own breathing and posture, and that all movement should emanate from the *hara,* a point below the navel that is deemed to be the centre of gravity and the seat of vital energy. This, in turn, brings a calm and meditative quality to the mind, which imparts itself through the contact of touch as a healing force.

Shiatsu is a truly holistic therapy, working on body, mind, and spirit which are perceived as indivisible. It can bring tranquillity to the mind and emotions, and can alleviate many physical conditions, such as back pain, muscular tension, headaches, and digestive problems. Shiatsu seeks to heal the patient at the source of energy rather than focusing purely on the symptoms that the illness or condition presents.

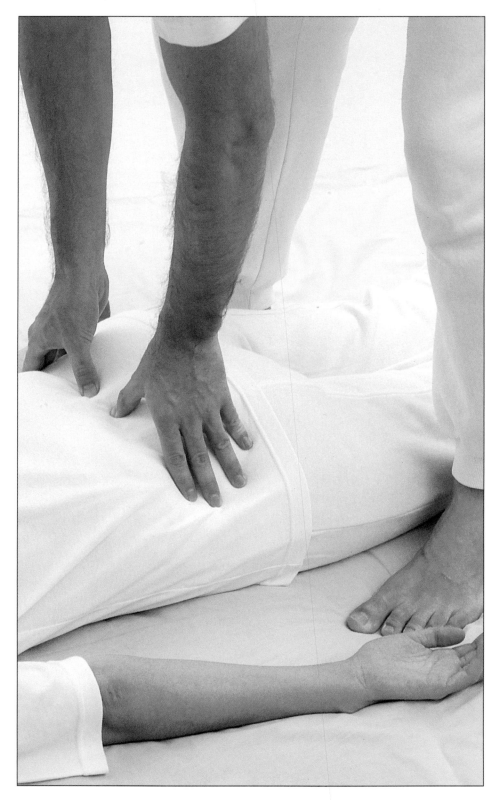

Palm Pressure

By relaxing the hands, the Shiatsu therapist shifts the weight into the palms and heels of the hands to press firmly but gently along the bladder meridian points.

▼

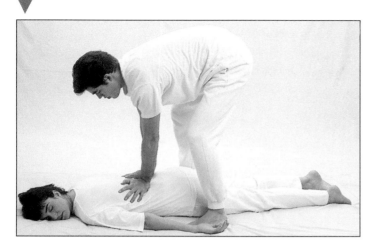

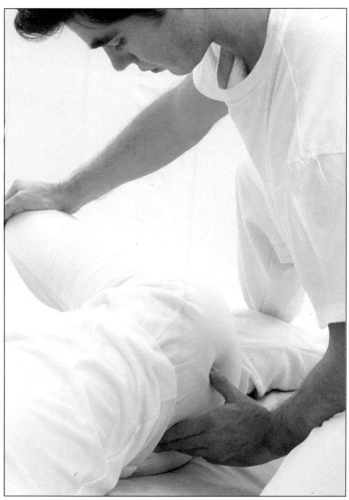

Gall Bladder Point ▲

Pressure on this gall bladder meridian point can release congestion in the pelvic area; it is particularly effective in relieving genito-urinary conditions in women, as well as easing lower back pain.

Shiatsu Stretches

Passive stretch movements increase the effects of Shiatsu treatment by relaxing the joints and unblocking congested energy meridians.

▼

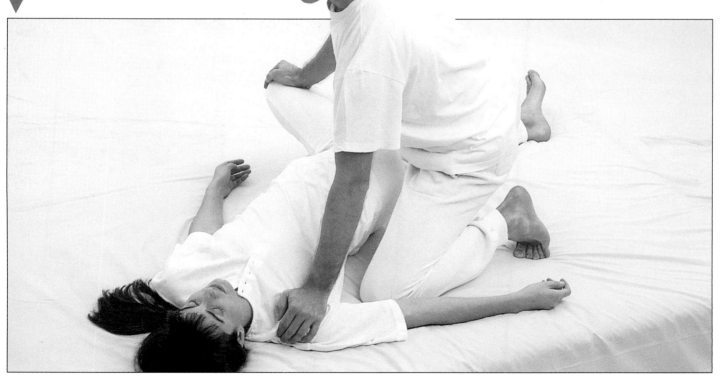

The Basic Techniques of Massage

The following sequence introduces the basic techniques of massage, which will help you build up a flowing sequence of strokes and enable you to bring a harmonious state of relaxation and invigoration to your partner.

Effleurage

Effleurage is the first and main stroke of massage. It prepares the body's soft tissues and warms the muscles for all deeper movements. It is also used to follow up more vigorous strokes such as kneading and friction, in order to soothe and relax an area that has just been massaged. Effleurage simply means "stroking", and is a free-flowing, continuous movement made with the flat of one or, more usually, both hands at a steady pressure.

Effleurage strokes have a calming and almost hypnotic effect on the body, allowing a sense of trust to develop so that the recipient can relax both physically and psychologically. The strokes can be applied with a light to medium pressure, with the whole hand in contact with the skin. When applied in a movement up towards the heart these strokes benefit the cardiovascular system (the heart and network of blood vessels) and the lymphatic system (the lymph vessels) by boosting the circulation of blood and lymph around the body. A lighter movement has a calming effect on the function of the nervous system.

While making the strokes the hands should be completely relaxed so that they mould themselves into the body's contours and define its shape and structure. Effleurage has a fluid quality so that the strokes flow around the body and never finish abruptly.

The Preparation

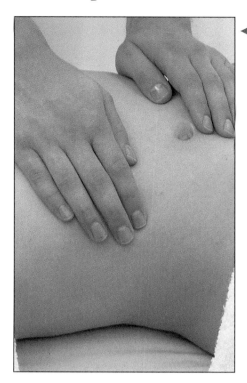

◀ *1* Applying the oil. Rub a little of the essential oil into the palms of your hands and spread it over the area you intend to massage with the flat of the hands, in smooth, flowing motions. This is the best method of spreading oil on any part of the body during the first stages of massage.

2 The integration stroke. It is important with effleurage to let your hands mould into the contours of the body shape. When applied as an initial preparatory, or integration, stroke the flowing sequence of motions should define the contours of the area you intend to massage. While integrating the whole surface of the body this stroke also warms the muscles and prepares them for subsequent massage techniques. The integration stroke is usually a large, flowing and continuous motion, which is repeated three to five times for full effect. ▶

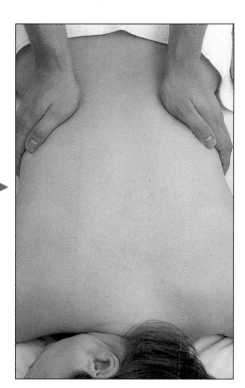

Fanning

Fanning is an effleurage motion that can be applied to many areas of the body, including the back, chest, legs, and arms. It is an excellent stroke to follow on from larger preparatory movements and can be used to stretch and manipulate tension away from the muscles. Fanning can be applied either as a series of shorter movements for remedial benefit or in larger, more flowing motions for sensual and soothing effects.

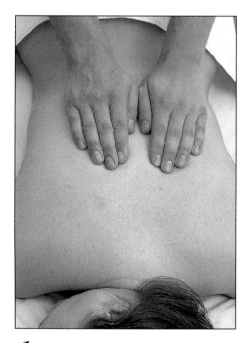

1 Place both hands flat on either side of the spine, with the fingers close together and pointing to the head. Stroke with an even pressure for about 15 cm/6 in up the back.

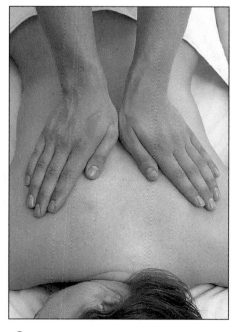

2 Let your hands flow outwards in a fanning motion, moving towards the sides of the ribcage.

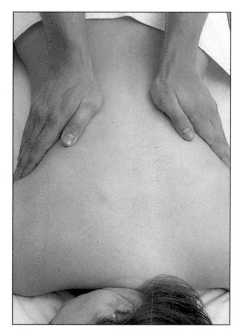

3 Shape your hands to the sides of the body, then draw the hands down before sliding them lightly around and towards their original position alongside the spine. Now stroke further up the back.

Continuous Circle Strokes

Continuous circle strokes add a sensual, relaxing, and soporific element to the massage. If applied at a more vigorous pace and with slightly firmer pressure, they are excellent for warming the superficial layer of tissue and for releasing tension. These effleurage strokes can be used on any broad expanse of the body, such as the sides of the ribcage, the back, and the thighs, when they are applied in a flowing unbroken motion. Continuous circle strokes also form the main preparatory stroke on the abdomen.

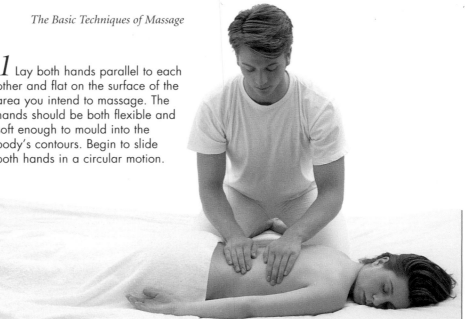

1 Lay both hands parallel to each other and flat on the surface of the area you intend to massage. The hands should be both flexible and soft enough to mould into the body's contours. Begin to slide both hands in a circular motion.

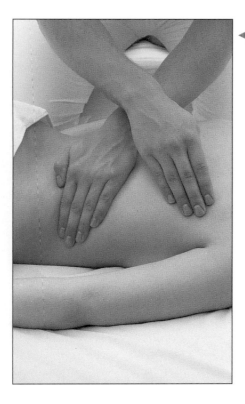

2 While your left hand continues to make a full circle, the right hand lifts up and passes over the top of the moving left hand.

3 The right hand returns to the body to perform a half-circle stroke before lifting off again to let the left hand complete the next full circular motion.

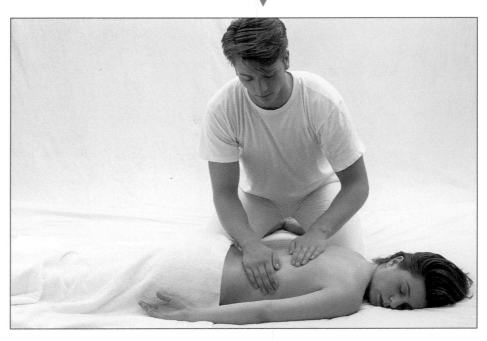

Kneading

Kneading is one of the most satisfying strokes in massage both to give and receive, because it takes hold of the muscle and moves it about, creating greater flexibility and suppleness. To knead well the hands should be dextrous and pliable; the motion is similar to the action of a baker kneading dough. Kneading is a lifting, squeezing, and rolling movement that passes the flesh from one hand to the other. It has a rhythmic, circular motion and should be applied with the wrists and shoulders relaxed, and the arms held at a distance from the body.

Kneading is a suitable stroke to apply on muscular and fleshy areas such as the calves, thighs, buttocks, and waist after they have been relaxed and warmed by effleurage. It benefits the muscles by releasing underlying tension, breaking down fat deposits and toxins trapped in the tissues, and aiding the exchange of tissue fluids. Always follow up kneading with effleurage strokes to soothe the area and boost the blood and lymph circulation so that releasing toxins can be properly eliminated.

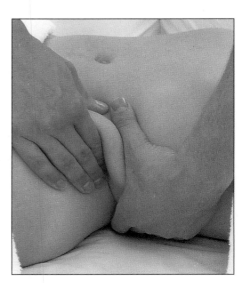

Friction and Pressure Strokes

Friction and pressure strokes work on releasing tension from a deeper level of muscle by pushing the tissue down towards the bone and then stretching it. Apply after kneading on fleshy areas, or following effleurage wherever the bone is close to the surface of the skin, such as on the hands, feet, face, or alongside the spine. A pressure stroke is made by leaning your weight steadily into a particular part of your hand or arm in order to sink into muscle or connective tissue (tissue that holds organs and other structures in place). The heel of the hand, thumb pads, finger pads, knuckles, and forearm can all be used. The pressure must always be applied and released slowly and sensitively. The grinding or stretching action can be a firm, sliding motion, circles, or a series of alternating circular motions.

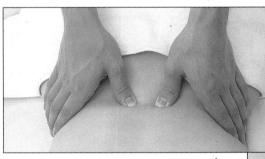

1 The heel of the hand provides a broad, flat surface with which to add pressure during massage, and it is particularly effective in stretching and draining muscle in tight areas such as the lower back and thighs. Shift the weight in the hands into the heels and use in alternating, circular motions – one hand following the other in a continuous flow of movement. The pressure should be applied in the upward and outward half of the slide but decreased in the last half of the circle as the hands glide softly around to repeat the stroke.

2 By keeping the whole hand relaxed, but applying direct pressure into the heel, these circular motions will ease tension from the muscles of the buttocks.

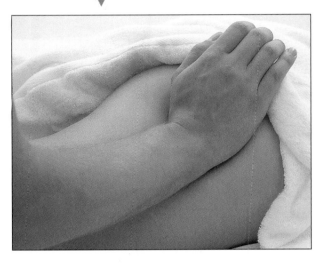

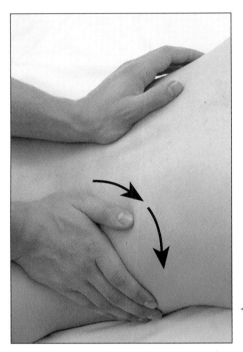

3 The small surfaces of the thumb pads are able to penetrate into those areas where muscles and tendons are attached to bone, for example alongside the spine. Painful tight spots can be eased by leaning weight into the thumbs while the hands remain relaxed on the body, and then making a good firm sliding motion up each side of the spine.

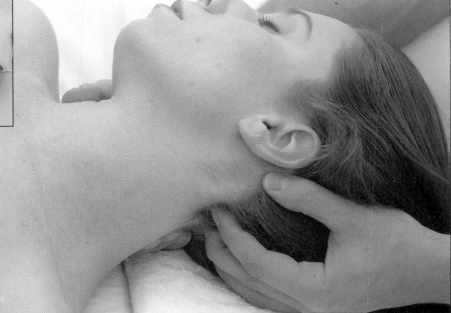

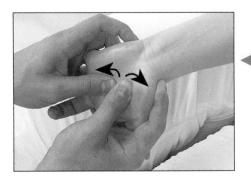

4 Support the back of your partner's hand with your fingers, and use small and continuously alternating thumb circles over the palms and wrists to remove stiffness. To achieve the correct movement in these strokes you must rotate the thumbs from their base joint.

5 Finger pad pressure can be applied to release tension from under bone, such as the ridge of the skull. The pressure must be applied slowly to allow your partner time to relax. Slowly rotate your fingertips on one area at a time. Then release the pressure gradually before moving to the next spot.

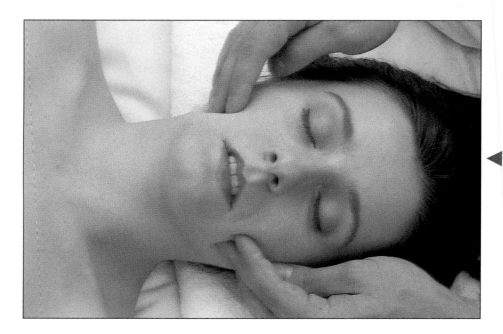

Vibrating

Vibration helps to free muscle from a habitual pattern of tension. It is particularly effective on small muscles such as in the cheeks of the face or those alongside the spine.

◄ Sink the fingertips into the fleshy area of the cheeks of the face and vibrate with rapid movements. Move to another spot and vibrate again. This will help the mouth and jaw to relax.

Percussion

Percussion strokes include a variety of invigorating movements that briskly strike fleshy and muscular areas of the body to produce a toning and stimulating effect on the skin. They are performed with one hand following the other in a series of rapid and rhythmic movements, helping to draw the blood towards the skin's surface and leaving it with a warm and healthy glow. The rapid action also dispels tension and rids the tissues of excess fluid and fatty deposits. To achieve the best results, keep your shoulders, wrists, and hands relaxed, and bounce your hands immediately back off the skin the moment they make contact.

The invigorating effects of percussion help to enliven the body after the euphoric effects of other massage strokes, but they may not be suitable to use if your partner is in a particularly sensitive or vulnerable mood. Percussion strokes should never be applied over varicose veins or directly on top of bone.

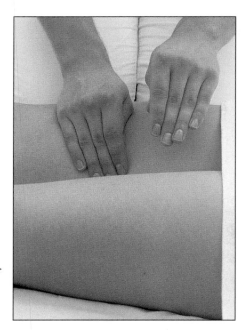

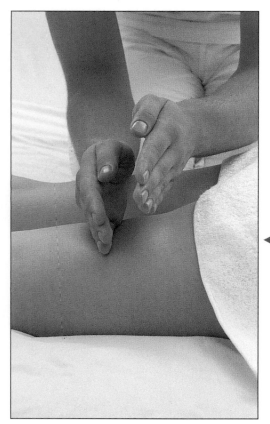

To perform the cupping movement, ► form both hands into a softly cupped shape by keeping your fingers straight but bent at the lower knuckles; at the same time draw the thumbs close into the palms. This should create an airtight vacuum in the centre of your palms, which works as a suction on the skin during the rapid cupping action. Using the palms to make contact, briskly strike and flick off the skin, one hand following the other in quick succession over fleshy areas.

◄ Hacking uses the same fast rhythmic motion as cupping, but contact with the skin is made from the sides of the hands, one following the other in quick succession. The wrists and fingers should be relaxed and the palms of each hand should face each other with only about 25 mm/1 in distance between them. Hacking tones and stimulates all fleshy areas, and works particularly well on the buttocks, thighs, and tops of the shoulders.

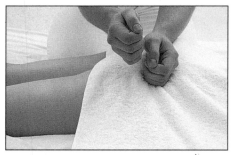

For the pummelling stroke, keep your shoulders and wrists relaxed and make loose fists in order to pummel over the fleshy parts of your partner's body. Contact with the skin is made with the sides of the hands. Apply the stroke in the same brisk fashion as the previous percussion strokes, letting one hand after the other pummel over the area you are massaging. This stroke, applied to the thighs and buttocks, is excellent for helping to breaking down cellulite.

Applying the Correct Sequence of Strokes

The following sequence of strokes on the calf muscles of the leg show the order in which the basic techniques of massage should be applied to create a relaxing and invigorating effect. This sequence can be used, as appropriate, on any part of the body.

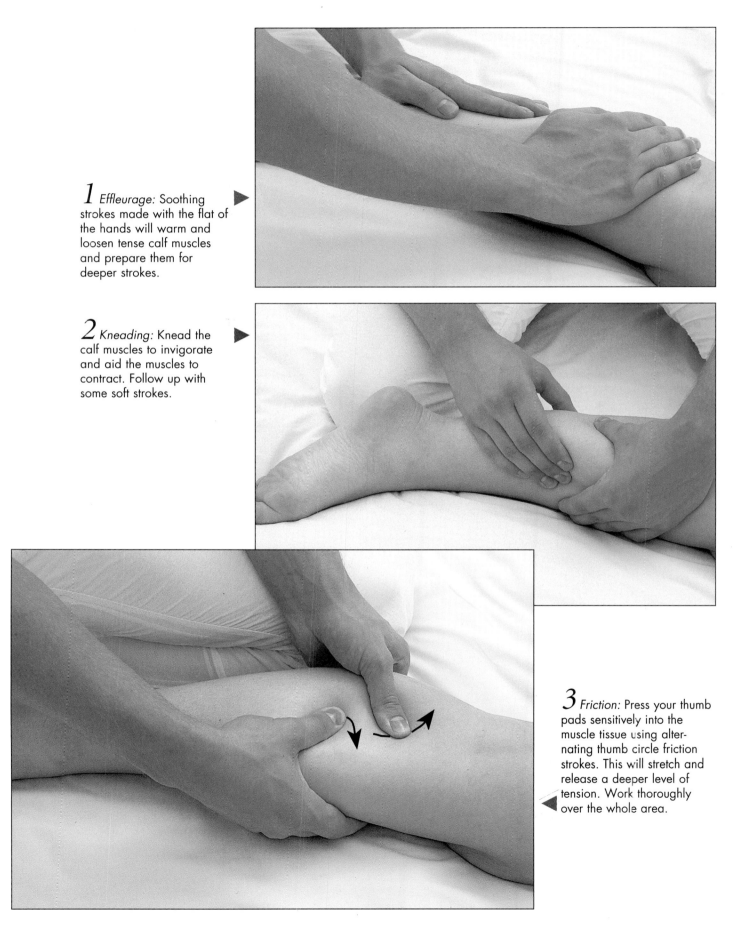

1 Effleurage: Soothing strokes made with the flat of the hands will warm and loosen tense calf muscles and prepare them for deeper strokes. ▶

2 Kneading: Knead the calf muscles to invigorate and aid the muscles to contract. Follow up with some soft strokes. ▶

3 Friction: Press your thumb pads sensitively into the muscle tissue using alternating thumb circle friction strokes. This will stretch and release a deeper level of tension. Work thoroughly over the whole area. ◀

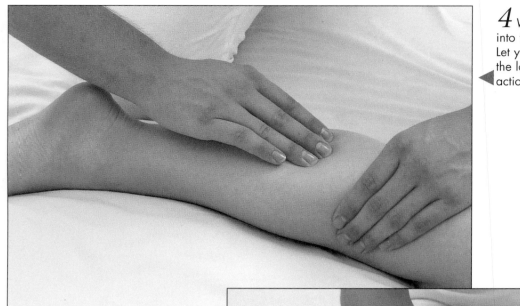

4 *Vibrating:* Gently sink your finger tips into the calf muscle and vibrate it rapidly. Let your hands mould into the shape of the lower leg as you follow the vibrating action with flowing effleurage.

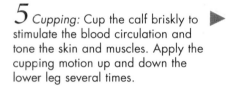

5 *Cupping:* Cup the calf briskly to stimulate the blood circulation and tone the skin and muscles. Apply the cupping motion up and down the lower leg several times.

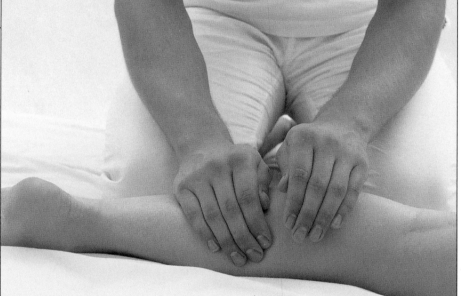

6 *Hacking:* Use the hacking stroke over the bulk of the calf muscles for further toning, and to aid the elimination of excess tissue fluids. Do not strike the back of the knee.

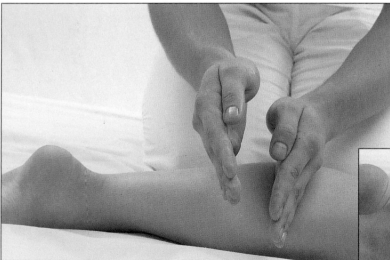

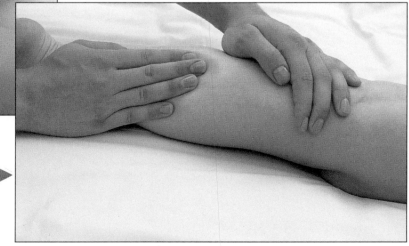

7 *Stroking:* Gently stroke over the calf to harmonize the previous massage movements and to boost both the blood and lymph circulation towards the heart.

The Correct Use of Towels

Use warmed, fresh clean towels to cover your partner during massage. The towels will prevent the loss of body heat once the oil has been applied and the person is lying still. They also ensure your partner's modesty. Move the towels as needed while applying your strokes, leaving uncovered only the area on which you are working during the massage.

1 Ideally you should use one large bath towel to cover the whole body, and two medium-sized towels to add further warmth to the upper body and the feet. Tuck the towel snugly around both feet.

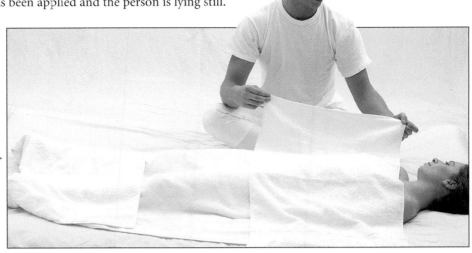

2 When massaging the abdomen, peel back the large towel and cover the breasts with a folded towel. Do not leave the chest and breasts exposed.

3 Once you are working on the legs, ensure that the upper body stays warm by covering it with an extra towel. Fold the large towel over so that only the leg on which you are working remains exposed.

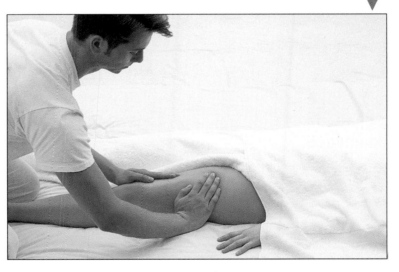

4 When your partner turns over, hold the towel up between you both, and then let it drop softly down on the other side of the body.

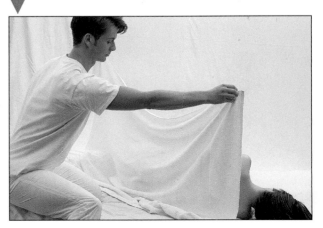

Part Two
The Aromatherapy Massage

To give a whole body massage with essential oils is both an art and a skill. The following pages explain how to carefully prepare your tools and equipment, and to select the aromatic oils most suitable for the individual needs of the person who is to receive the massage. There is an emphasis on breathing, posture, and self-massage techniques, which will enhance your own body awareness prior to a massage session. Having made your preparations, the final section takes you step-by-step through the sequence of strokes that is needed to give a truly satisfying whole body massage.

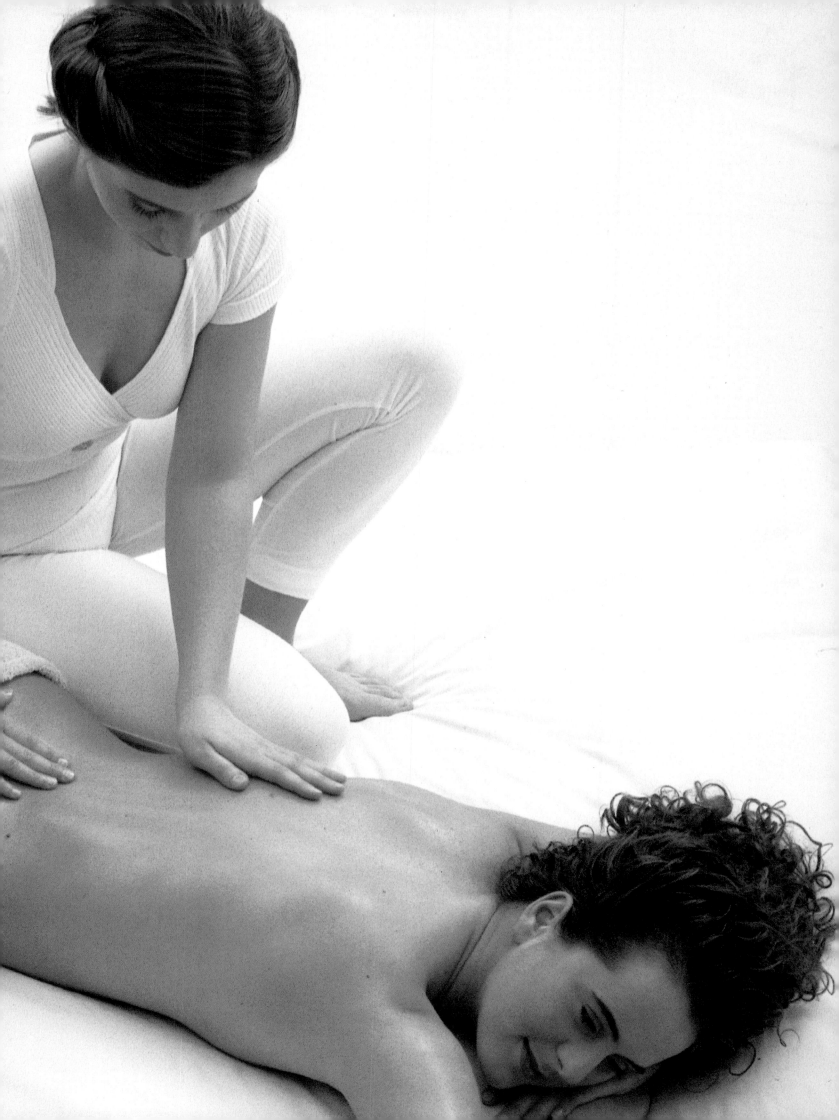

Preparation, Tools, and Equipment for the Whole Body Massage

A successful massage benefits and relaxes both body and mind, and careful preparation prior to the session helps you to achieve this aim. This involves creating a natural and nurturing ambience, as well as having to hand the necessary tools and equipment. Your preparation will give you confidence and trust in your abilities, and your friends will instinctively feel safe in your hands, knowing that you value and respect their comfort and needs. In an atmosphere of mutual relaxation, your massage can proceed in a calm and serene manner.

Most rooms can be easily converted into a peaceful setting. Ensure that the room you choose is adequately heated and draught-free, so that the person receiving the massage feels warm and cosseted at all times. Body temperature is likely to drop rapidly while lying still, especially when the person is covered in oil. As the giver of massage, be aware of the discrepancy between your body temperature and that of your friend. A humidifier will help to keep the atmosphere fresh, and good ventilation is necessary to prevent the room from becoming stuffy and airless. Wear light, comfortable clothing while giving the massage.

Under some circumstances it may be preferable to use the selected essential oils in a burner, or vaporizer, rather than blend them with the massage oil.

Privacy and quiet is essential to relaxation during massage. Pick a time when you will not be disturbed. It is extremely disconcerting for the person receiving the massage if the session is interrupted. A massage can last between one and one-and-a-half hours, so you will have to dedicate yourself totally to your partner for this length of time.

Avoid bright overhead lights. Soft, diffused lighting will enhance the tranquillity of your setting. You can use natural light, low lamps, or even candles, although the last must be placed a safe distance away from the massage bed.

Have a pile of fresh, clean towels and sheets ready for use. Keep a selection of these items specifically for the purpose of massage, so they can be laundered and stored away in preparation for the next session. Warm, pastel colours of uniform or complementary shades will be soothing to the eye and mind. Cover the surface your partner will be lying on with a sheet, and when your partner is lying down, place a large bath towel over the length of the body, both to protect modesty and to keep them snug and warm. Have several pillows or thinly folded towels ready at hand to place beneath the body to ease areas of tension. If the massage will take place at floor level, use cushions to kneel or sit on for your own comfort.

The massage base must be firm, comfortable, and supportive. A futon or foam rubber mattress is ideal or you can provide adequate padding with folded blankets. Beds are generally too soft and therefore not suitable locations for massage unless you are stroking very lightly. (As your skill develops, you may want to buy or build a massage couch for your practice. Ensure that the area surrounding the massage base is uncluttered so you have maximum freedom of movement while keeping your equipment within easy reach.

Once you have selected the essential oils most appropriate to your partner's needs, decide whether you wish to use the essential oils in a burner or add them to your carrier oil. Have your aromatherapy materials and equipment ready for use before your friend arrives. Tissues or small towels should be available for wiping oil from your hands, or for your partner's convenience. If you are concerned about oil stains, place a thin rubber sheet under the massage sheet, or a beautician's tissue couch roll or a bath towel over the top of the sheet.

Finally, personal hygiene and body care for both people is of the utmost importance. Make certain you come to the session freshly showered, and with clean nails, hands, and feet. Cover any minor cuts with a plaster, and check the list of contra-indications for massage before starting. Wipe your hands after massaging the feet before proceeding with strokes on other parts of the body. Always wash your hands thoroughly at the end of each massage session.

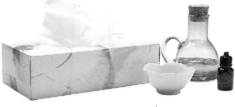

Have all materials and equipment ready well in advance of the massage, including tissues and oils. All sheets, towels, and pillow cases should be freshly laundered for each session.

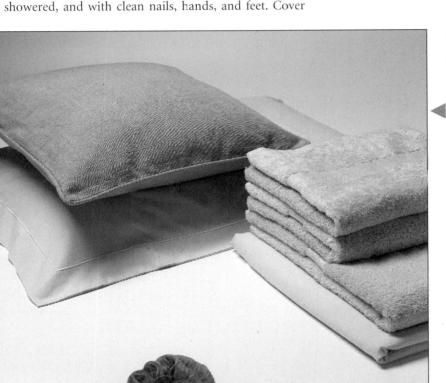

Massage tools are particularly useful for the self-massage.

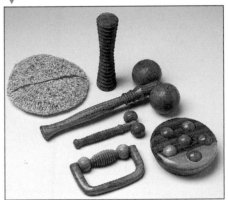

A futon is ideal for massage, but a foam rubber mattress placed on the floor is a suitable alternative. Wear clean, comfortable clothing that is not tight and keep this specifically for giving a massage. Both you and your partner should arrive at the session freshly showered or bathed.

Aromatherapy Blends for the Whole Body Massage

The nurturing touch of a massage is considerably enhanced by the aroma of essential oils. A selection of blends appropriate to everyday circumstances is given below. These few suggestions are to be used as a guide. If you are already familiar with some of the essential oils and have a favourite blend, there is no reason why you should not use it.

Choose up to four oils to make the blend appropriate to your needs. Mix them with a carrier oil as described in the section on choosing and blending oils.

A Blend to Aid Relaxation

Relaxation is particularly important following a stressful day at work. A massage with any of the following oils is a most effective way to encourage relaxation. Choose three or four oils from this list: bergamot, German chamomile, clary sage, lavender, rosewood, or sandalwood. To add an uplifting note choose one of the other citrus oils, which will produce a blend that is relaxing and uplifting at the same time.

A Blend to Dispel Gloom

When everything seems grey, an enlivening massage with some of the invigorating oils could help turn the day around from one of gloom and despair to a more energetic one. Try a blend of three or four of the following oils: black pepper, cypress, eucalyptus, fennel, ginger, grapefruit, jasmine, juniper, lemon, nutmeg, peppermint, rosemary, tea tree.

A Blend for Stiff Muscles

Everyone can suffer from minor muscular aches and pains from time to time. They may be brought on by unusual physical exercise – from gardening or dancing to sporting activities – or simply by remaining in an uncomfortable position too long. At such times the warming oils that bring blood back into the aching muscles are the most helpful. Choose your oils from the following list: benzoin, black pepper, clary sage, eucalyptus, ginger, grapefruit, jasmine, juniper, lavender, lemon, marjoram, nutmeg, orange, peppermint, or rosemary.

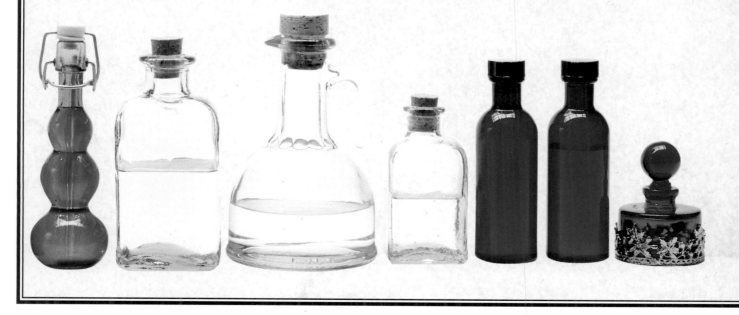

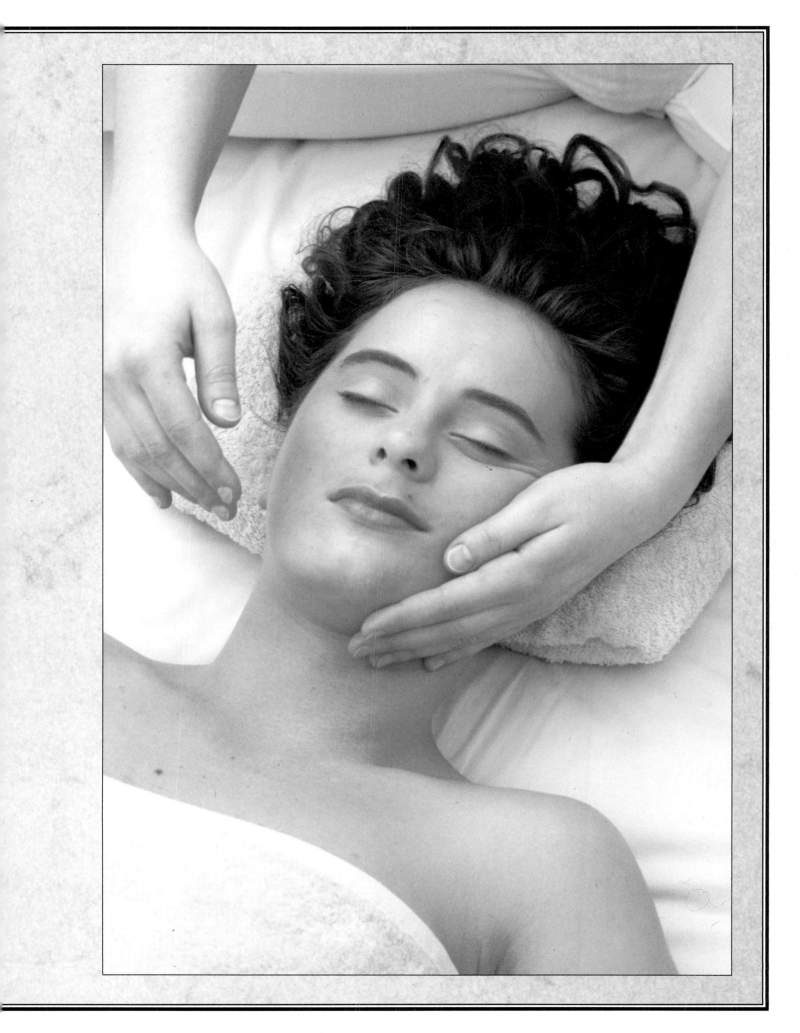

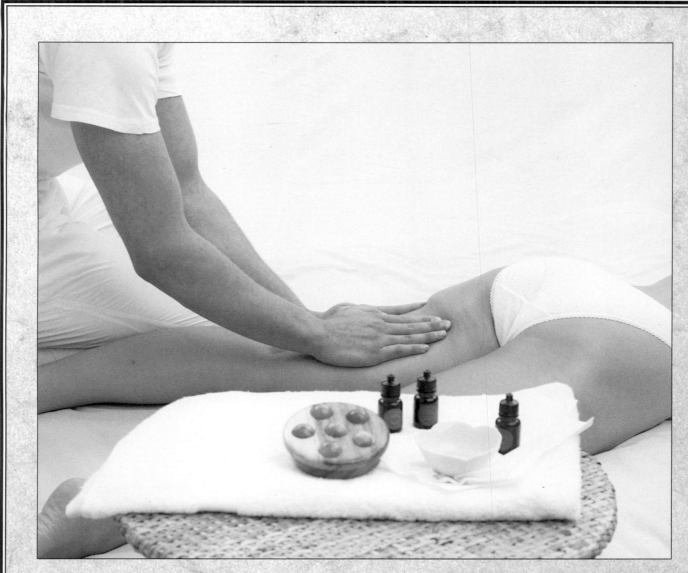

A Remedy for Over-indulgence

If you have over-indulged in alcoholic drinks, try to drink several glasses of water before sleeping, in order to help alleviate the dehydration caused by an excess of alcohol. Drink plenty of water and orange juice at breakfast to help detoxification and, if possible, eat some wholemeal toast with a yeast spread. A gentle massage, using three or four of the following oils, may help restore normal good health after eating or drinking too much: black pepper, fennel, geranium, ginger, juniper, orange, or peppermint.

A Blend for Raising the Spirits

For the days when the ordinary activities of life seem too difficult there are a number of oils that can help raise the spirits: benzoin, bergamot, cedarwood, clary sage, frankincense, geranium, grapefruit, jasmine, mandarin, nutmeg, orange, rose, rosewood, or ylang ylang. A blend of three or four from this list, and the comforting quality of a massage, can give you back a zest for life.

A Blend to Bring Warmth and Comfort

After struggling with bitter winds and the cold of winter the idea of undressing for a massage may seem foolish. However, there are some warming and comforting essential oils that can be very nourishing when you are feeling emotionally, as well as physically, cold. Blend benzoin, ginger, orange, and rosewood, together and allow them to envelop your body in their special aroma.

An Aphrodisiac Blend

In a long-term relationship the intimate physical bond between partners may weaken or cease to exist. A long illness, overwork, or emotional crises can also contribute to a lack of sexual interest. At such times the non-sexual but loving touch of massage can play an important part in rediscovering the sexual intimacy that has been missing. Essential oils that may help are: black pepper, cedarwood, clary sage, fennel, frankincense, ginger, jasmine, rose, and sandalwood. Note that this is an area where it is particularly important to take in each individual's personal preferences for fragrance.

Seasonal Blends

To create the mood of the festive season, make use of the scents that are the very essence of Christmas: frankincense, ginger, and mandarin. You could also try experimenting with benzoin, neroli, and orange.

Easter, occurring at the time of renewal and refreshment, is a good time to try a blend of geranium, palmarosa, and rosewood.

A Nuptial Blend

There is only one choice of blend for a pre-wedding massage: jasmine and rose, respectively the king and queen of fragrances, and neroli, to calm the nerves. This luxurious blend will bring the essence of calm to the beginning of married life.

A Blend to Instil Peacefulness

Frankincense, sandalwood, neroli, and ylang ylang blend together to create a rich perfume of peace. This blend can help recreate feelings of tranquillity and reduce feelings of fragmentation. It can be valuable in helping to reconnect someone to their strong inner core. Give or receive a massage with this mixture and help yourself regain peace in your life.

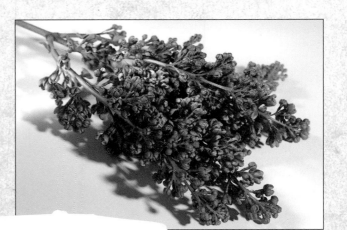

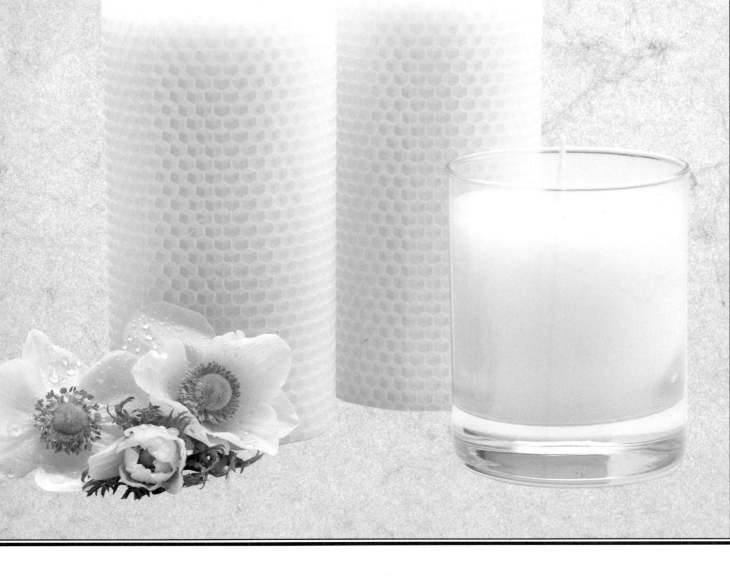

Breathing and Posture

Correct breathing and posture are fundamental to learning the art of massage. It is essential to know how to relax within your own body in order to pass the same vital message on to another person through the medium of your strokes.

An awareness of your own breathing and posture helps you to remain energized and comfortable while giving a massage, so that the massage experience is wholly beneficial for both you and your partner. The following sequences introduce you to the fundamental techniques.

While massaging at floor level, kneel with one foot on the ground so you can ease your body back and forth with the longer strokes. This will allow movement from the lower body, so your torso, spine, neck, and head remain relaxed.

Posture

Posture refers to the way in which you hold and move your body. A good posture enables the whole physical structure to achieve graceful and flexible motion. In massage, it will help you to perform fluid strokes and allow you to remain relaxed throughout the session, without exhausting yourself or straining your own body. This ease and grace within you will be imparted through your hands, carrying the message of relaxation to the person on whom you are working.

There are several main points to remember about posture while giving a massage. Always establish a good, firm contact with the ground, whether you are kneeling or standing during a session. This means letting the lower half of your body, your pelvis, legs, and feet, support your weight and movement. Ease your body back and forth with your strokes by using your leg muscles. Keep your knees flexed and tip forward from your hips, so that your spine is straight and extended upwards. Try to keep your neck and head in line with your spine so they don't hang forward.

Constantly remind yourself to relax your shoulders so there is width in your chest, and let your arms hang loosely downwards so that your shoulders, elbows, and wrists are flexible at all times. Keep a space between your arms and your body to avoid hunching in your shoulders. Each time your hands apply strokes to ease tension from a certain part of your partner's body, check that the same area is relaxed in your own body.

Breath

Deep and easy breathing assists in bringing oxygen to the cells of your body and allows tense muscles to open and relax. Breath is the basic fuel of your vital life force, and will constantly replenish your energy. Full and easy breathing will allow you to be more present and attentive in your massage, bringing a vitality to your hands and your strokes. It will also enable you to be more connected with your feelings, thereby enhancing the loving quality of your touch.

Synchronizing your breath with your strokes will deepen the effects of your massage, so that it flows over the body like a wave of energy. The ease of your breathing and the relaxed vitality that it brings to you will transmit itself to your partner, enabling her to let go of tensions and breathe more fully.

Co-ordinating Breathing and Movement

This simple exercise helps you to deepen your breathing and to synchronize it with your movement, with each breath lasting for the length of each movement. This practice will allow you to remain calm but energized while giving a massage, increasing the vitality in your hands and bringing fluidity to your strokes. Repeat the cycle of movement and breathing up to ten times.

1 Stand in the basic stance of good posture, with your feet parallel and a hip-width apart, the knees slightly bent and the arms dropped loosely to the sides of your body. Lengthen your spine and keep your neck and head balanced lightly above it and extended away from your shoulders. ▼

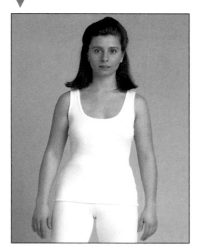

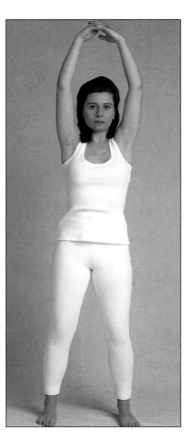

◄ *2* As you inhale, let both arms float out from the sides of your body until they meet above your head, then clasp your fingers lightly together.

3 As you slowly ▶ exhale, press your palms down towards the floor until your arms are straight. Unlock your fingers, and repeat the cycle of breathing and movement.

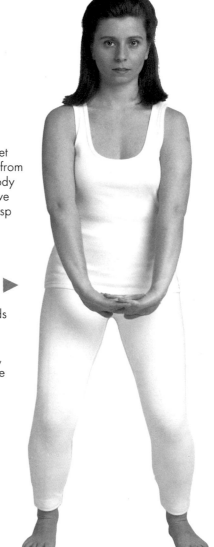

Breathing to Increase Stamina

This exercise is more complex than the previous one and is adapted from the Chinese martial art form Chi Kung. It helps you to build up stamina and vital energy, while controlling and deepening your flow of breath. It also brings you in contact with your *chi*, the source of vital life energy in your belly, which is the centre of gravity in your body. Practice will help you to maintain a relaxed strength while giving a massage.

1 Begin with the basic stance, but place one hand, palm facing outwards, at the front of your forehead, and the other hand, palm facing downwards, in front of your navel. Let both hands remain relaxed.

2 As you breathe in, straighten your knees and push up with one hand and down with the other hand, until both arms are vertical to the body.

3 Continue with this long inhalation of breath as you rotate your arms like a windmill to move into the opposite positions.

4 Once you have switched the positions of your arms, flex your wrists and flatten your palms, pushing one hand up towards the sky, and the other hand down towards the ground.

5 Now slowly release your breath and sink your weight down into your knees, while bending your arms at the elbows so that, once again, one hand is in front of the forehead and the other is in front of the navel.

Massage Instruments

Nothing feels better than the touch of hands on the body, but massage instruments can be used successfully in self-massage to reach awkward areas. This two-ball roller is ideal for working on sore points on the back.

Relaxing the Face

One area of the body most likely to suffer from tension is the face. Emotional tension becomes trapped in the facial muscles as we try not to expose our feelings to other people when we are under stress. A daily self-massage of the head and face will help you to look and feel more relaxed.

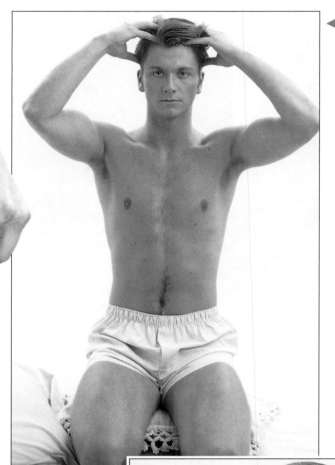

1 Loosen the muscles covering the skull using a motion similar to that used when washing your hair. Rotate the fingertips of both hands on one area at a time so that you can feel the scalp move. Massage thoroughly over the front, sides and back of the head.

2 Rubbing the temples can help to soothe an over-active mind. Using the first two fingers of both hands, gently smooth the temples in an anti-clockwise motion until you feel relief.

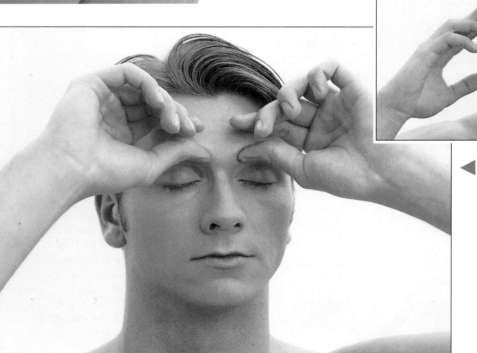

3 The feeling of having a "thick head" often results from blocked or congested sinus passages caused by excess mucus, or the start of a cold. Gentle pressing on these sensitive cavities can help to relieve this uncomfortable sensation. Begin by steadily pushing your thumbs into the tiny hollow on the inner edge of the eyebrow. Continue the motion along the ridge of the brow and back along the bone under the eyes. Then press up into the sinus cavities under the ridge of the cheekbones, moving out from the edge of the nose to the side of the face.

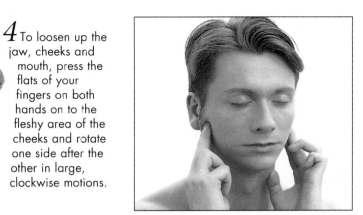

4 To loosen up the jaw, cheeks and mouth, press the flats of your fingers on both hands on to the fleshy area of the cheeks and rotate one side after the other in large, clockwise motions.

5 Tension builds up in the jaw whenever anger or fear are repressed. To loosen the jaw, use the first two fingers of both hands to work each side of the face, circulating and freeing the jaw joint.

6 A relaxing ear massage is a pleasant way to complete the self-massage on the head and face. Support the back of the ear lobes with your thumbs, then use your index fingers to massage in tiny rotations. Reverse the position of thumb and finger to stroke around the top rims of your ears.

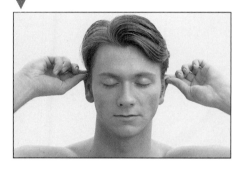

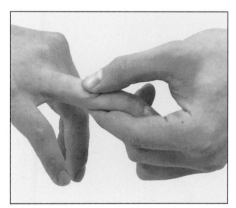

The Hand Massage

Keeping your hands supple and relaxed is an important part of massage. While practising the strokes, you may find yourself using certain hand movements for the first time, so it is a good idea to exercise the hand joints frequently to increase their flexibility. Use one hand to gently squeeze all over the other. Repeat for the other hand. Rub the palms together briskly to increase warmth and vitality.

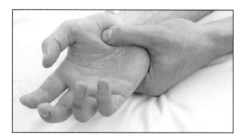

1 Release tension in the muscular pad at the base of the thumb by pressing into it with the thumb of the other hand and then rotating it on one spot at a time. Support the back of the hand with the fingers. Work over the entire palm in a similar way.

2 Sink and rotate your thumb into the web between the thumb and index finger of the other hand. You will find a tender spot that can bring relief from toothache, headaches and digestive problems.

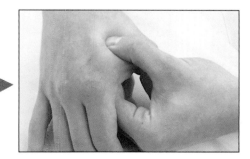

3 Pinch the base of a finger on one hand between the thumb and index finger of the other hand, then pull the thumb and index finger in alternate short, firm slides along the length of the finger to its tip to stretch it. Repeat this movement on all the digits. Repeat the whole hand massage sequence for the other hand.

The Whole Body Massage

Creating an atmosphere of confidence and trust is an important element in giving a successful whole body massage. It will help your massage partner relax if she knows that you are carefully prepared and in control. Make sure that the room is heated and all of your equipment and oils are ready. Take time to compose yourself so that your whole attention is focused on the massage. Give your partner privacy to undress, and clear directions on how to lie down on the mattress. Use the towels correctly to cover the body, both to keep it warm and to protect modesty. By following these suggestions, your partner will immediately feel safe and secure in your hands.

The whole body massage discussed in the following pages starts on the back of the body, with special focus on main areas of tension. Once your partner has turned over, the massage continues on the feet before moving up the entire front of the body, finishing with soothing strokes to relax the face.

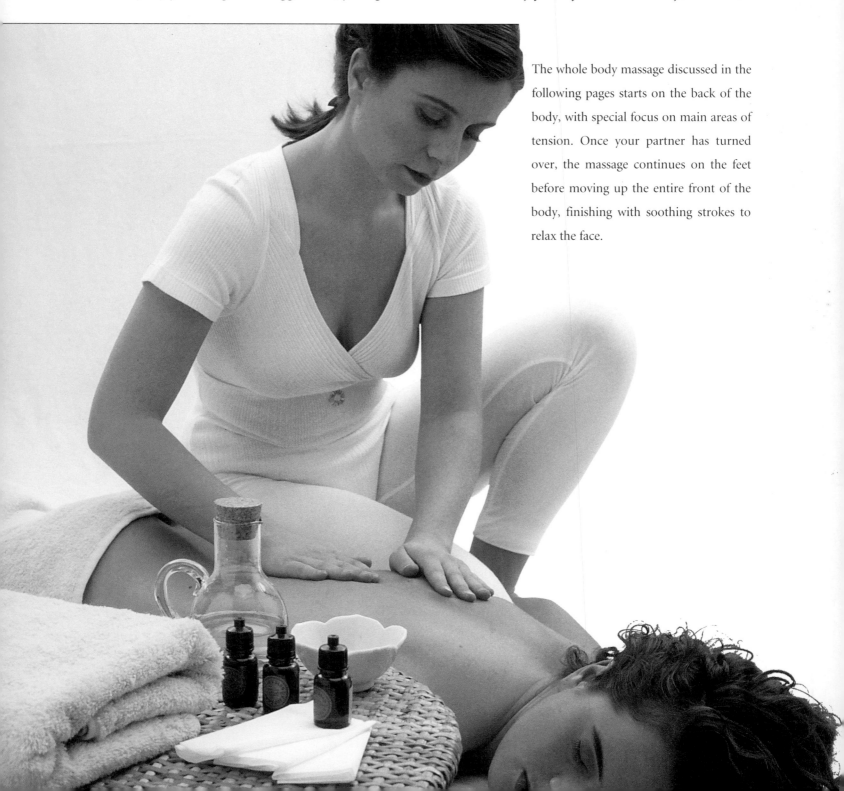

The Back Massage

There are several good reasons for starting a whole body massage on the back. Some people need time to relax sufficiently to allow the process of massage to work properly, and the back presents a broad surface that does not feel as immediately intimate or as vulnerable to touch as, for example, the chest or belly. At the same time, the muscles of the back are especially prone to tension resulting from stress, uncomfortable posture, and injury. A thorough back massage can take the strain out of the whole body. Combine your strokes so that they prepare, soothe, warm, and relax the whole back, while working therapeutically on the main areas of tension, such as the spine, the lower back, and the shoulders.

◀ Establishing Contact

Establish contact with your partner by placing your hands gently down on to her body, so that one hand rests on the top of her spine and the other at its base. Check that your own body is relaxed while suggesting to your partner that she takes a few moments to settle herself comfortably on to the mattress.

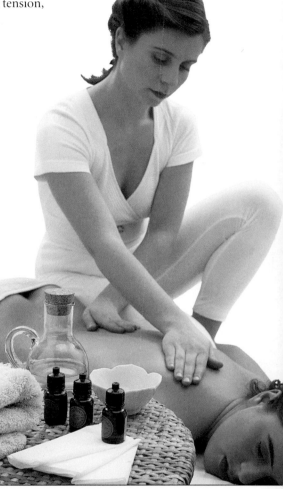

Applying the Oil ▲

Fold the top towel over the lower half of her body. Pour 2.5 ml/¹/₂ tsp of your blended oils into the palm of one hand, then rub your hands together to warm them and the oil. Apply more oil as appropriate. Using smooth and flowing effleurage strokes, spread the oil over the back, taking time to allow your hands to become familiar with the shape and feel of the body. Relax your hands so they become pliable and are able to mould into the body's curves.

Focus on the Spine

The first stage of the back massage focuses on relaxing the spine and the muscles that support it. Begin from a position behind your partner's head so that you can make a series of effleurage strokes over the whole back, followed by some deeper pressure strokes to release tension from alongside the spine.

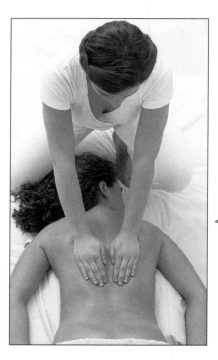

The Initial Integration Stroke

This initial main effleurage movement embraces the whole shape of the back, warming the muscles and tissues. It can be applied up to five times as the preparatory stroke in a continuous sequence of motions.

◀ *1* To start, place your hands flat on each side of the spine, fingers pointing towards the lower back. Lean your weight into your hands and slide them steadily downwards to stretch the long muscles beside the spine.

◀ *2* As your hands reach the lower back, swing them out and around the hips to enfold the sides of the body. Your fingers should slip slightly under the front of the body.

3 Draw your hands gently but firmly up along the sides of the waist and ribcage until they reach the shoulder blades. Turn your wrists so that your hands glide in and around the edges of the shoulder blades.

▼

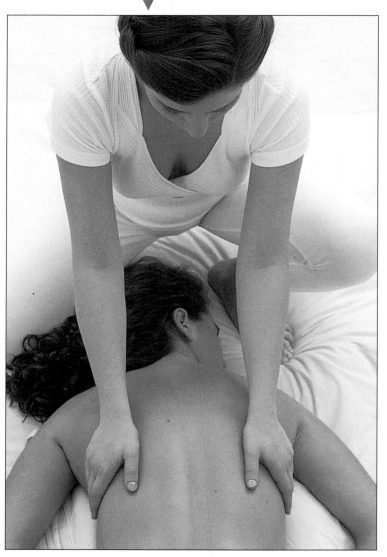

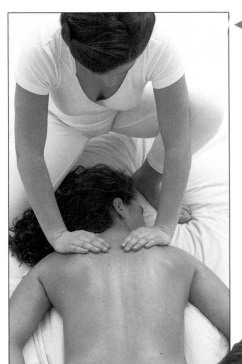

4 As your hands draw out across the top of the shoulders, shift the pressure into their heels to give a good stretch to tense shoulder muscles.

5 Slip your hands softly around the shoulder joints and swivel your wrists to glide them lightly back in across the top of the shoulders. Take the stroke up the back of the neck and out through the head and hair.

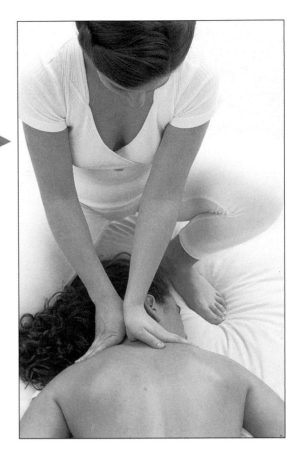

Rocking the Body

Some variation can be added to the above stroke to bring extra vitality and movement to the body. Complete both rocking sequences with a sweep around the shoulders, drawing your hands towards the neck and up over the head.

1 After your hands have curved around the sides of the lower back, draw them in towards the base of the spine. Slip your left hand on top of your right hand to add support. Slightly cup your right hand to create a suction effect and rock gently and rhythmically up over the length of the spine.

2 Separate your hands at the top of the spine. Put pressure into the heel of each hand to create an alternating press-and-release movement, which works out towards the shoulders. This rocking motion is similar to the way in which a cat paws on a soft surface.

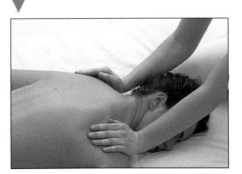

Fanning

To enhance the overall relaxation of the back, perform three sequences of fanning strokes. Massage towards the lower back, and then return your hands by sweeping them out and up along the sides of the body in the same manner as the initial effleurage stroke.

1 Place your hands flat on each side of the spine at the top of the back, fingers pointing downwards. Stroke down below the shoulder blades before sliding your hands out to the sides of the body.

2 Mould your hands to the sides of the body, gliding them up the ribcage for a short distance before flexing your wrists to draw them very lightly towards the centre of the back.

3 Turn your hands so they are once again lying flat against each side of the spine, fingers pointing to the lower back. Stroke down another hand's length to repeat the fanning motion.

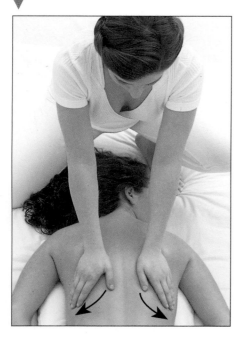

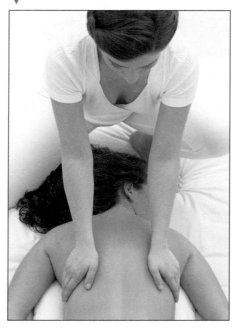

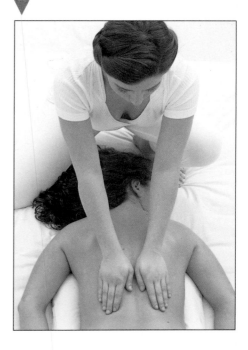

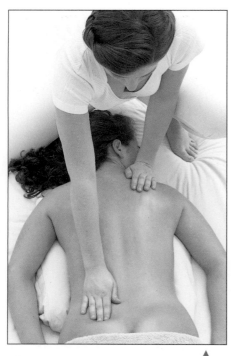

Double Stretch Stroke

This stroke focuses specifically on the long muscles, or erector spinae, which give support to the spine and help it extend and rotate the trunk of the body. Its stretching and rubbing effect releases tension and brings heat to the muscles, creating greater flexibility and movement in the back.

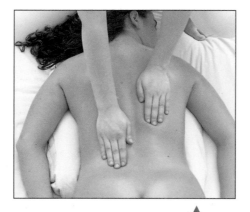

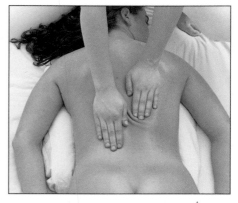

1 Place both hands over the top of the shoulders and close to the spine, fingers pointing down the back. Using a firm and steady pressure, slide the right hand down over the long muscles while keeping the left hand in its original position.

2 When the right hand reaches the small of the back, curve it around the hip and back to the base of the spine, before drawing it back up the long muscle on the left side of the spinal column. At the same time, slide your left hand down to repeat the motion on the right side of the spine.

3 Continue to move both hands back and forth over the long muscles for up to five sequences. Increase the speed and pressure to create a heat-producing friction and rippling effect in the tissue as the hands pass each other. Complete the stroke with both hands resting by the shoulders.

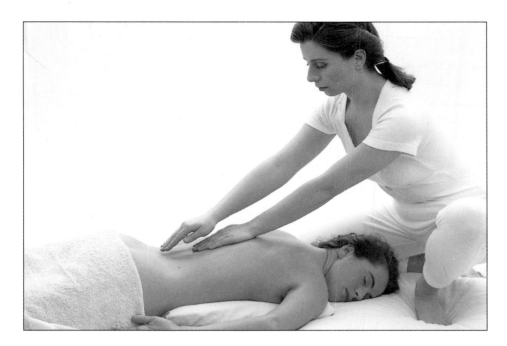

Overlapping Strokes

Following the vigorous action of the double stretch stroke on the long muscles, soothe the area with soft, gentle movements. Stroke up over the spine with one hand following the other in short overlapping motions, with the fingers relaxed and spread apart.

Pressure Strokes On The Spine

Now is the time to increase the pressure of your strokes alongside the spine in order to ease tight spots and bring relief. Sink the weight slowly into the underlying level of muscle tissue at the top of the shoulders before starting the stroke, remaining sensitive to your partner's response to the pressure. Keep the strokes close to the spine, but avoid pressing directly on the bone. Once your stroke has reached the base of the spine, open out your hands to sweep them around and up the sides of the body so that each sequence can be repeated.

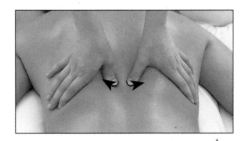

1 Starting at the top of the back, place your thumb pads on either side of the spine. Shift the weight into your thumbs while your fingers rest on the body. Massage in small circular motions close to the edge of the bone.

2 Deepen the pressure as your thumbs rotate towards and away from the spine in the first half of the circle, and release the pressure to glide softly back and around. Work down the length of the spine in a spiralling motion. Repeat the stroke, increasing the pressure.

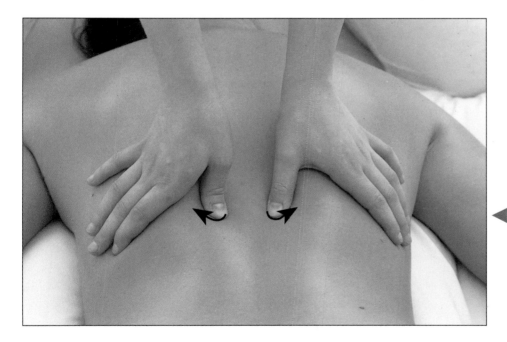

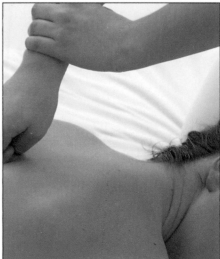

Knuckle Stretch

Crook the index and middle fingers of your right hand and sink the flat edges of the knuckles into the furrow on either side of the spine. Raise your own body so that you can lean your weight steadily into the arm, keeping it straight and slightly ahead of your body. Clasp your right wrist with your left hand to add pressure and support. Wait until your knuckles have settled comfortably into a deeper level of tissue, and slide them slowly and steadily alongside the spine to give a good stretch. Remain aware of your partner's breathing.

To integrate the different strokes and to complete the spine massage from this position, make several large effleurage strokes to encompass the back, and finish by placing your hands softly over the spine for several moments.

Focus on the Lumbar Region

Change your position so that you are kneeling beside the hip and facing towards the head. Spread a little more oil on the skin if necessary. Your focus is now on relaxing the lower half of the back, known as the lumbar region. This area is particularly prone to aches and pains which are the result of compression and strain caused by uncomfortable posture, awkward movement or prolonged sitting. Many of the following strokes also benefit those muscles that cross over the sides of the body from the abdomen to the back. These muscles, known as abdominus obliques, support abdominal organs and flex the spine.

Start with a series of relaxing effleurage movements over the whole back before working specifically on the muscles between the pelvic girdle and the shoulder blades. To avoid twisting in your own posture, you can straddle your partner's body while doing these strokes. Keep one foot on the mattress, and use your leg muscles to lever yourself back and forth, and to support your own weight. Ensure that you remain at some physical distance from your partner.

3 Moulding your hands to the body, glide them over the shoulders, down the sides of the ribcage and waist as far as the lower back.

Soothing with Effleurage

1 Begin the large effleurage stroke from the lower back. Place both hands flat on each side of the spine, fingers pointing to the head. Leaning your weight into your hands, stroke firmly up the back towards the head with a steady pressure. ▶

2 As your hands reach the top of the back, fan them out towards the shoulders in a continuous flow of motion. ▼

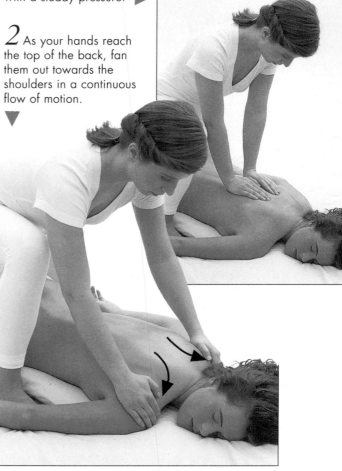

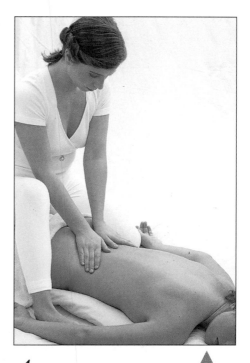

4 Swivel your wrists and softly stroke towards the centre of the back in order to repeat the stroke two more times.

Fanning Upwards

A firm fanning motion towards the heart can give a boost to the blood circulation. Massage with smaller fanning motions, moving up the back until your hands reach the shoulder blades, and then adapt the stroke to encompass the broad surface of the upper back before gliding back down the sides of the body.

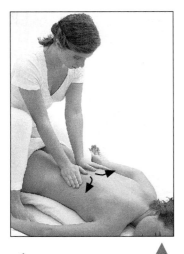

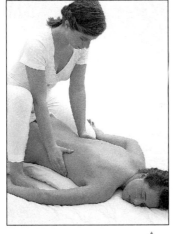

1 Place your hands on each side of the spine, fingers pointing to the head. Stroke upwards with a steady pressure before fanning your hands outwards.

2 Sculpting the sides of the body, pull softly but firmly downwards. Flex your wrists to stroke very lightly back into the body.

Pressure Circles on the Lower Back

Pressure circles are excellent strokes for removing tension from a tight lumbar region. Start the stroke softly, and as the tissue warms increase the pressure into the heels of your hands. Build up speed to massage vigorously on the small of the back. Use firm pressure on the upward and outward half of the circle, flexing your wrists to glide your hands very lightly around to the start of the stroke. Complete the sequence with a full and soothing effleurage stroke over the back.

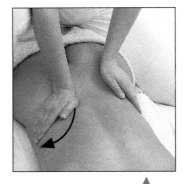

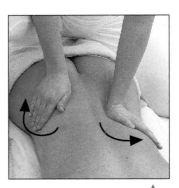

1 Place both hands flat on each side of the base of the spine, with the fingers slightly tilted towards the sides of the body. Stroke your right hand up a short distance, fanning it outwards into a circular motion.

2 At this point the left hand begins to stroke upwards. As the right hand decreases pressure and glides lightly back in a circular motion towards the start of the stroke, the left hand fans up and outwards.

Soft Circle Strokes

To accomplish the next series of strokes, turn to face into the back. Once you have finished the sequence, change position to repeat the whole sequence from the opposite side of the body. Flow from stroke to stroke without breaking the movement of your hands.

Soft circle strokes feel wonderful on the skin, with their overlapping and fluid motion easing and stretching tension out of the body's soft tissue. They are a perfect stroke for the broad yet rounded dimensions of the back. Begin circle stroking up the side of the body opposite to you, spiralling from the hip to the edge of the shoulder blade. Without breaking the flow, swing the stroke out to cover the spine and massage down towards the sacrum. Repeat three times.

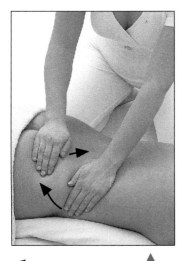

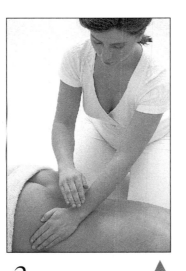

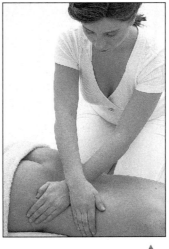

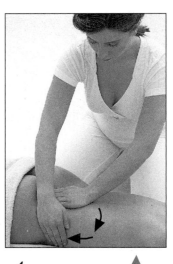

1 Lay your hands over the opposite side to you, keeping the hands about 10 cm/4 in apart. Circle both hands in a clockwise motion.

2 Lift up the right hand as it completes the first half-circle to allow the left hand to pass underneath it in an unbroken motion.

3 As the left hand continues to circle over the side of the body, cross the right hand over it, dropping it lightly back on to the skin.

4 Let the right hand form another half-circle stroke before lifting off as the left hand completes it full circle, spiralling upwards.

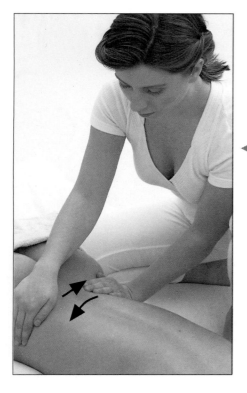

Wringing The Back

The wringing action on the lower back is done by crossing your hands from side to side, creating a warm friction on the muscle fibres. Work the stroke across the back, from the hips to the shoulder blades, and down again three times, always making sure that your hands fully encompass both sides of the body. Increase the speed and tempo of the wringing for an invigorating effect and then slow it down for a soothing finish.

1 Place your right hand over the hip opposite to you, with your fingers wrapped slightly under the belly, the left hand cupped over the hip closest to you. Slide your hands towards each other with enough pressure to lift and roll the flesh on the sides of the body.

2 Decrease the pressure as you stroke across the back, hands passing each other to the opposite sides of the body. Without stopping, immediately begin to slide them back. Continuously stroke your hands back and forth while you wring up and down the lumbar region.

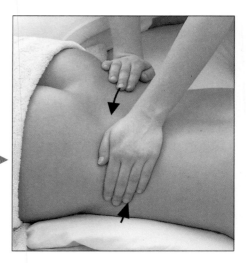

Kneading

Invigorating kneading on the buttocks, hips, and along the flank of the body will help to release weight and tension from the back, bringing relief to the whole area. Scoop, squeeze, and roll the flesh with your right hand and then roll it towards the left hand. Without breaking the motion, repeat the action with the left hand so that it passes the flesh back. Keep the stroke moving back and forth in a rhythmic and circular manner. Take care to relax your own shoulders, wrists, and hands. Knead thoroughly from the hip to just below the arm and back down again. Repeat once more.

1 Knead over the top of the buttock and beside the hip on the side of the body opposite to you. Work the kneading stroke up alongside the waist and rib cage. The amount of flesh on this area varies considerably from person to person.

2 Thorough kneading beside the shoulder blade will help the upper back to relax and the shoulder to drop.

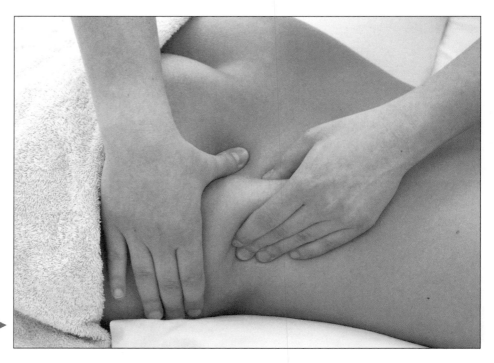

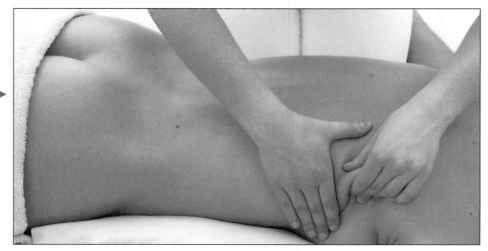

Hip, Shoulder and Spine Stretch

This stretch stroke brings a lovely sense of integration to the body as the hands move diagonally from the hip to the opposite shoulder, fans around and over the shoulder blade several times and then finishes with a soft stretch over the length of the spine.

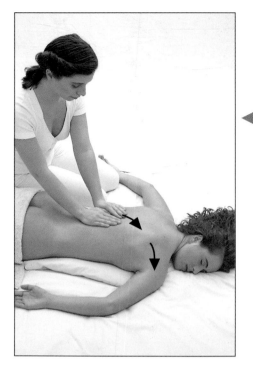

1 Place your hands close together, fingers pointing towards the opposite shoulder, over the hip nearest to you. Stroke across the body to make a sweeping diagonal stretch.

2 When your fingers reach the tip of the opposite shoulder joint, mould them to curve into the shape of the shoulder blade. Draw your hands outwards to surround its circumference until the fingers of both hands meet at the centre of its inner ridge.

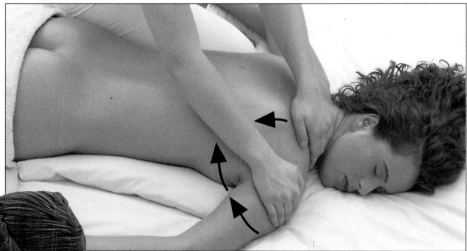

3 Sweep your hands several times over and around the bone, keeping your hands supple and wrists loose in order to fully enfold its flat triangular shape. Feel the muscles warm up beneath your touch.

4 Now pull both hands back towards the spine and draw your hands in opposite directions over the vertebrae, one towards the neck and the other towards the lower back. Stop briefly to rest your hands in a calm, still hold over each end of the spine. Move to the other side of your partner and repeat these strokes, following up with harmonious effleurage strokes to cover the whole surface of the back.

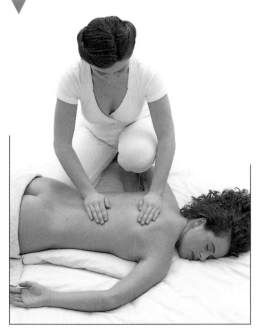

Focus on the Upper Back

The upper back tightens under stress, and most people welcome the therapeutic touch in this region. The following strokes will help to disperse the tension, allowing a greater sense of freedom and vitality.

Criss-cross and Squeeze

This criss-cross stroke requires co-ordinated movement. It combines effleurage with a squeezing action and follows the line of the diamond-shaped trapezius muscle that lifts and lowers the shoulder girdle and helps to raise the head.

1 Place your hands over the spine at the mid-point of the back. Both hands should be slightly angled towards each other, with the fingers of your right hand resting lightly over the fingers of the left hand. Stroke both hands directly out towards the opposite shoulders in a cross-over action.

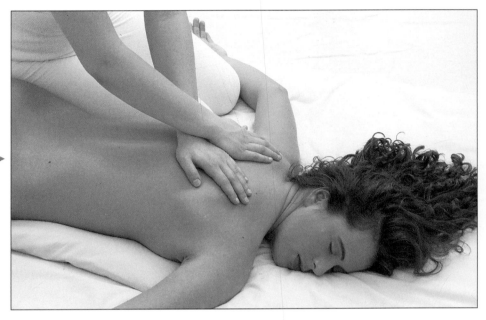

2 Without breaking the motion, wrap your fingers slightly over the front of the shoulders, then, adding pressure to both your fingers and heels of the hands, lift, roll, and squeeze the flesh. Release the pressure and pull your hands back towards the mid-point so that your arms are no longer crossed

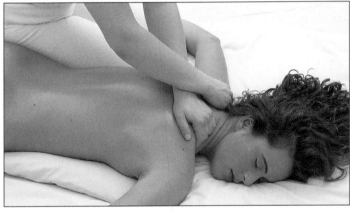

3 Now glide your hands out again to the shoulders, so that the hands form a V shape. Again let your fingers wrap over the top of the shoulder, but this time slide your hands back without squeezing the muscles. Repeat at least two more times.

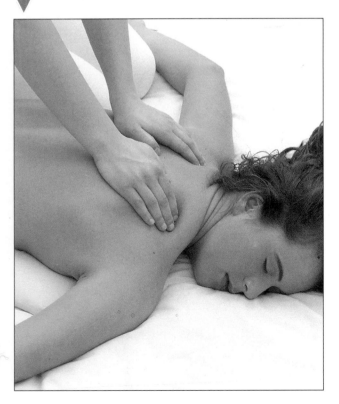

Kneading the Shoulders

Use a kneading action to roll and squeeze the muscles between the thumbs and fingers to ease tight spots at the base of the neck and over the shoulder. Work on the shoulder opposite to you and ask your partner to turn her head towards you so that the shoulder's surface is fully exposed.

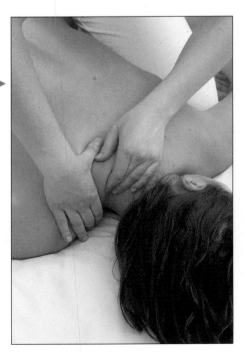

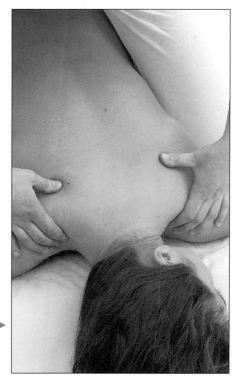

Friction Strokes

Thumbs and fingers are the perfect massage tools with which to penetrate deeper tissue around the shoulder blades and spine. These following two friction strokes will bring relief to sore, constricted muscles.

Easing the Vertebrae

1 Anchor your fingers gently but securely in front of the shoulders, placing your palms on either side of the spine. Apply pressure into your thumbs and sink them into the tissue alongside the vertebrae. Begin to slide firmly up towards the top of the shoulders.

2 Without releasing your fingers, circle your hands lightly back to their original position. Repeat the thumb slide several times.

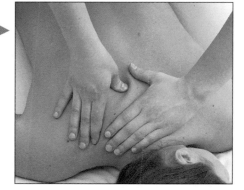

Thumb Friction

Another deep friction stroke can be achieved by using firm pressure in the thumb pad to grind tissue against the bone, helping to dispel toxic build-up in muscle fibres. Using one hand to push the muscle towards the stroke, make a series of short slides with the other hand, using the thumb pad to stretch and ease tense areas. Always remember to sink into and release pressure slowly and gently from a friction stroke.

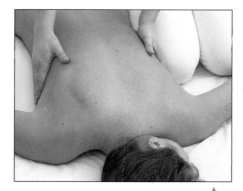

A Soothing Finish

The deeper tissue work of kneading and friction strokes should now be followed by soft and soothing effleurage strokes to bring a sense of overall relaxation and integration to the upper back.

1 Place your hands on the mid-back, flat against each side of the spine with the fingers pointing to the head. Sweep your hands up towards the top of the shoulders.

2 Forming your hands perfectly to the curve of the body, spread them out to the edge of the shoulders, then glide them around the joints.

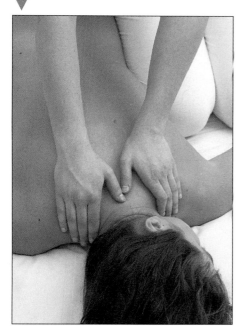

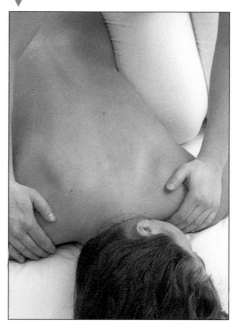

3 Draw your hands down the sides of the ribcage until they are once again mid-back. Turn your hands so they can slide lightly to the centre of the back and repeat the effleurage stroke two more times.

To complete the back massage, do three full integration strokes, and then place your hands on the neck and base of the spine in a restful hold.

Massaging the Back of the Legs

The following sequence of massage strokes focuses on the lower half of the body – the legs, buttocks, and feet.
This is an area of primary importance to the body's posture, weight, and locomotion. By combining the techniques of
effleurage, kneading, friction, percussion, and passive movements, this programme of massage will help to warm and
stretch the muscles, improve the circulation of blood and lymph, ease tension from the large strong muscles, and free
contracted joints. Begin the massage on the left leg before repeating all the strokes on the right side of the body.

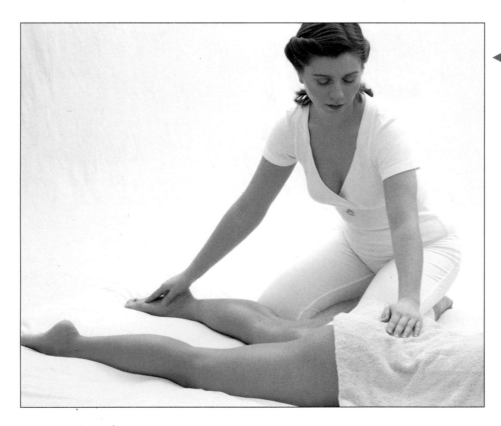

Preliminary Strokes

◀ *1* Connecting the leg and back: Bring your partner's awareness to the leg with a connecting hold on the sacrum and foot. The gentle presence of your hands begins the process of relaxation.

2 Integration stroke on the leg: Spread the oil smoothly down the whole leg, from the buttocks to the foot, then begin with the initial integration stroke. Repeat the stroke three times, increasing the pressure with each upward movement. Be sure to mould your hands to the shape of the leg and to adopt a posture that enables you to stroke upwards and pull back with ease. Place one foot on the mattress ahead of your body to lever your position back and forth.
▼

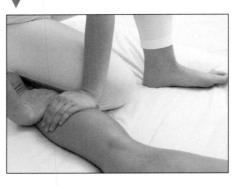

The Back of the Leg

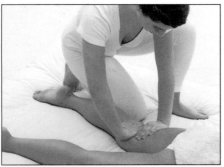

◀ *1* Starting on the left leg, wrap both hands over the back of the ankle, little fingers leading, with your left hand taking the top position. Slide with a steady pressure up over the calf. Continue to stroke both hands towards the thigh, sliding lightly over the back of the knee. Then use enough pressure to create a ripple in the strong thigh muscles.

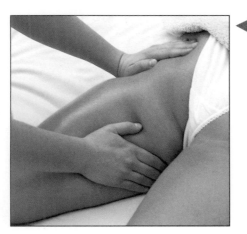

◀ *2* As your hands approach the top of the leg, glide the lower one on to the inside of the thigh to rest for some moments while stroking the upper hand over the buttock and out around the hip joint.

3 When the moving hand descends to the outer thigh and is parallel with the waiting hand, slip your fingers slightly under the front of the leg so that you are holding it securely. ▶

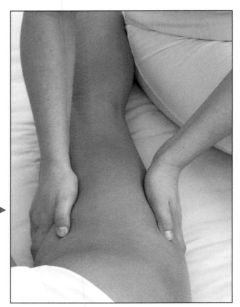

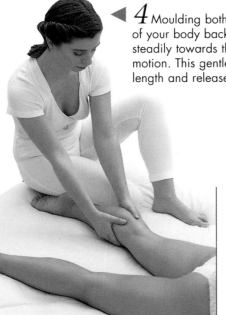

4 Moulding both hands to the leg, lean the weight of your body backwards, returning the stroke steadily towards the ankle in a long unbroken motion. This gentle stretch will bring a feeling of length and release to the leg.

5 As your hands reach the ankle, slip the hand on the outside of the leg over the back of the heel of the foot and, lifting the foot slightly, pass the other hand over the instep. Stroke out over both sides of the foot.

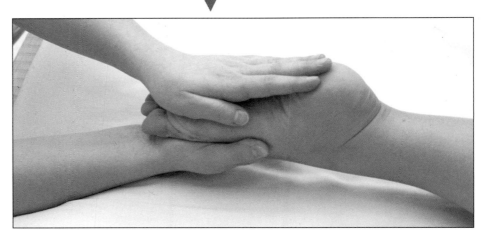

Focus on the Calf

The function of the calf muscles is to flex the knee and ankle joints, while the Achilles tendon flexes the foot and provides leverage for body movement. Keeping this area supple is important for general health. Muscle stiffness causes a sluggish blood circulation and poor lymphatic drainage, which results in low energy levels. The purpose of this sequence of strokes is to bring relief and relaxation to sore calf muscles.

Begin the sequence with some integrating effleurage strokes, which cover the lower leg from the ankle to just below the back of the knee.

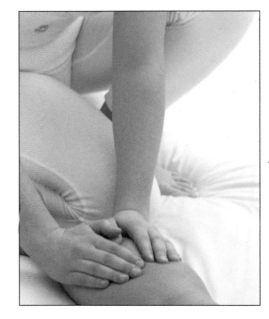

2 Fan both hands out to wrap around the sides and front of the leg, before sliding down and back towards the original position. Stroke further up over the calf to repeat the motion.

Fanning to the Knee

Perform a series of fanning motions on the lower leg, moving up from the ankle to just behind the knee. Then glide your hands back down the sides of the leg and repeat the sequence.

1 Softening your hands to the shape of the leg, place them side by side so that the fingers tilt towards each other but point to the back of the knee. Stroke a hand's length up over the calf muscles.

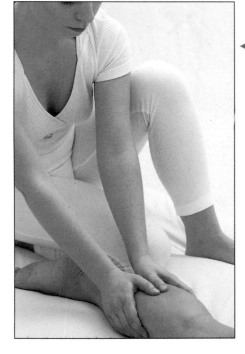

Relaxing the Achilles Tendon

Cup your fingers under the front of the ankle, so the heels of both hands fit snugly on each side of the heel of the foot, and your thumbs rest on the lower calf. Flex your wrists to rotate your hands in steady circular motions, soothing away strain from the heel and the Achilles tendon.

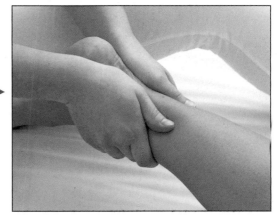

Draining the Lower Leg

This stroke drains blood and lymph from the extremity of the body. It also creates a long, firm stretch on the lower leg muscles.

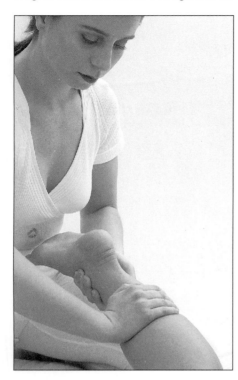

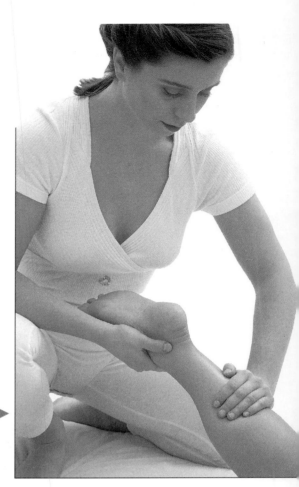

1 Raise the foot and lower leg off the mattress by lifting and supporting the front of the ankle with your left hand. Wrap your right hand over the back of the ankle so that the palm and heel of the hand folds over the inner half of the leg.

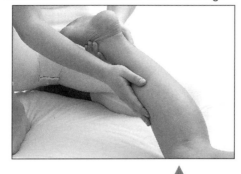

2 Stroke with a firm and steady pressure up the leg towards the back of the knee. Swing the hand to glide down the front of the leg to the ankle.

3 Pass the leg to the right hand and repeat the motion with the left hand up over the outer half of the leg; return the stroke to the ankle. Repeat the sequence two more times.

Kneading the Calf

Kneading strokes will revive fatigued or aching calf muscles resulting from poor circulation, prolonged standing, or excessive exertion. Position yourself to face the calf and knead thoroughly from the ankle to just below the back of the knee and down again. Follow up with effleurage strokes.

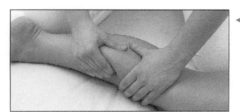

1 Keeping both hands slightly apart, place them over the leg with the thumbs angled away from the fingers. Scoop, lift, and squeeze the muscle by applying pressure between the thumb, heel, and fingers and push it towards the left hand.

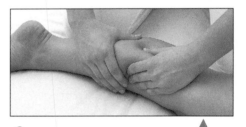

2 Pick up and squeeze the flesh with the left hand and push it back to the right hand. Keeping both hands on the leg, pass the muscle back and forth in a rhythmic and circular movement.

Deep Friction

These deep friction strokes use the thumbs to penetrate and stretch a deeper level of muscle tissue, freeing it from underlying tension. Sink into the muscle slowly, always remaining aware of your partner's response to the pressure. Both strokes are achieved by rotating the thumbs from their base joints. Once your hands have reached to just below the knee, glide them back down the sides of the leg and repeat the sequence.

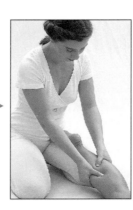

1 Clasp the front of the leg with your fingers and stroke one thumb after the other up over the calf. Using short sliding movements, press firmly into the upward movement and then swing each thumb out and glide lightly back to perform the next upward stroke. At the same time gently roll the leg from hand to hand, squeezing the sides of the calf muscles with the heels of your hands.

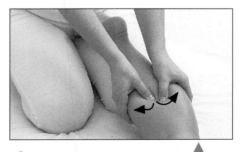

2 Focus the pressure into your thumb pads, and rotate them in alternate and tiny outward flowing circles. Soften the stroke on the last half of the circle. Move up over the calf in three separate lines from above the back of the ankle to just below the knee. Follow up with several flowing integration strokes to cover the whole leg from the ankle to the top of the thigh.

Focus on the Thigh

A thorough massage of the thighs brings relief to this ample area of powerful body muscle, which provides essential support to the body's posture and mobility.

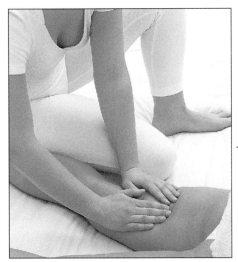

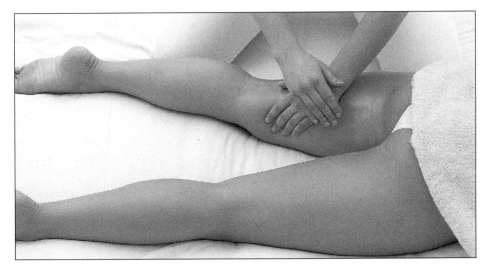

Fanning the Thigh

Start with a series of short, flowing fanning motions, stroking up from the back of the knee to just below the buttock. Then glide your hands down the sides of the leg, swivelling around on to the back of the knee. Repeat the sequence two more times.

Soft Circle Strokes

Turn your body so that you face into the thigh and cover the top of the leg with continuous circle strokes to relax and soften the tissue. Pay special attention to the inner thigh muscles, which draw the leg towards the centre of the body.

Draining the Thigh

Boost the lymph drainage and blood circulation in the thigh by leaning your weight into the heels of both hands for a series of firm, alternating pressure circles, one hand following the other. Lessen the pressure of the stroke as each hand fans out to the sides of the leg and glides back and around.

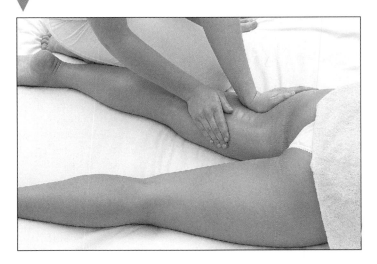

Kneading the Thigh

Vigorous kneading of the thigh muscles will enliven the upper leg, helping to break down excess fat deposits and boosting the exchange of tissue fluids. Lift, squeeze, and roll the flesh from hand to hand, working first up along the inner thigh and then over the bulk of the muscles. Follow the kneading with soothing fanning motions and other effleurage strokes.

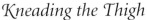

Wringing the Thigh

This wringing action massages across the bulk of muscle fibres and connective tissue that surrounds them on the thigh.

1 Wrap your right hand over the inner edge of the thigh so that your fingers slip slightly under the leg. Place your left hand over the outer side of the leg so that the fingers rest on the thigh. Pull firmly to scoop up the flesh before crossing your hands over the top of the thigh to the opposite sides.

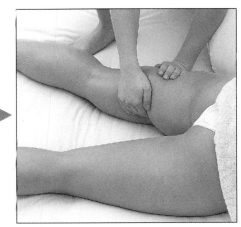

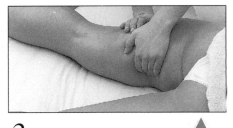

2 Continue to pass your hands rhythmically back and forth over the thigh, creating a slight twist in the movement to produce a wringing effect in the muscles. Stroke from above the knee to the top of the leg and back down again. Repeat once.

Focus on the Buttocks

The powerful muscles of the buttocks help to elevate the trunk of the body and move the thighs. Massage will contribute to a relaxed posture, as the body's weight will be more able to drop down into the support of the lower half of the body, taking the strain off the lower back. After massaging the thigh, focus your strokes on the buttock on the same side of the body. Begin with some flowing integration strokes that cover and connect the thigh and buttock and mould into its contours. The strokes below are shown on the right side of the body for clearer instruction.

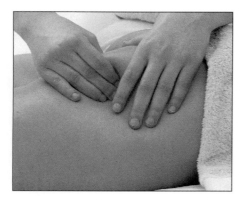

Kneading the Buttocks ▲
Release tension from the buttocks by thoroughly kneading this fleshy area. You may find it easier to knead from a position on the opposite side of the body; stretching your arms will enhance the squeezing and rolling action of the stroke.

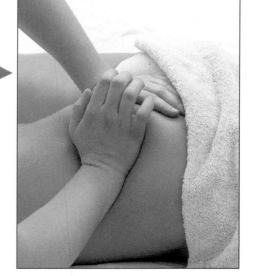

◄ Thumb Rolling
Continue the massage from the left side of the body, and use your thumbs to work around and under the bones at the base of the pelvic girdle. Placing both hands over the buttocks for support, roll one thumb after another in short firm slides into the crease at the juncture of the buttocks and thigh.

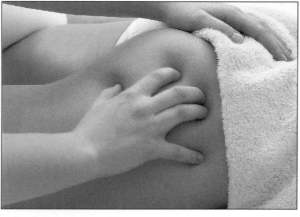

Shaking Out ▲
Shaking the buttocks can loosen any remaining stiffness and tension in the muscles. Place one hand softly over the sacrum to add support. Sink the fingers of the other hand into the muscle and vibrate rhythmically.

Heel Pressure
To press deeper into the muscle, sink the heel of your hand into the buttock and rotate. Lean your weight into the first half of the circular motion and release the pressure on the return. Place your other hand close to the stroke and push the muscle towards the action. Apply these heel-pressure rotations over the whole area. ►

Stimulating the Whole Leg

After applying all the strokes on the leg and buttocks, return to a position beside the ankle and repeat the initial integration stroke several times. Now begin a series of percussion strokes on the leg to enliven the skin and tone the muscles.

Cupping the Leg
Turn to face into the leg and briskly cup it, working from the calf up to the thigh, one hand following the other in rapid succession. Form a vacuum in the palms of your hands by bending the base knuckles and holding the fingers straight and close together while pulling the thumb in tight to the palm. As the hands cup the leg, flick them off the skin at the moment of contact. This creates a suction of air, drawing the blood supply up to the surface of the skin and leaving it with a healthy glow. ►

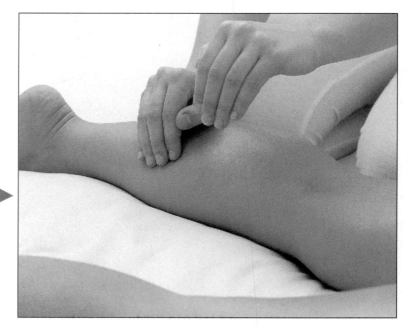

Hacking on the Leg ▶

Now use the hacking stroke, moving up the leg from the calf to the thigh, but taking care not to strike the delicate area on the back of the knee. Keeping your shoulders and wrists relaxed, hold your hands straight with the palms facing. Briskly strike the flesh with the sides of your hands, one hand following the other in quick, rhythmic succession so that they bounce off the skin immediately.

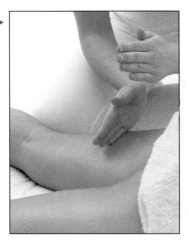

Enlivening the Skin

Complete the percussion strokes on the leg by stimulating the sensitive nerve endings in the skin with soft feather touches. Starting at the top of the thigh, use your fingertips to brush down the leg in short strokes with one hand at a time. Lift each hand off the leg to cross above the other in a continuous stream of downward overlapping motions.

Passive Movements on the Leg

Once the leg muscles are relaxed, you can introduce passive movements to gently stretch and ease tension from the joints, ligaments, and tendons. The most important thing to remember while making passive movements is never to move a part of the body beyond its point of resistance, and always to work within its natural range of movement. Your hands should impart sufficient confidence to encourage your partner to relax completely and allow you to lift, move, and stretch that part of the body

Gentle Hip and Knee Stretch

This passive movement helps to stretch the muscle attachments around the hip and knee joints by gently pushing the lower leg towards the thigh.

1 Kneel beside the foot and slip your right hand under the ankle to give it support, at the same time placing your left hand just above the back of the knee. Begin to raise the lower leg off the mattress so that the knee is flexed.

▼

2 Move your left hand to rest securely on the sacrum and lean forward to ease the raised part of the leg down towards the top of the thigh. Bounce the lower leg in tiny movements, gently against the point of resistance, and then lower it slowly back down to the mattress, keeping it in a straight line with the thigh. ▶

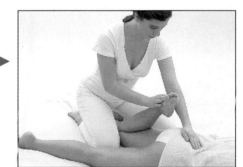

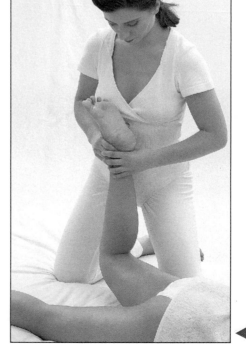

Lifting the Leg

Take care of your own posture while doing this passive movement. Ensure that your back is straight, and elevate your own body from the muscles in your haunches during the upward lift. Do not attempt this movement if you have a weak back or the leg is too heavy.
 Raise the lower leg so the knee is flexed and then clasp the ankle firmly with both hands. Lift the leg slowly upwards to take the thigh slightly off the mattress. Bob the leg up and down a little ◀ before lowering the thigh.

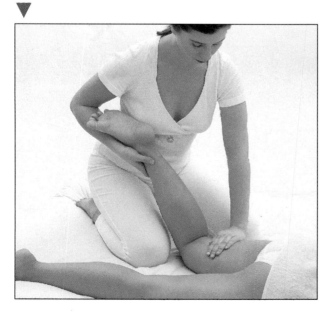

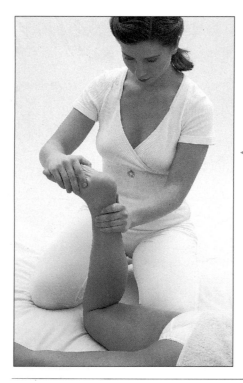

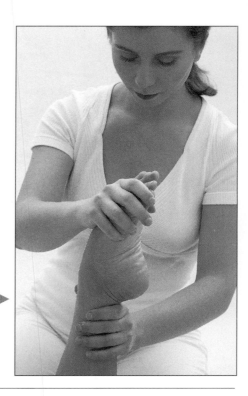

The Ankle Stretch

Ankle stretches should be made while the lower leg is raised and the knee is flexed. The flexion and extension movements will ease the tendons and the ligaments surrounding the ankle joints.

1 Hold the lower leg with your left hand while placing your right hand over the ball of the foot. Gently and slowly depress the foot to extend the back of the heel and ankle, creating a stretch in the Achilles tendon. Do not push beyond the point of resistance.

2 Slip your right hand over the instep and move the foot backwards to stretch and extend the front of the ankle. Repeat both movements on the ankle to encourage greater flexibility. Then lower the leg to the mattress.

The Feet

The function is to provide support and locomotion. While walking, the entire weight of the body is shifted into different areas of the feet. The bones form into two arches, which are able to yield to the body's weight and provide leverage in motion. A good foot massage can benefit the whole body, not only by taking the strain and tension away from the tendons and many bones, but by stimulating the nerve endings and boosting the entire physical system.

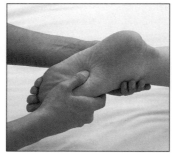

Relaxing the Heel

1 The heels of your hands fit perfectly into the sides of the foot's heel so that you can ease away strain with firm flowing circles. Raise the foot slightly with your left hand. Clasping the front of the ankle with your right hand, rotate the heel of your hand just below the ankle bone. Change hands and repeat the massage on the other side.

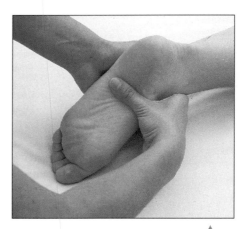

2 Holding the foot with your left hand, stroke your right thumb firmly back and forth under the inner ridge of the heel to release pressure and tension.

Easing the Sole

The following strokes on the base of the foot are made by sinking a thumb pad sensitively into a depth of tissue and rotating it slowly, on one spot at a time, before slowly releasing the pressure. Work down the sole in bands, from the heel to the base of the toes, starting on the arch and moving across to the outer edge of the foot. Keep the foot slightly raised and supported by your hands.

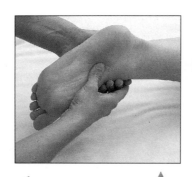

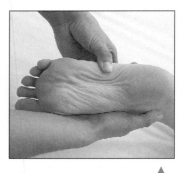

1 Bring greater flexibility to the arch of the foot with the thumb rotations. Press gently with your right thumb on this sensitive area, starting at the edge of the heel.

2 Stimulate the nerve endings and ease away stiffness by pressing and rotating your right thumb carefully into the tissue, taking care to cover the entire surface.

3 Start using your left thumb to press and rotate down the outer edge of the sole to increase the overall relaxing effect of the foot massage.

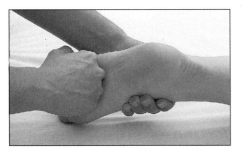

Knuckling the Sole ▲
Make a loose fist with your right hand, and hook the knuckles into the tissue just below the heel. Draw steadily down over the sole to the base of the toes to create a deep, satisfying stretch.

Soothing Strokes
Follow up the pressure and stretch movements with soothing effleurage strokes.

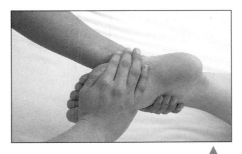

1 Cup the foot in the palm of your left hand and stroke over the sole with your right hand.

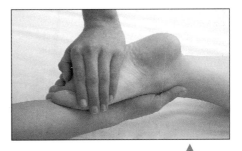

2 As your stroke glides around the ankle and down over the instep, repeat the movement with your left hand. Repeat steps 1 and 2 several times.

Rotating the Toe Joints
Exercise the toes with passive movements to loosen tight joints. Work across the foot from the little toe to the big toe. Start by holding the left foot in your right hand, then change to the left hand when necessary. The photographs shown here illustrate the right foot for clearer instruction.

1 Clasp the toe just above its base joint between your thumb and index finger; circle it three times to the right and then to the left. Now squeeze gently along the toe to its tip. ▼

2 Repeat all the movements on the big toe, using the thumb and index finger of your other hand. Relaxing the big toe will bring substantial relief to the whole foot. ▼

Stroking the Instep
By raising the lower leg so the knee is flexed, you can massage the front of the foot while your partner lays on her belly. Hold the foot with both hands, fingers resting across its sole. Stroke over the instep with alternating thumb slides, working down towards the ankle from the base of the toes. ▼

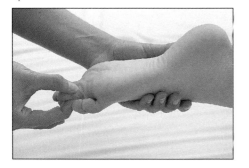

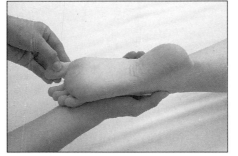

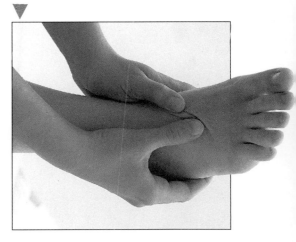

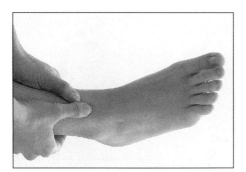

Relaxing the Ankle Joints ▲
Grip the back of the leg and rotate one thumb after the other so that their pads grind against the tiny ankle bones to relax the ligaments and joints.

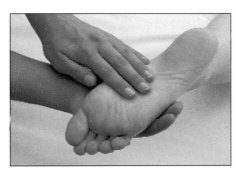

Warming the Foot ▲
Clasp the foot between both hands and rub briskly back and forth across the sole and instep to create heat and vitality. Then hold the foot softly for several moments.

Lay your hands over the soles of both feet to bring a sense of balance to the body. You can now repeat all the above strokes on the right leg, buttocks, and foot to complete the first half of this wonderful whole body massage.

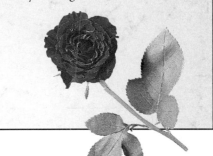

Massaging the Front of the Body

When your partner has turned over and you are ready to apply your strokes to the front of the body, take a few moments to compose yourself and relax your own body, so that you can again focus your full attention on the massage. You will now be touching the more vulnerable areas of the body, such as the face, chest, and belly, so you need to bring a great deal of sensitivity, confidence, and care into your hands. Give your partner a few moments to settle into her new position, and reassure her with a calm and tender hold.

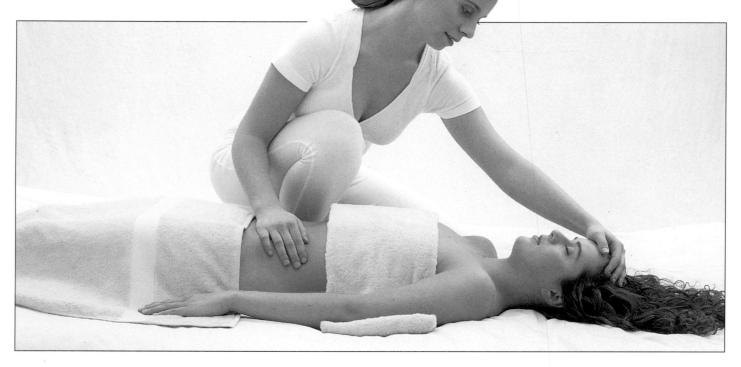

Focus on the Front of the Leg

Begin working on the front of the body by continuing the leg massage. Most of the strokes are similar to those used on the back of the legs. Specific strokes are required for the shin and knee as the bones are closer to the surface of the skin.

Balancing the Body
Hold the feet for several moments to bring a sense of balance to both sides of the body. Then begin your massage on the left leg.

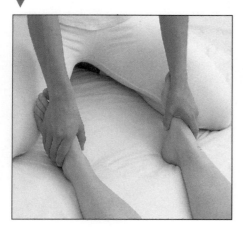

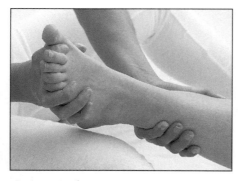

Joint Release
▲

1 Take the opportunity to create more space in the ankle joints with passive movements. Support the back of the lower leg with one hand, and place your other hand over the sole so that your thumb and fingers lightly clasp the foot.

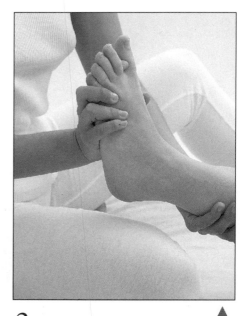

2 Slip the index finger between the first and second toes to maintain a secure grip. Circle the ankle three times to the right and then three times to the left to rotate its joints.

The Main Stroke

Spread your essential oil on the front of the leg, stroking it down from the hip to the foot. Begin with the main integration stroke, using the same flowing effleurage motion as you applied to the back of the leg. Glide gently over the knee before taking the stroke up to the thigh.

Fanning

1 Warm and stretch the muscles that cover the shin with a series of fanning strokes, moving up from the ankle to just below the knee before gliding your hands back down to the lower leg.

2 Glide one hand after the other over the shin in a series of alternating fanning motions, slipping your fingers under the leg on the return movement to stroke back down over the calf.

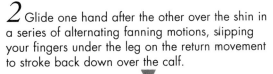
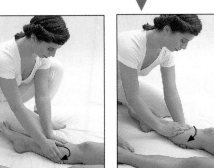

A Long Stretch

This friction stroke stretches and eases the tissue between the two long bones that form the shin. Secure the back of the leg with your left hand and pull gently on the leg to create a slight traction. Wrapping your right hand over the inside of the lower leg, sink the right thumb sensitively between the two bones at the point where they join the front of the ankle. Slide the thumb slowly and steadily along the edge of the large bone until your hand reaches the knee. Lighten the pressure and glide your hand around the knee-cap and back down the side of the leg. Follow this deep stretch with some effleurage.

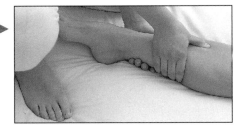

Relaxing the Knee

The knee, like the ankle, plays an important part in the support and mobility of the body's weight and structure. The knee-cap itself is bound by tendons and ligaments, which attach to the muscles and long bones in the thigh and lower leg. Strain and injury in the knee are common complaints, and it is important to include this area in your massage strokes to help keep it flexible. When working on and around the knee-cap, settle your fingers beneath the knee to give it support.

1 Using the heels of both hands at the same time, rotate them firmly around the sides and above the top of the knee-cap.

2+3 Place both thumbs, one above the other, across the base of the knee. Slide them over the bone and then draw them out in opposite directions to encircle the edge of the knee-cap until they return to their first position. Repeat the stroke several times as a continuous motion.

4 Face towards the leg and knead thoroughly just above the knee. This will increase suppleness and circulation to the ligaments, tendons, and the muscles that attach to the joint.

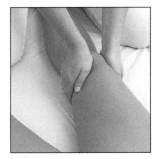
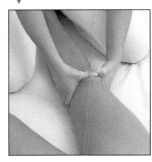
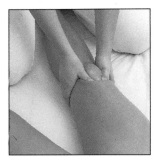
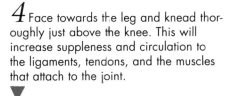
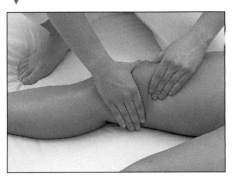

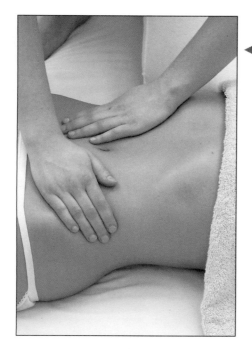

Circling the Belly

◀ *1* Circle strokes are a lovely way of soothing and relaxing the abdomen, and fit perfectly to its shape. Repeat the continuous circles with the whole surfaces of your hands, moving in a clockwise direction until you feel the belly becoming soft and warm.

2 As the abdominal muscles relax, sensitively shift the pressure into your fingertips as you make the circular strokes. Decrease the circle so that you are stroking around the navel, then widen the circular movement outwards to cover the belly, shifting the weight back into the full surface of your hands. ▼

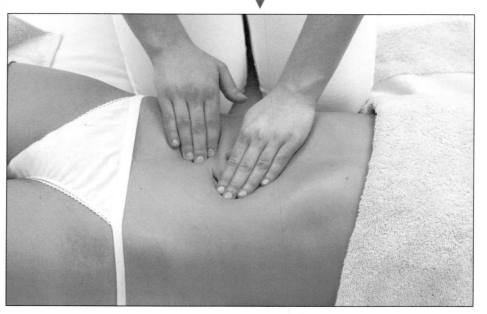

Relaxing the Sides of the Belly

The muscles that cross from the back of the body to the front of the abdomen help to support the vital organs and rotate the spine. Make the following milking and kneading strokes on both sides of the body to increase suppleness.

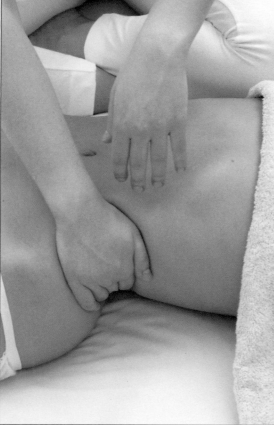

◀ *1* Using one hand after the other in a milking action, pull firmly over the sides of the abdomen from just under the back. Glide lightly to the centre of the belly before lifting the hand off to repeat the stroke. Stroke in this way from the hip to the ribcage.

2 Lift, squeeze, and roll the flesh from hand to hand in a kneading stroke along the sides of the abdomen from the hip to the base of the ribcage. ▼

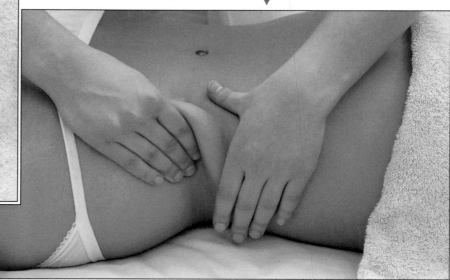

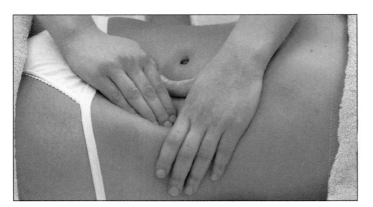

1 Sink the first three fingertips of one hand slowly into the abdominal muscles of the belly surface. Place the other hand close to your fingers, with the thumb at an angle in order to anchor the muscle and push it slightly towards the stroke. Rotate the fingertips in tiny circles on one spot at a time, moving in a clockwise motion around the belly. Pay specific attention to the areas close to the wings of the pelvic bone.

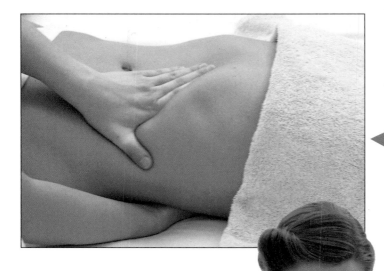

Deeper Belly Strokes

If your partner is responding well to the belly massage and the area is relaxing, you can begin to apply the deeper abdominal strokes. Be very sensitive and alert to your partner's responses, applying and releasing pressure slowly, ensuring that she is ready to receive the deeper strokes at any given time.

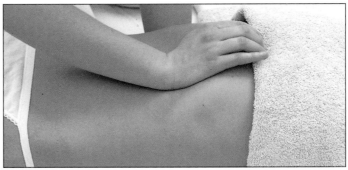

2 The upper abdomen can become particularly tense during times of stress, as the diaphragm muscle that separates the chest and belly tightens, and the solar plexus, a nerve centre, becomes hyperactive. Once the area has been relaxed by softer strokes, and the breath deepens, slip your left hand under the body to rest below the spine. This creates a sense of support as you use the heel of your right hand to massage gently, but with increased pressure, in circles around the base of the ribcage.

3 Ease constriction from under the ribcage with a firm, steady slide of one hand, while the other hand rests parallel and just beneath the body for support. Keeping your fingers close together and your thumb at an angle, sink the side of the index finger and hand gently under the edge of the lower rib. Slowly slide your hand down to the side of the body, lightening the pressure towards the end of the stroke. Repeat this stroke on the other side of the body.

Hands on the Belly and Chest

Repeat the flowing, soft, circular motions on the belly to bring an harmonious finish to the deeper strokes. Then complete this part of the massage by placing one hand over the abdomen and the other on the chest so that it rests over the heart. This peaceful hold will bring a calming sense of equilibrium and unity to the body.

Focus on the Arms

Muscular tension forms in the arms and hands for a number of reasons. Poor posture can cause the shoulder girdle to stiffen and inhibit the flexibility of the upper limbs. Repetitive movements at work put strain, wear and tear on the muscles, tendons, and ligaments. On an emotional level, the arms and hands represent the ability to reach out and contact the outside world, or the means of expressing creativity. Arm and hand massage feels wonderfully relaxing, bringing relief and ease to the upper body and renewing vitality. Using the following strokes, work first on one arm and hand, and then on the other.

Opening Out

This first movement helps the upper chest and shoulders to open out to create freedom from contraction in the shoulder joint and a feeling of length in the arm. The oil remaining on your hands from the previous strokes should be sufficient for this opening stretch but, if necessary, add just a little more to your hands as you work.

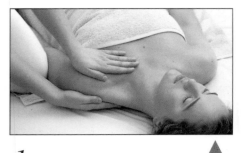

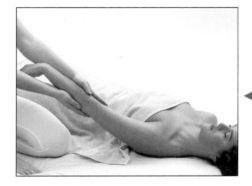

1 Face in towards the shoulder to lift it, and slip the hand furthest from the body under the top of the back so that the fingers point towards the spine. Place the other hand across the top of the chest, fingers pointing towards the breast bone. As you feel the shoulder relaxing between your hands, pull firmly and steadily out towards its edge.

2 Keeping one foot on the mattress, manoeuvre your position so you are able to sandwich the top of the arm between both hands, and then pull steadily down its entire length to give a gentle stretch to the shoulder joint.

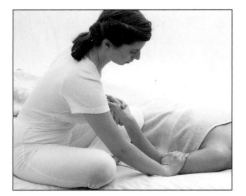

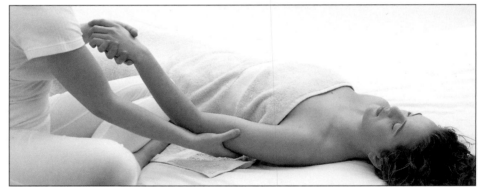

The Integration Stroke

1 Spread some oil down the arm, moulding your hands to its shape and using overlapping strokes. Hold your partner's hand with the hand closest to the body. Wrap your other hand across the wrist, to lead the stroke with your little finger. Glide your hand firmly up the arm towards the shoulder.

2 Forming your hand to the curve over the shoulder, glide it around the joint.

3 Lifting the arm slightly off the mattress, stroke lightly down the back of the arm to the wrist.

4 Pass your partner's arm to your other hand and clasp it by the wrist. Stroke up along the inside of the arm with the hand closest to the body, the little finger leading. Swivel your hand around just below the armpit and glide it back down the arm. Repeat the sequence two more times.

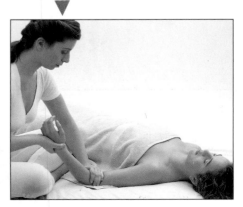

Relaxing the Forearm

1 Relax the lower arm with a series of alternating fanning motions, one hand following the other and moving up from the wrist to the elbow. Squeeze the muscles gently between the heel and fingers as the hand curves outwards, stroking firmly with your fingers on the under-side of the arm as your hand glides back round. Glide your hands from the elbow back to the wrist to repeat the sequence two more times.

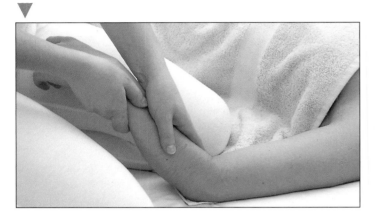

2 Secure the wrist with the hand closest to the body, and pull very gently on the arm to create a slight traction. Wrapping the other hand around the outer side of the forearm, sink the thumb slowly into the groove where the long bones of the forearm join the wrist. Stroke firmly and slowly up the arm, between the bones, releasing the pressure at the elbow. Slip your hand around the joint and glide it back down to the wrist.

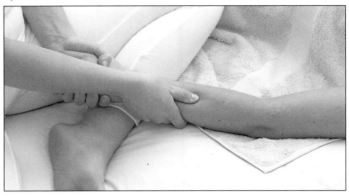

Draining Strokes

Boost the circulation towards the heart with the following strokes, which drain the lower arm.

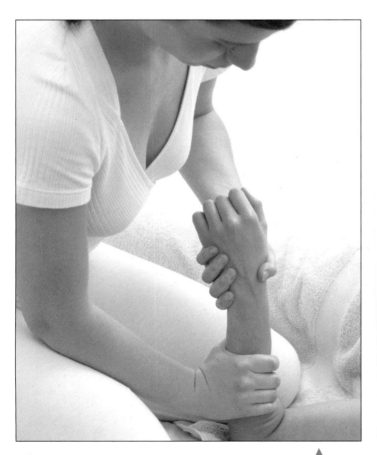

1 Raise the forearm vertically so that it rests on the elbow. Clasp your partner's hand with your left hand and wrap your other hand around the top of the wrist, the little finger leading the stroke. Slide firmly down the arm as if to drain it. Open your hand to glide softly around the elbow joint and lightly back up the forearm.

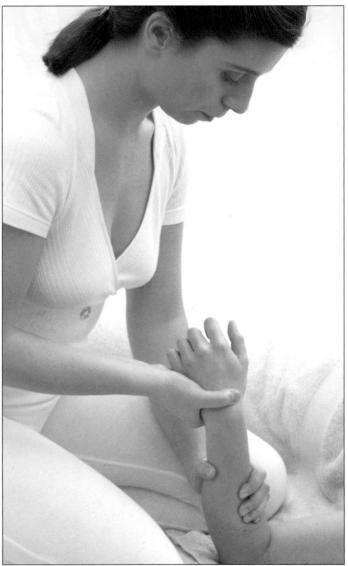

2 Repeat the same draining motion on the inside of the arm, changing the position of your hands.

Loosening the Upper Arm

The position and narrow structure of the arm can make the application of strokes more difficult than usual, so be sure that the limb is supported comfortably before massaging the upper half of the arm.

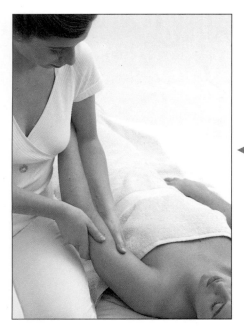

◀ *1* Start with a series of alternating fanning motions, one hand following the other, from just above the elbow to the shoulder. Squeeze the muscles gently between your fingers and heels of the hands as each hand fans outwards. When your hands reach the top of the arm, sweep them around and back down towards the elbow. Repeat once. To keep the arm in a raised position, secure its lower half between your own body and arm.

2 Cradle the shoulder joint between both hands, placing the hand furthest from the body beneath the shoulder, and the hand closest to the body on top. Slide both hands back and forth over the top of the shoulder several times, making a see-saw motion for a warming effect.
▼

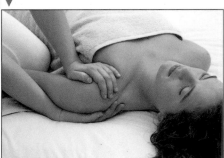

3 Keeping the elbow flexed, lift the arm and place it across the body, asking your partner to clasp her other shoulder so that the upper arm remains steady and vertical. From this position, it is easy to apply your strokes. Holding the inside of the arm with your fingers, work around the back of the elbow joint with
◀ tiny alternating thumb circles.

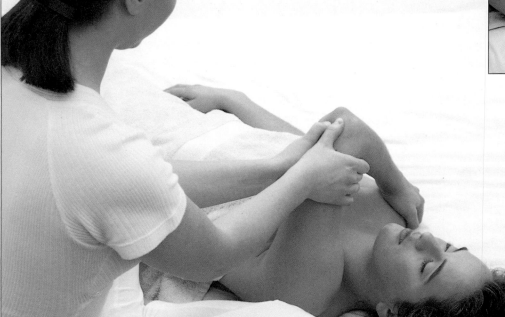

4 Clasping the upper arm firmly with the thumbs placed centrally next to each other, slide both hands steadily downwards in a draining action. Complete by gliding the right hand softly around the back of the shoulder and then repeating the stroke.
▼

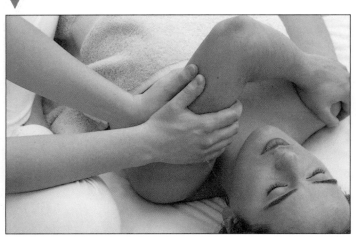

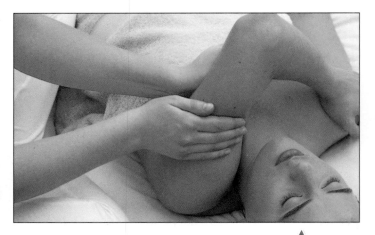

▲
5 Wrapping your fingers around the inside of the arm, squeeze and knead down the upper arm muscles with circular fanning motions, applying pressure from the heels of the hands as they move outwards, and then gliding them back around more lightly.

Passive Movements on the Arm

These passive arm movements create a sense of length and space in the upper body and shoulder girdle by gently stretching the joints. Do them slowly and sensitively, working with the natural movement of the shoulder joint. Never force the arm or shoulder beyond its point of resistance or tension.

1 Kneel behind the shoulder to remove the arm from its previous position. Support this movement by wrapping your right hand around the wrist and the left hand under the elbow. Begin to circle the arm slowly in a low arc-shaped motion, compatible with the movement of the shoulder joint, until it is stretched out behind your partner's head.

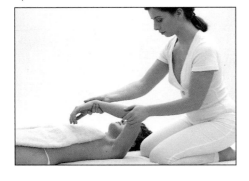

2 Tuck the arm into the side of your body and change the position of your hands to support the elbow with your right hand. Pull very gently on the arm to create a slight traction.

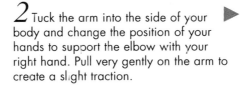

3 Lean forward to mould your left hand to the waist, and then slide it firmly up along the side of the body and softly under the shoulder joint in a steady stretching motion, bringing the feeling of length to the upper body.

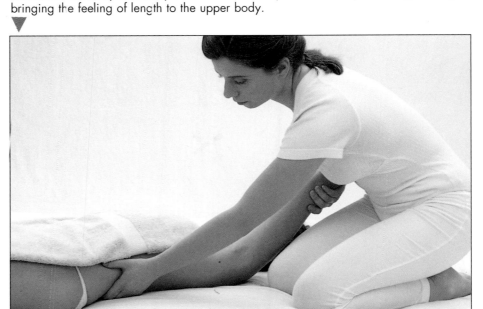

4 Continue sliding your left hand up the back of the arm towards the elbow to increase the stretch in the shoulder joint. Now relax the shoulder and move yourself slowly back to the side of the body, taking the arm with you in a fluid arc-shaped movement. Ensure the arm is properly supported by your hands and the elbow stays flexed until the whole limb has relaxed back on to the mattress.

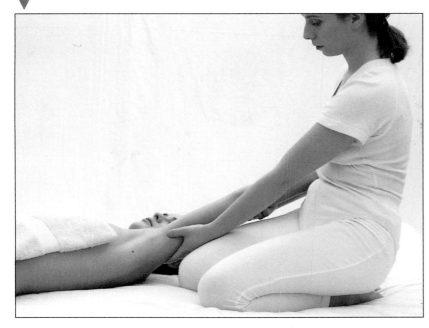

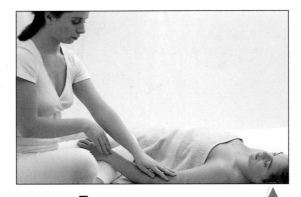

5 Complete the passive arm movement with soft feathering touches, letting your fingertips sweep over the whole limb, one hand following the other in overlapping strokes.

Focus on the Hands

Once the arm is relaxed, turn your attention to the hand. Your strokes will ease away tension from the tendons, muscles and bones to increase suppleness and dexterity. They will also stimulate the hand's many sensory nerve endings. A hand massage soothes away the stress of a day's activity: it is an essential part of a whole body massage, or can be done as a session in itself.

Kneel or sit below your partner's hand so that it can rest comfortably on your lap with the forearm slightly elevated. Change hands when necessary to complete the strokes on both sides of the hand. Use only a small amount of oil in order to secure a firm slide with your strokes.

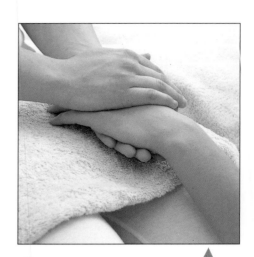

1 Cradle the hand gently for several moments to allow the warmth radiating from your palms to melt away tensions. The stillness of this calming hand-to-hand hold will enhance the deep sense of connection between you.

2 Support the palm with your fingers and place your thumbs side-by-side over the centre of the top of the hand. Draw your heels and thumbs firmly out to the edges of the hand in a stretching motion, to create space between the bones and tendons. Repeat the stroke higher on the hand.

3 Support your partner's palm and wrist with one hand, and use the heel of your other hand to make firm circular motions over the near-side of the top of the hand. Apply pressure in the heel on the outward fan of the circle, while stroking the palm firmly with your finger-tips on the return slide. Perform the same stroke over the other half of the hand.

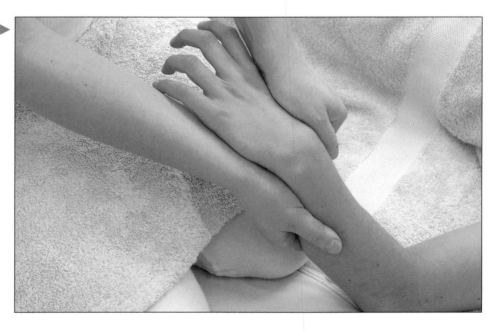

4 Keep the hand supported and slide your thumb firmly in a straight line between each tendon and bone on the top of the hand, lightening the pressure as the stroke reaches close to the wrist.

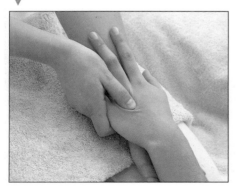

5 Place your fingers under the wrist and make small, alternating thumb circles to ease the strain away from the tiny bones and surrounding ligaments on the top of the wrist joint.

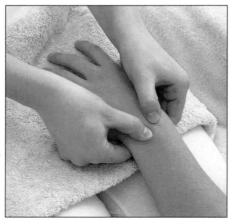

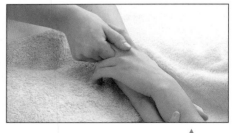

6 Relax the fingers and thumb, starting with the little finger and working across the hand. Begin by massaging the base knuckle with gentle circular motions using your thumb and index finger.

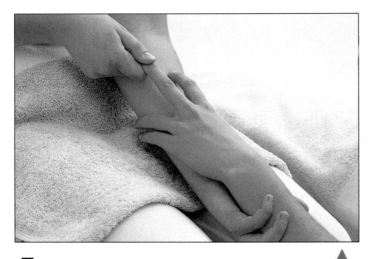

7 Now pull firmly but gently along the top and bottom of each digit and out of its tip as if you are releasing tension away from the extremities of the body. Use smooth actions as the joints in the fingers are relatively delicate.

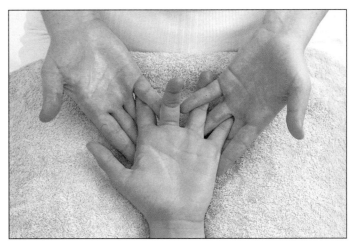

8 Turn the hand so the palm is facing upwards. Interlock your fingers between those of your partner's hand, as shown, so that they rest against the back of the hand. Push them gently upwards, using enough pressure to open up and spread out the palm.

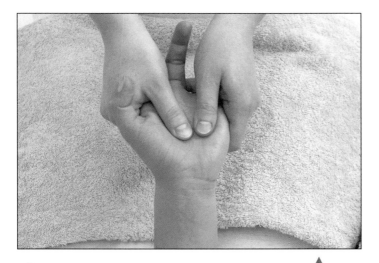

9 Use both thumbs to make short, alternate sliding strokes over the surface of the palm to stretch and release tension from the muscles. Be sensitive to your partner's reactions.

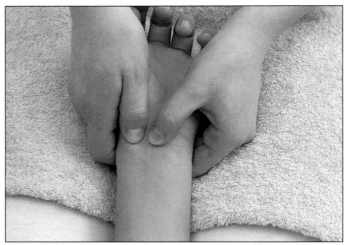

10 Once the palm is relaxed, unlock your fingers and place them behind the back of the wrist. Massage over the inside of the wrist with small, alternating thumb circles.

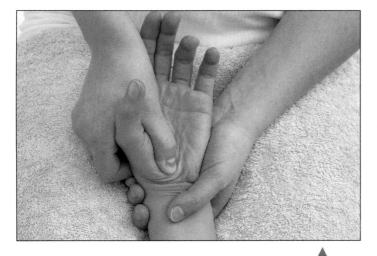

11 To massage more vigorously on the palm, support the back of your partner's hand with your hand, and use your other thumb to apply stronger pressure circle strokes, working on one spot at a time. Focus particularly on the area at the base of the thumb.

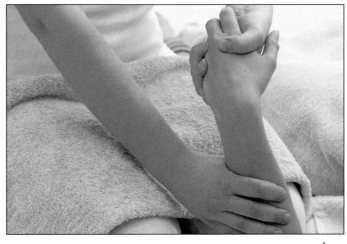

12 Apply some passive movements to loosen the wrist joints. Raise the forearm by flexing the elbow and supporting it with one hand. Firmly clasp your partner's hand with your other hand. Rotate the wrist several times first in one direction, and then in the other.

Focus on the Chest, Neck, and Head

Prepare for the chest, neck, and head massage with an opening out stroke, to increase width and relaxation in the shoulders, and length in the neck.

Kneel behind your partner's head and rub a little oil into the palms of both hands. Place them side by side, fingers pointing down, flat over the top of the breast bone. Slide both hands steadily up and then outwards over the pectoral muscles towards the shoulders. Swivel your wrists to glide your hands softly behind the shoulders and, once more, turn your hands to rest parallel but cross-ways to each other in a gentle clasp of the base of the neck. Ensuring the neck is fully supported, pull both hands towards the head, lifting it slightly as your hands pass under the hairline, and out behind it. Repeat this movement two more times.

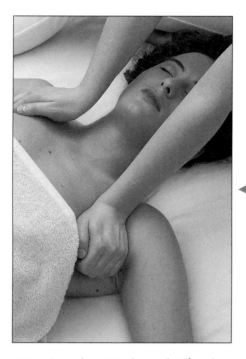

Kneading the Pectorals

The pectoral muscles often tense up during times of stress. This can inhibit a full inhalation of breath and cause a feeling of tightness around the heart. These kneading strokes will loosen the area, helping both the chest and the shoulders to expand and relax.

◀ *1* Hook your fingers into the edge of both armpits so that the heels of your hands rest at an angle under the collar bone. Applying pressure to the heels, slide one heel and then the other towards the fingers (thereby making a fist) to stretch and squeeze the muscles. Lift the heel slightly off the body to return it to its original position before making the next slide. Create a rhythm between the alternating movements of both hands.

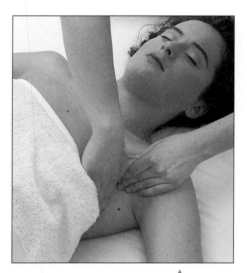

2 Lift, squeeze, and roll the flesh between the thumb and fingers of your hands to knead the pectoral muscles on both sides of the chest. ▲

Freeing the Neck and Head

Carrying the heavy weight of the head can cause neck muscles to shorten, especially if the body's structural line is out of balance. The following movements will encourage extension in the upper spine and free the neck and head from constriction. While performing these movements, take care of your own back and posture. Place one foot on the mattress so you can lever yourself forwards and backwards with your leg muscles while keeping your own spine lengthened and relaxed.

1 Scoop your hands under the back so they rest, palms facing upwards, between the shoulder blades and parallel to each other on either side of the spine. Wait for your partner to relax into your hands. Lean your own weight backwards as you pull both hands steadily up along the spine towards the back of the neck.
▼

2 Continue to slide both hands ▶ steadily up behind the neck to gently extend it away from the shoulders. Lift the head slightly as your hands mould to its shape and pass beneath it, while your thumbs stroke up behind the ears.

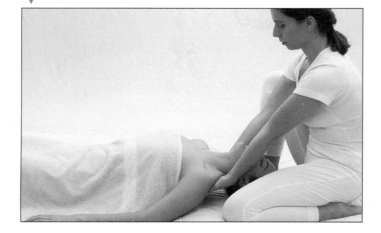

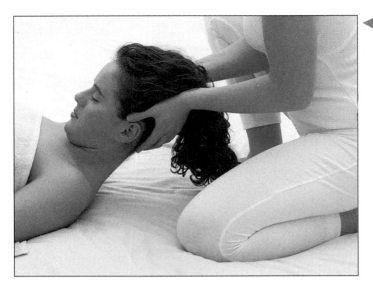

Lifting and Lowering

During this passive movement, you lift and lower your partner's head to encourage her to release its weight into your hands. As the head is elevated in direct line with the spine, the neck muscles are also subtly stretched. As the head is lowered down with the safe support of your hands, your partner can release its weight and tension. Repeat the motion several times, noticing how the head becomes heavier in your hands the more your partner relaxes.

Slip both hands behind the head to cup it safely in the palms. To secure the hold, rest your fingers against the top of the neck and your thumbs beside the ears. Raise the head slowly upwards until it reaches its natural point of resistance, and then lower it equally slowly back down to the mattress.

Rolling the Head

Rolling the head slowly from side to side will induce a further release of tension in the neck muscles and attachments at the ridge of the skull. Apply this passive movement sensitively to ensure the head pivots from the vertebrae at the top of the spine.

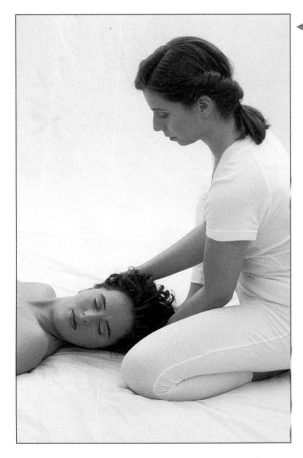

1 Cradle the head securely in your hands and roll it towards the left side of the body.

2 Reverse the movement, tilting the head towards the right side of the body. Roll the head several times encouraging your partner to allow you to take control of the movement.

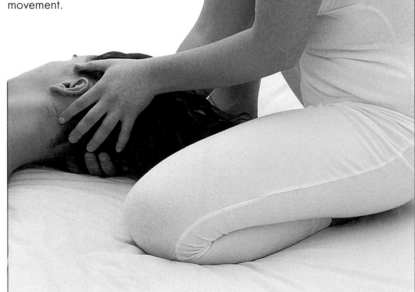

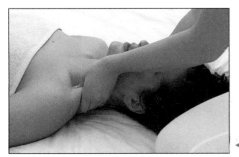

Kneading the Base of the Neck

Unlock the tension at the base of the neck by kneading the muscles at the top of the shoulders. Hook your thumbs over the shoulders while slipping your hands behind the upper back to rest, fingers pointing downward, beside each side of the spine. Using the fingers, and using one hand after the other in an alternate, rhythmic kneading motion, scoop and roll the flesh upward towards the waiting thumb. Release the flesh and slip your fingers back to their original position while the other hand is in motion. Repeat the action once more.

Relaxing Neck and Head Strokes

Now apply a sequence of strokes to further relax the neck and head. Work first on one side and then the other. Begin with a stroke that encircles the side of the neck and shoulder. Then add circular pressure strokes under the rim of the skull and over the scalp to ease tension from the head.

1 This stroke stretches neck and shoulder muscles that elevate and rotate the head. Turn the head to rest against one hand, while moulding your other hand over the exposed side of the neck just under the hairline.

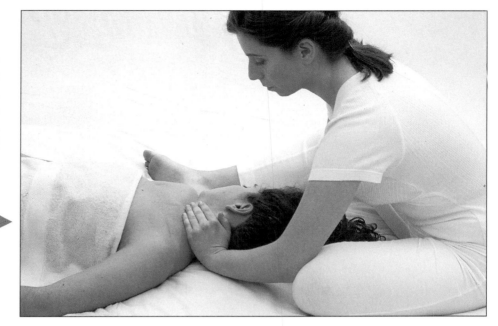

2 Slide your hand firmly down the side of the neck. Add a slight traction to the movement by lightly gripping the back of the neck with the fingers of your other hand.

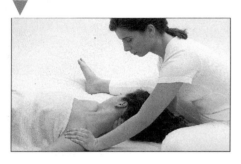

3 Soften the pressure in your hand to glide it around the shoulder joint, flexing your wrist to let your fingers stroke up the back of the neck.

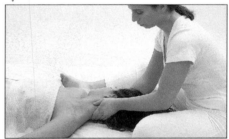

4 Forming your hand into the neck's contours, sweep up towards the hairline, ensuring that the heel of your hand and your thumb stroke behind the ear.

5 Continue to draw your hand up over the head and out of the hair before repeating the whole stroke twice more.

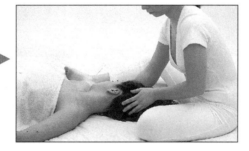

6 Indent your fingertips slowly under the edge of the bone where the skull joins the neck. Rotate them and, as the muscles relax, deepen the pressure. Release the pressure gradually before working on the next area until you reach the side of the spine. Remain aware of your partner's responses, as this is a sensitive region.

7 Continue to rotate your fingers on one area at a time over the side of the scalp you are presently massaging. Use your thumb and little finger to anchor your strokes, applying pressure circles from the three middle fingers.

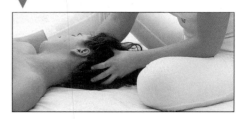

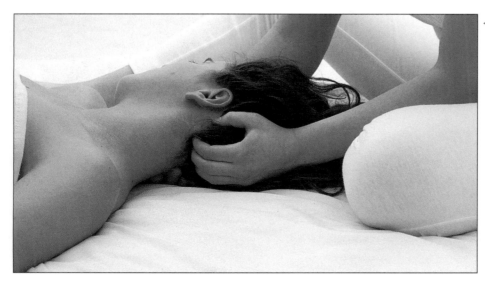

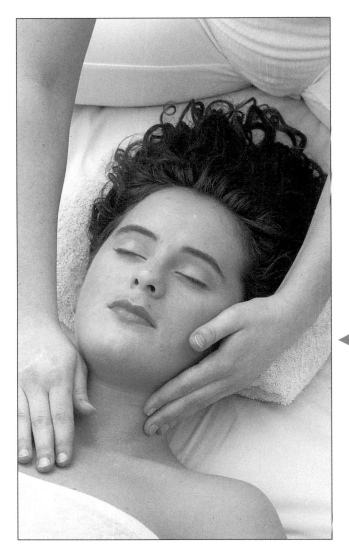

Focus on the Face

Complete your whole body session with a tender face massage. When applying strokes to the face, focus your total attention on to your hands and fingers so that each touch is made with great sensitivity. Let your strokes be firm but gentle, following the natural symmetry of the facial features and bone structure.

A face massage dissolves anxiety and stress, eases away headaches, and enhances relaxation. It is a wonderful way to finish your massage, or combined with the chest, neck, and head strokes, it can be a deeply satisfying and effective session in its own right. Add a very small amount of oil to your hands to ensure a smooth glide over the skin.

Gentle Strokes

1 Softly stroke your hands, one following the other, up over the neck and sides of the face, moulding them to the natural contours.

2 A gentle caress of the jawline will comfort your friend. Slightly cupping your hands, stroke one after the other in alternating movements on both sides of the face, moving from the point of the chin towards the ears.

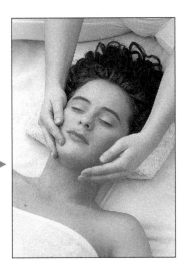

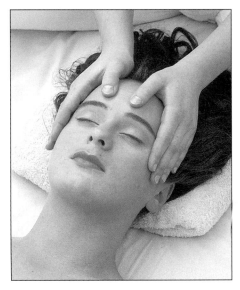

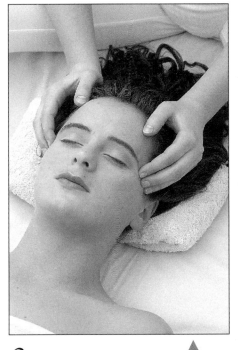

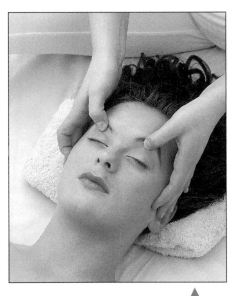

Relaxing the Forehead ▲

1 Place your thumbs side by side on the centre of the forehead, while your hands cradle the sides of the face. Draw both thumbs out towards the side, finishing with a gentle sweep around the temples. Lift your hands away from the head to settle your thumbs on a higher level of the brow. Repeat the stroke over the forehead and up to the hair-line.

2 Keeping your hands relaxed and cupped, use your fingertips to circle-stroke the temples softly several times in a clockwise direction.

3 The hollows under the ridge of the brow are sinus passages. Gentle pressure on these points can help to release tension headaches. Placing your hands on each side of the face, press sensitively up under the ridge, on one spot at a time, with your thumb pads. Hold the pressure for a count of five before releasing it slowly. Move from the inner to outer edge of the eyebrows.

Circling the Cheekbones

This stroke encircles the nose and cheekbones, finishing with a soothing sweep of the head and hair before being repeated.

1 Slip your thumbs each side of the bridge of the nose, while wrapping your hands softly against the sides of the cheeks. Slide both thumbs firmly down each side of the nose to the edge of the nostrils.

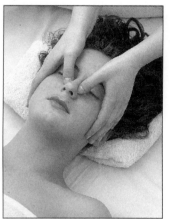

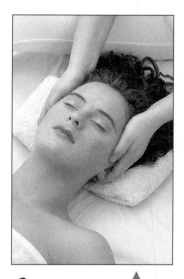

2 Without breaking the flow of motion, draw your thumb pads out under the cheekbones, indenting them slightly up under the ridge of the bone.

3 Soften the pressure in your thumbs as they reach the sides of the face, and begin to pull both hands soothingly up towards the top of the head.

4 Continue by drawing your hands and fingers out through the head and hair in a steady motion until they pull away from the body. Float your hands lightly back to the first position of the stroke. Repeat the whole movement twice.

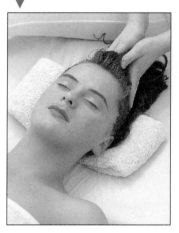

Easing the Cheeks and Jaw

Tension causes the cheeks, mouth, and jaw to stiffen. The following strokes relieve tightness from this area, allowing it to soften and relax.

1 Relax your hands and sink your fingertips into the cheek muscles. Rotate them, counter-clockwise, several times on one area before moving to the next fleshy area.

2 Gently press and rotate the heels of your hands in continuous but alternate movements on the cheeks to increase suppleness and to loosen the muscles surrounding the mouth.

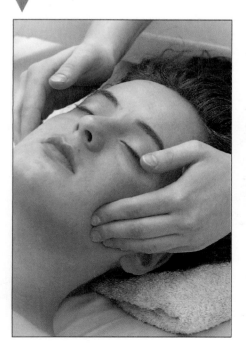

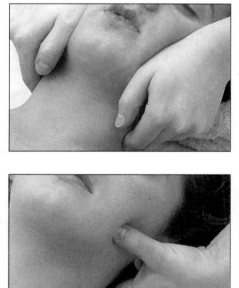

3 The strong muscles at the side of the jaw assist in biting, chewing, and forming words, in addition to moving the mouth. To reduce tension, slip your fingers behind the neck, and sink your thumb pads gently into the muscle before rotating them firmly on one spot at a time.

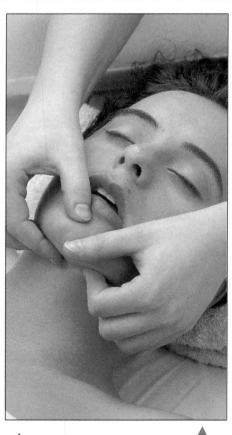

4 Grip the jaw bone gently with your fingers and use your thumbs to stroke over the chin in small alternating circles, applying more pressure on the down and outward slide, before lightly gliding back. Complete with soothing caressing strokes over the jaw line.

Massaging the Ears

Ear massage is especially rewarding as it induces deep relaxation and is very pleasurable. Support the back of the ears with your index fingers, and circle-stroke thoroughly over the lobes and along the rim with your thumbs.

Completing the Face Massage

Comb your fingers comfortingly over the scalp and out of the hair as if you are drawing away any residual tension from the head and face. A very gentle pull of the hair will also stimulate the scalp.

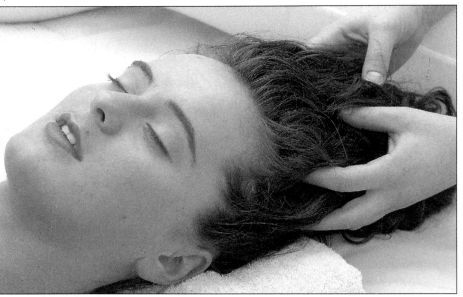

The Calming Hold

A perfect way to finish your whole body massage and the strokes on the face is by applying a restful and calming hold. Link your thumbs together over the centre of the forehead, and tenderly lay your hands over the cheeks. Bring your full attention to your touch, allowing both of you time to assimilate the beneficial effects of the session.

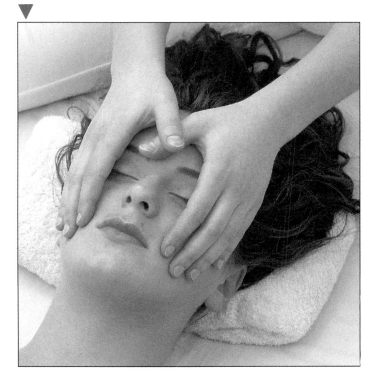

Contra-indications to Massage

Certain medical conditions require the exercise of caution concerning the advisability of giving or receiving massage. If you are in any doubt, or if you or your partner are under medical supervision, check with your family doctor or other qualified medical practitioner before the session. This advice applies particularly in the case of cardiovascular conditions and heart disease, especially in cases of thrombosis, phlebitis, and oedema.

Never apply pressure under or over varicose veins. Never massage directly over infected skin, for example where there are warts, herpes, or boils, or where there is inflammation, unexplained lumps, bruises and open cuts. While giving a massage, take care to cover any open cuts or scratches on your hands with a plaster or other dressing.

Massage on the abdomen is best avoided during the first three months of pregnancy when the risk of miscarriage is highest.

The causes of acute back pain should first be diagnosed by a doctor or osteopath before receiving massage treatment. Consult a qualified medical practitioner in cases of raised temperature, infections, or contagious disease.

For contraindications for essential oils, see pages 16-29 and the special programmes in Part Three. pages 124-157.

How to Finish Your Whole Body Massage

Once you have withdrawn your hands from your partner's body, stand silently by her side for several moments so she remains aware of your presence. Cover her with a sheet or blanket to ensure she stays warm, then tell her to relax completely while you go to wash your hands. When you are ready, help your friend to get up from the mattress and offer her a towel to wrap around herself. Encourage her to stretch and move a little so that she adjusts to the standing position.

Deeper Strokes on the Back

Deeper tissue strokes can be integrated into a back massage to bring greater relief to areas most commonly associated with back pain. These strokes focus on the sacrum, pelvic girdle, either side of the spine, and the shoulder blades.

The art of deeper tissue strokes, also known as friction or petrissage, is to apply steady pressure to the tissue before stretching the muscle with a sliding, grinding, or circular motion. Never force a muscle with undue pressure, as not only is this unpleasant, it is also counter-productive. Apply pressure by leaning your body weight into your hands, rather than by using muscle power. Ask your partner to focus her attention and breathing on her back throughout the massage so that she can consciously help the deeper penetration of the stroke. The following strokes should be applied to both sides of the back.

Deeper Strokes on the Pelvis

Postural tensions can cause compression in the lower back, thereby creating inflexibility at the base of the spine and around the pelvic girdle. Relax the area with effleurage and kneading, then use the deeper strokes to stretch the underlying tissue.

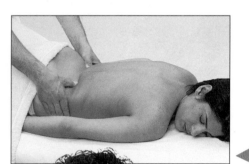

1 Place your hands on either side of the body just above the buttocks, so that your thumbs are resting at the base of the sacrum. Gently sink the pads of your thumbs into the muscle and stroke them firmly up over the sacrum. Then draw both thumbs out over the top of the pelvic crest to eliminate tension along its ridge. Relax the pressure slightly as your thumbs move towards the sides of the body. Repeat the stroke.

Stretching the Long Muscles

The flexibility of the body is impeded whenever the long sheath of muscles that run beside the length of the spine become tense or rigid. This also puts a constriction on major nerves branching out from the spinal column, and this has a detrimental effect on the entire physical system. A deep stretch stroke moving steadily along these muscles from the spine to the shoulder will lengthen and relax the back and vertebral column.

1 If you are standing on the left side of your partner, use your right hand to make the long stretch stroke. Place your right hand on the base of the back, directly alongside the spine, with your fingers pointing towards your partner's head. Place your left hand over your right hand to give it added weight, then lean your body into your hands and slide them slowly and steadily up over the long muscles, transferring the pressure into the heel of your hand so that it hooks into the muscle to create a rippling effect.

2 Half-circle slides over the sacrum help to alleviate pain from a tight lower back. Slowly sink and hook the fingertips of one hand into the tissue and then apply pressure to stretch it with a slow, upward, and outward slide, using your other hand to anchor the stroke. Gently release the pressure, and allow your fingertips to glide back to their first position before stretching into another area of the muscle.

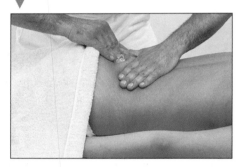

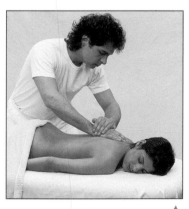

2 Tip your body forward as you continue this deep stroke up to the top of the spine. Then soften the pressure of your hand as you sweep it over the shoulder and down the length of the arm to release the tension from the body.

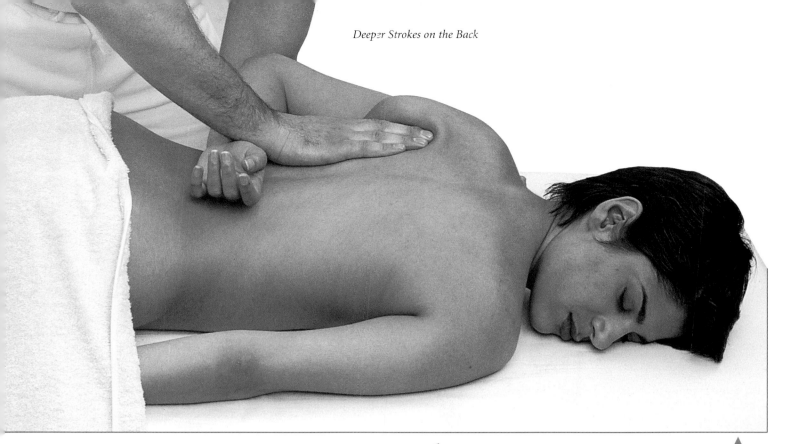

Relaxing the Shoulder Blades

Tight shoulder blades can cause pain and discomfort, and are often the result of a tense posture or prolonged inactivity such as sitting at a desk.

Once the lower back and spine have relaxed, create space for the shoulder girdle to drop its weight downwards. You can alleviate tension from beneath the ridge of the shoulder blades and surrounding areas using the following deeper tissue strokes.

1 Gently lift and lay the lower arm across the back with the elbow flexed. This will raise the shoulder blade and create more slack in its underlying muscles, enabling your stroke to penetrate to a deeper level. To increase the effect, lift the shoulder slightly with your left hand. Keeping your fingers close together to add weight, sink the sides of your index finger and hand into the tissue beneath the lower end of the raised shoulder blade.

2 Slowly slide your hand beneath the ridge of the bone towards the top, inner corner, carefully manoeuvring around any bulky bundles of muscle attachments. Release the pressure of your hand, and stroke firmly out over the top of the shoulder and down the arm.

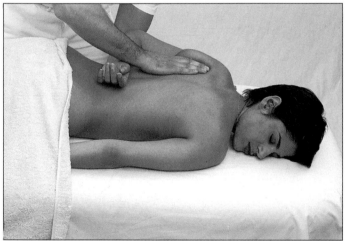

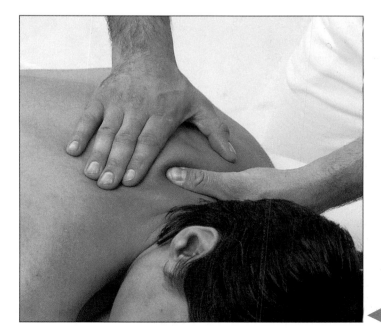

Loosening the Knots

Once the shoulder blade has relaxed, there will be more space in the area between the edge of the bone and the spine, as well as around the base of the neck. Friction strokes with your fingers and thumbs can now loosen up the remaining sore 'knots' caused by contraction or deposits of toxic granules in the muscles. Stand by the shoulder joint so that you are facing into the area, then, using one hand to push the muscle towards your stroke, work on specific points with a grinding, circular motion of your thumb or finger pads. Remember to follow up the deeper strokes on the back with effleurage to soothe the area, boost the circulation, and to integrate them into the whole massage.

Part Three
The Specific Programmes

Once you have attained the basic skills of aromatherapy massage you will naturally want to broaden your knowledge and technique. The real beauty of this healing art is that it is a never-ending process of discovery of the body, how it functions, and the way in which it responds to treatment. Part Three takes you into a deeper and more intuitive understanding of the oils and how they can be combined with strokes to treat a whole range of conditions. Your enhanced skills will enable you to bring greater relief, relaxation, invigoration, pleasure, and comfort to your friends and family.

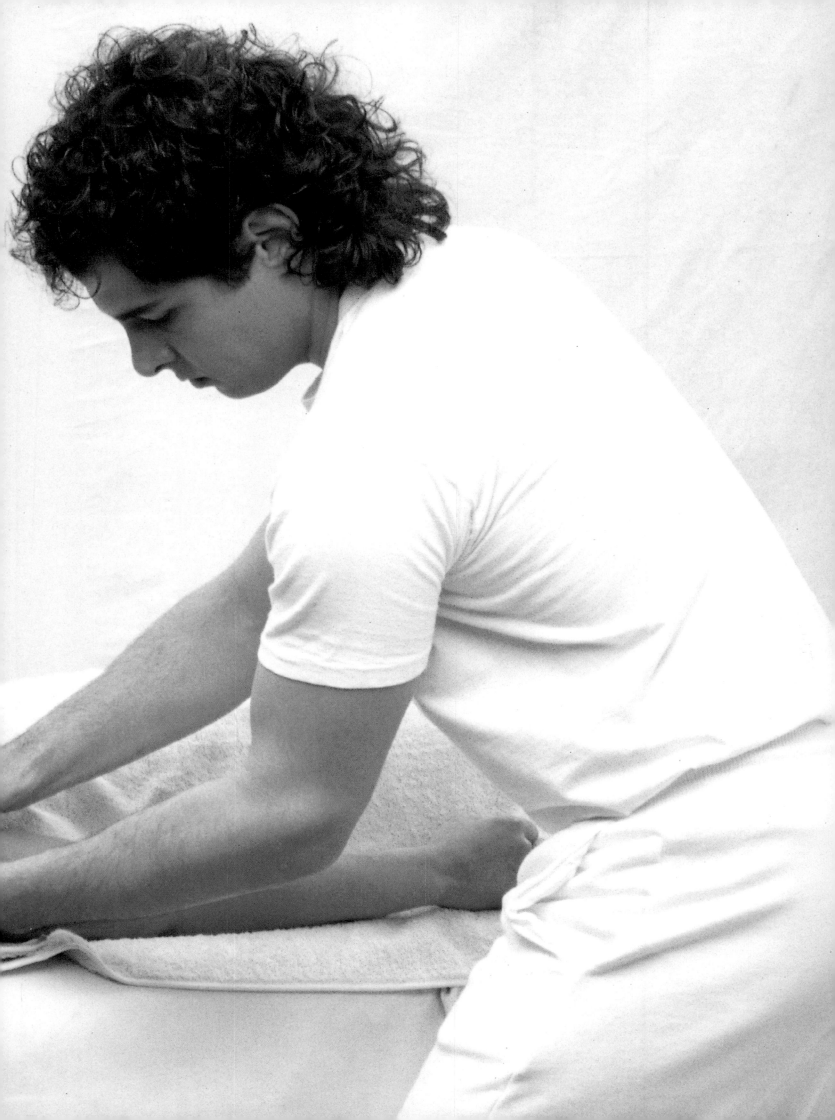

Developing Your Knowledge of Aromatherapy

Once you have become familiar with essential oils and with the practical benefits they offer, you may wish to gain a deeper understanding of the nature of these aromatic substances.

Most people begin to collect essential oils slowly, one by one, as they can afford them. They usually choose these oils to answer a particular need, or because they find a scent especially appealing. Having used the oils for a while they may become aware that their understanding of the use and benefits of a particular oil has deepened. This may become apparent with the realization that the aroma of the oil will relieve a painful or disquieting emotion or a physical symptom time after time. For those who would like to explore this situation further, there are several exercises that may help. Two of them are given here.

Exercise One

The first exercise uses the power of your imagination to take you on a journey inspired by an oil of your choice. You will need to choose a period of at least half an hour when you will not be interrupted, and to assemble the following items for the exercise: a comfortable upright chair, or a cushion on which you can seat yourself comfortably on the floor; the essential oil of your choice, preferably one that you have used frequently for a reasonable period of time; and a handkerchief or paper tissue.

Put one or two drops of the chosen essential oil on to the handkerchief or paper tissue and place it within easy reach. Seat yourself comfortably. If you are sitting in a chair you may want to put a cushion under your feet to help you relax your body. Once you are in a comfortable position place your hand lightly, palms down, on your thighs. Concentrate on the rise and fall of your breath and become observant of your breath as it enters and leaves the body. If any thoughts of daily activities come into your head, acknowledge them and then allow them to pass away.

After a few minutes have passed take the scented tissue and inhale from it deeply for one or two breaths. Try to observe which parts of the body you

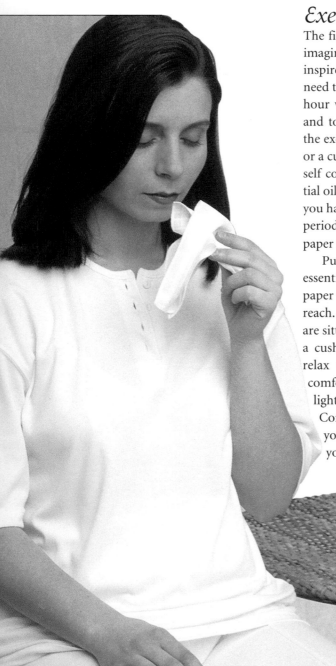

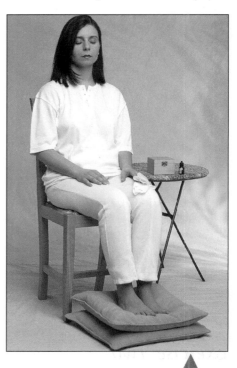

Choose a time when you will not be disturbed. Make sure you adopt a comfortable position, and put everyday concerns out of your mind.

When your mind is clear take the hankerchief or tissue with the essential oil on it and inhale for one or two breaths.

The stress that is often associated with studying for an exam may be eased by using an essential oil such as ginger or cedarwood.

▼

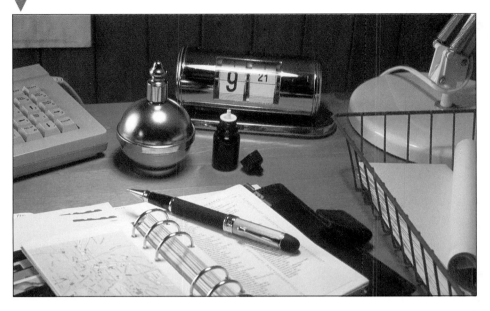

Specific Recipes

- Essential oils for a special occasion: Clary sage, grapefruit, orange
- Oils to try in preparation for an exam or an interview: Bergamot, black pepper, ginger, grapefruit, lemon, peppermint, neroli, orange, rosemary, sandalwood, rosewood, cedarwood, frankincense
- Essential oils to help when preparing to study: Bergamot, eucalyptus, frankincense, ginger, lemon, peppermint, rosemary, grapefruit, juniper, nutmeg, jasmine
- Oils for cleansing after difficult situations: Cypress, eucalyptus, juniper, lavender, lemon, peppermint, rosemary
- Essential Oils to aid meditation: Cedarwood, clary sage, frankincense, jasmine, palmarosa, sandalwood, rosewood

become aware of and what feelings are there – for example, it may be a warm sensation or a tingling one. Colours may come to mind, specific pictures, or perhaps a dream-like story. Allow the inspiration of the scent to transport you in your imagination, and as far as possible allow yourself to really trust what you imagine and feel. When the images begin to fade, gently bring your attention back to your own breathing, observing the rise and fall of your belly.

Become aware again of the comfortable armchair in the room and, when you are completely ready, slowly open your eyes. You may feel a little dreamy after completing the exercise, and a glass of water or juice can help regain a solid, present feeling in your body. The activity of writing down any thoughts and feelings about the experience will also help achieve this.

By making this journey into the imagination several times with different essential oils it is possible to develop your confidence and intuitive knowledge. As a guide, the whole process should last approximately 15 minutes.

Exercise Two

The second exercise provides an alternative way of getting to know each essential oil in greater depth. The power the essential oils possess to affect our state of mind is available to all of us if we actively choose to use them for one of these specific purposes. A suitable occasion

might be prior to a very special social event, an interview or exam, or a period of study. You may also want to refresh yourself after an unpleasant experience such as an argument or an unwelcome visitor.

For the exercise you will need to gain access to your bathroom for half an hour or more. You will also need: the essential oils of your choice, previously blended and ready to put into the bath; a candle securely fixed in a holder; and some matches. Some people like to listen to a relaxing piece of music while bathing, and for this you should have a battery operated cassette player and the music of your choice.

Try to do this exercise at a time when you don't need to cleanse yourself thoroughly, so that the bath is something special. Run as deep a bath as you can, making certain the water is at a comfortable temperature. Meanwhile, prepare the essential oils in a carrier oil.

When you are ready, concentrate on the purpose of the bath and light the candle. Put the blended essential oil into your bath just before you get into it. Remain in the bath for as long as you feel like it, or until the water is no longer comfortably warm. Allow any thoughts

that float into your mind to gently come and go, and concentrate on any dream-like images or colours inspired by the aromas rising in the steam.

This type of bath can be tremendously restorative as well as developing a heightened awareness of each of the oils used in this way.

Body Awareness and Visualization

Massage is a never-ending process of learning about the human body in all its holistic aspects.
The more you know, the more there is to discover about the relationship between body, mind, and spirit.
The best place to explore these mysteries is within your own body.

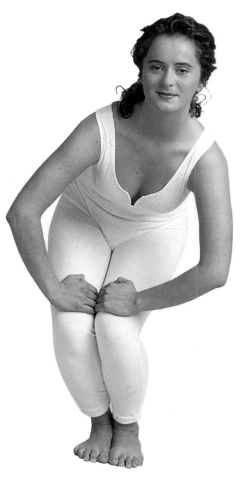

If you are giving massage on a regular basis it is very important that you maintain a strong and flexible physique. Exercise regularly to relax and strengthen your muscles and, in particular, to provide good support for your spine and back. Learn how to breathe deeply and synchronize your flow of breathing with movement, so that your strokes become fluid and you remain energized. Practise visualizations, which will help you contact your energy resources and cleanse and relax your body, mind, and spirit. The more you learn about your own body, the better able you will be to pass on that knowledge through your massage to help others.

Exercises for Strength and Flexibility

Your legs help you to maintain a balanced and stable posture while you are giving a massage. They provide you with a firm but flexible foundation to support your body weight and to connect you to the ground, so that you will be able to release tension away from your spine and back as you work. This exercise helps you gently to warm and loosen the ankle and knee joints, areas which are vital to structural support.

Creating a Stable Foundation ▲

1 Rest your hands on your knees without straining your shoulders. Place your feet together and, bending your knees, rotate them in circles, first in one direction and then in the other. Begin with small circular movements and gradually make larger ones as your joints and muscles warm up.

◄ *2* Straighten the knees slowly and gently press your abdomen down in the direction of the floor to create a stretch in the hamstrings at the back of your legs. Alternate this step with the knee circles in step 1, repeating them two more times.

Breath and Movement

The next exercise is a series of continuous flowing movements adapted from the T'ai Chi form, a Chinese martial art. It helps to create stability and strength in the legs, while making pushing movements with the arms and hands. The complete motion is made in conjunction with your cycle of inhaling and exhaling. This makes the exercise particularly appropriate when learning how to apply long effleurage strokes with a graceful posture and synchronized breathing.

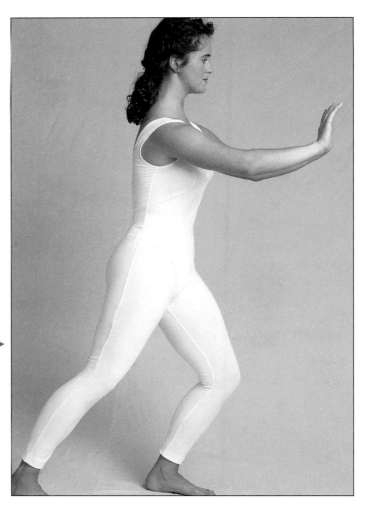

1 Begin with the basic stance of good posture, keeping both feet parallel and the knees slightly flexed. Step forwards with the front foot and turn the back foot out at an angle of 45 degrees. As you breathe in, bend your elbows and draw both hands to chest level, palms facing outwards.

2 Keeping both feet flat on the floor and the spine erect, transfer your weight to the front foot and push your hands away from your body while you exhale. Your torso should be facing in the direction of your front foot.

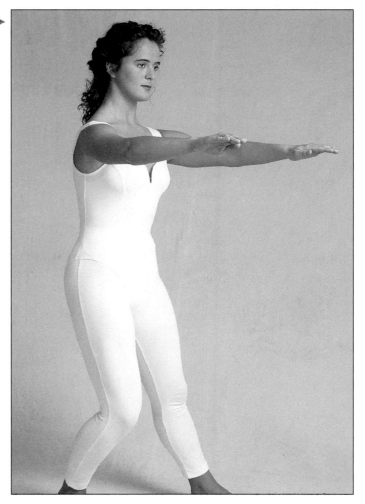

3 As you inhale, transfer your weight to the back foot, allowing your body and arms to swing around and face in the same direction. Draw your hands back to chest level. Continue moving as you breathe in and turn your body towards the front foot to repeat the full movement again. Repeat the exercise 10 times before changing the position of your legs and repeating the full flowing cycle of motion from the other side.

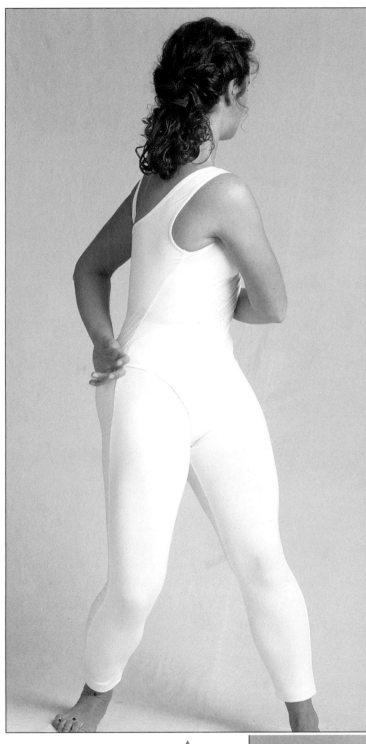

Swinging the Torso

Limbering up the spine and torso prevents strain and tension from gathering in the back while giving massage. It keeps the body supple, enabling it to turn easily while performing some of the longer strokes. The key to the following exercise is to transfer weight from one foot to the other as you swing around, leaving the other foot feeling "empty" and weightless. Flex both knees so your height never changes during the exercise, and your head rests comfortably on top of your spine. This gentle spinal twist will relax your muscles and nerves and stimulate your breathing.

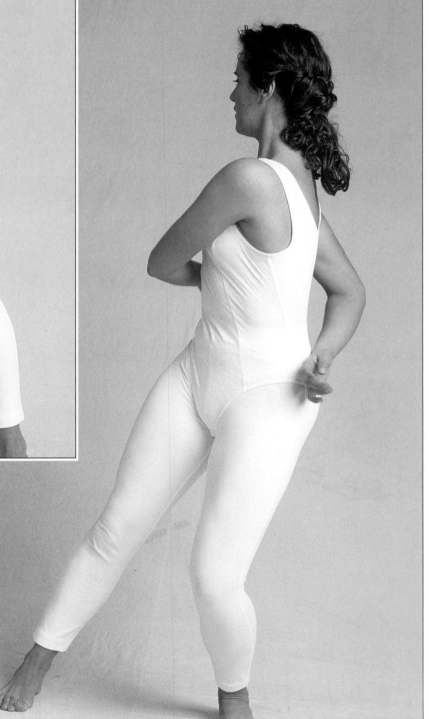

1 Begin the exercise with your feet parallel, and more than the width of your hips apart. Transfer your weight on to one foot, leaving the other weightless. Swing your torso and arms around to face the "empty" foot, letting your arms flop against the sides of your body.

2 Swing your torso back to the other side as you transfer your weight across to the other foot. As you turn, relax the gaze of your eyes so they take in a moving picture of your surroundings without fixing on any point.

Strengthening Abdominal Muscles

The abdominal muscles flex and support the spine, and it is important to strengthen them in order to safeguard your back while giving massage. A firm but relaxed abdomen will allow tension to sink away from the upper back and shoulders, while stabilizing the lumbar region. The belly is also the source of power and vital energy. These exercises will bring it strength and relaxation, helping you to gain stamina. Perform them slowly and carefully to avoid strain, and gradually build up to 10 complete movements for each exercise.

1 Lie on your back with your knees bent towards your chest and your feet flexed. Begin to make circles in one direction with your knees, making certain you keep them together. Gradually enlarge the circles, keeping the middle and base of your back in contact with the floor at all times, as this will activate the abdominal muscles. Remain lying down on your back and spread your arms to the sides of your body, palms facing downwards. Bend your knees towards your chest and flex your feet. Breathe in.

2 Breathe out as you take your knees to one side of the body as far as they will comfortably go, keeping them close together. At the same time, roll your head in the opposite direction. As you inhale, return both head and knees to their original position. Repeat the exercise, moving your head and knees to the other side of the body.

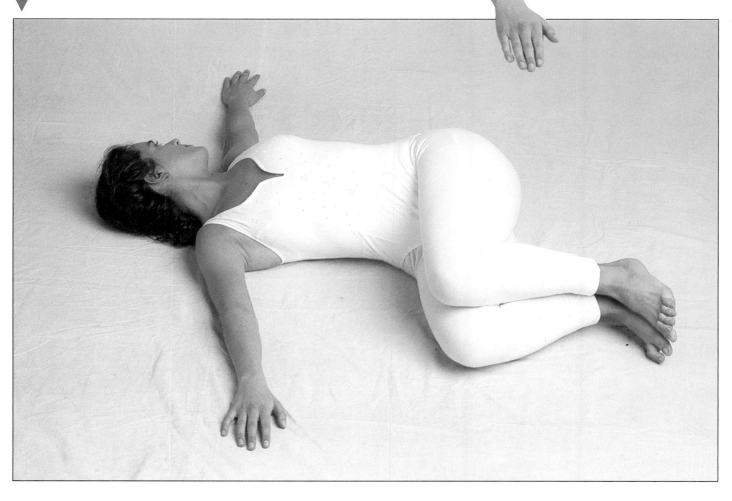

Visualization

Visualization is a powerful tool frequently used in healing work. It allows an intuitive use of the imagination to bring about subtle and beneficial changes in the body and mind. Within massage and body awareness work, imagery combined with "good intention" can be used in relaxation exercises as a means of directing the movement of energy within the body, or to "see" and heal its internal structure and physiology.

Tuning in to Light and Energy

When massage is performed with a relaxed posture and breathing, the experience can be equally as nourishing and invigorating for both people involved. If you believe, however, that you are using up all of your own energy while giving a massage, then the experience can sometimes leave you feeling tired or drained. This visualization exercise helps you to replenish your vital resources by opening you up to the idea of a constant stream of energy, or light, that passes through you to your partner. You can practise this during the massage, with or without a partner; it is an excellent way to start or finish a session.

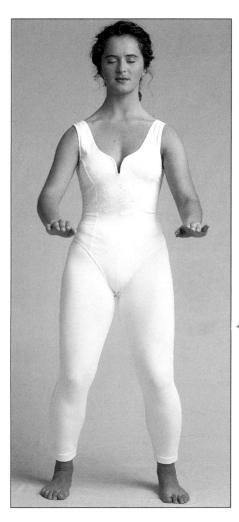

◀ Stand with your feet apart and with your arms slightly out in front of your body, palms facing downwards. As you breathe in, imagine a white light descending through the crown of your head and filling your body with vital energy. Breathe out and visualize the light flowing out of your arms and through your hands to the person beneath them, or towards the ground. As you continue to inhale and exhale, repeat this visualization several times.

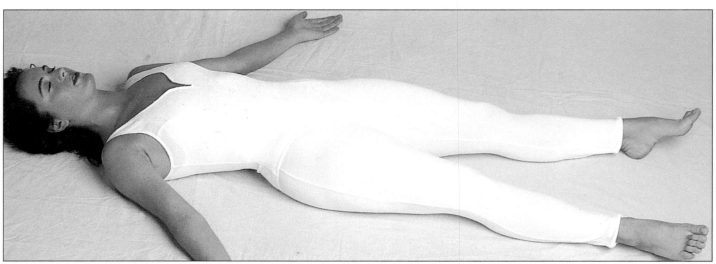

Bone Breathing

During massage, your hands are mainly in touch with the body's skin, soft tissues, and superficial muscles. However it is also beneficial to gain a sense of the skeletal structure, which is vital to the body's support and locomotion. Try this exercise on yourself to provide a mental image of the bones, and to encourage a sense of relaxation into the core of the physical body.

▲ Lie on your back. As your breathing deepens, focus your attention on your right leg and consciously relax the muscles from the foot up to the hip. Then try to visualize the bones as they link together from the toes, through to the ankle and knee joint and up to the hip socket. Now imagine that the bones are hollow, so that as you breathe in, a white light is drawn in through the toes and is pulled up through the bones to the top of the leg. As you breathe out, the light returns via the same pathway and out of the body.

Repeat this visualization several times with the right leg before repeating the exercise with the left leg. Finally, breathe in deeply and draw the white light up the right leg and into the belly. Hold your breath for a few moments and breathe out, before sending the light down through the left leg. Reverse the imagery so that you draw the light from the left to the right side of the body. The same visualization can now be applied to the arms and chest.

Opening the Heart Centre

Just as it is essential to connect through breath and awareness to your belly during massage – in order to work from your source of power and vital energy – it is also important to allow your heart and feeling centre to open and expand. By doing so, you can allow the essence of life to flow to your hands, enlivening them with a caring and healing quality of touch that is deeply nourishing. In this visualization, you imagine that your heart is like the bud of a flower. As you focus your breath towards your heart, allow the flower to open its petals until it fills the whole of your chest.

◀ To help you connect with the heart centre, sit and close your eyes while breathing, holding your hands just in front of your heart.

Enhancing Your Massage

Once you have achieved a good grounding in the basic massage techniques, you can further enhance your skills by using a specially-designed massage couch, and by familiarizing yourself with the use of additional pillows.

Working at a Couch

While some people prefer to kneel and give a massage at ground level, working at a couch increases your mobility, as you can use your feet and legs to move more freely around the body. This puts less stress on your posture, enabling you to bring length to your spine and neck and a relaxed width to your shoulders. In common with the kneeling position, your movement at the table should come from the lower half of your body, to prevent strain on your back.

There are many different types of massage couch to choose from that are designed for varying styles of massage. These are marketed in a range of prices. It is important to choose a couch built to the correct height for you to work at; if you stand with your fists loosely clenched, and let your arms hang down by your sides, you should be able to rest your knuckles comfortably on the surface of the couch. The width of a massage couch should be a minimum of 65-80 cm/26-32 in, in order to support the whole body securely and allow sufficient space for the arms to relax on the surface of the couch. The length is normally a minimum of 180 cm/72 in, although a few added centimetres will accommodate your taller clients. A comfortable padding of foam, covered with vinyl, should provide a supportive platform for the body.

A face cradle can be added to the table, or a face hole cut into its surface, to enable the massage recipient to keep the head and neck straight – some people find it difficult to lay in a prone position because it necessitates an awkward angle of the neck.

If you want to purchase a fold-up, portable couch, and plan to set up a mobile massage practice, then it is important to choose one that is easy to carry. You will need to find the right balance between the couch's stability and strength, and ease of transporting it.

Using Pillows and Towels to Ease Tension

Postural tension remains in the body even when a person lies down on the couch or mattress to receive a massage. A prolonged period of resting on a flat surface can even exacerbate physical strain, particularly in the major joints of the body. The more you massage, the more you will be able to visually detect where someone is holding their tension. For example, an individual may have a particularly swayed lower back, indicating stress in the pelvic region, or the neck may be contracted or sore, making it extremely difficult for the individual to lie comfortably. The use of pillows and towels to support key areas of the body can ease the structural tension, enabling your partner to relax and enjoy the beneficial experience of aromatherapy massage to its full potential.

A couch built with adjustable legs allows people of various heights to use it successfully. The height can also be adjusted according to the type of massage you are giving; for example, in a deep tissue massage a greater degree of pressure is applied to the strokes, and therefore a lower height is required than would be the case for a soft tissue massage.

When the person is lying in a prone position, place one pillow just below the knees. The benefit of taking the strain out of these joints will further relax the pelvis and lower back. A pillow under the front of the chest will allow the shoulders to fall forwards, opening up the upper back and creating space between the shoulder blades. The added support will also help lengthen and relax the neck.

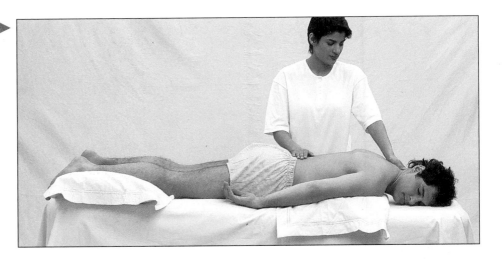

Pain in the lower back may be caused by an excessive curve in the base of the spine, or a chronic pattern of tension in the pelvic region. A pillow placed supportively under the abdomen can redress the postural imbalance during the massage, helping the lumbar region to relax under your touch.

Tension in the chest and rib cage can cause muscles to contract, pulling the shoulders forwards so that they are unable to rest on the table during massage. Ease this uncomfortable posture by placing a towel, folded into a thin strip, under and along the length of the spine. This will enable the chest to expand and the shoulders to fall back. Help your partner into the supine position so that the towel remains in the correct place.

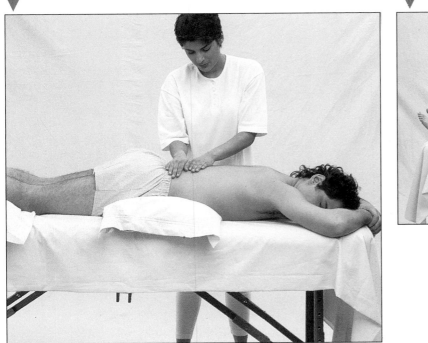

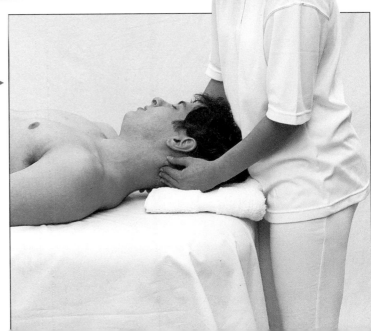

Constriction in the muscle attachments at the base of the skull will shorten the neck muscles, causing the head to contract backwards. Bring a sense of length and relief to this area by placing a thin, folded towel under the ridge of the skull to lift the head slightly upwards and to extend the neck.

Massage for Headaches

Generally headaches are caused by tension, but occasionally they are the result of an allergic reaction to food, or are a symptom of an ailment such as a digestive disorder or sinusitis. Massage, in combination with some of the essential oils suggested in this programme, will provide relief for most headaches.

A tension headache is often experienced as a "tight band" around the head. It is thought that such head pains are caused by a change in blood pressure, which occurs when the muscles tense and so restrict the normal flow of blood to the head and face. The pain is usually accompanied by muscular tension in a surprisingly large area of the upper body, as well as in the neck, scalp and facial muscles surrounding the jaw and temples.

Releasing Constricted Muscles

Focus your massage first on the shoulders, neck and below the ridge of the skull. These are the main areas that tighten and restrict the blood flow to the head and face.

1 Rest one hand on each shoulder for a few moments to make contact and to put your partner at ease. Then, anchoring your fingers over the top of the shoulders, begin to roll and squeeze the muscles in a kneading action, using the heels of your hands. Work out to the edge of the shoulders and down the top of the arms.

2 Place one hand across the forehead and the other across the nape of the neck. Ask your partner to drop the weight of her head into your hand and to breathe gently in and out, imagining that she is releasing the tension with each outgoing breath. Gently squeeze the neck muscles between the fingers and heel of your hand.

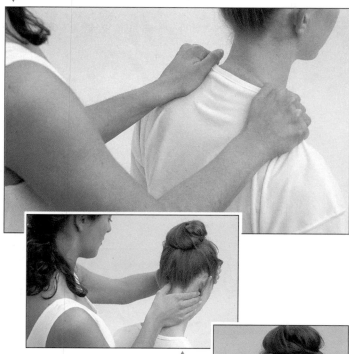

3 Still supporting the forehead, use the thumb pad of the other hand to press upwards into the hollow at the top of the spine beneath the skull. Apply gentle upward pressure for a steady count of five, then release.

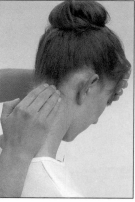

4 Loosen the constricted muscles under the base of the skull by massaging beneath the bony ridge, working from the top of the spine to the outer edge of the skull. Change hands to massage beneath the other side of the skull. Ease scalp tension by rotating the fingertips of both hands in small circles over the entire head.

Stretching the Neck Muscles

Ask your partner to lie down and relax for a few moments, then give her a gentle face massage to ease the headache. Tension can cause the neck muscles to contract as we "shrink" inside ourselves as a protection against stress. Gentle stretching and passive movements help to lengthen and relax the neck.

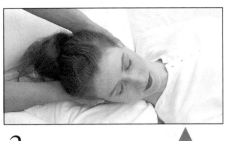

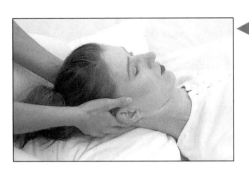

1 Slip both hands under your partner's shoulders, with your fingers resting at the top of the spine and with your palms securely supporting the back of the neck. Ask your partner to relax her neck into your hands, then pull them steadily upwards to stretch and lengthen the neck away from the shoulders. Raise her head slightly as your hands pass under the hairline and up the back of the head.

2 Cup the head in your hands, with your fingers resting on the neck and your thumbs lying gently against the sides of the face. Lift the head slightly, then roll it gently to the right and then to the left. Repeat several times, encouraging your partner to relax so that you have complete control of the movement.

Drawing Out the Pain

The following techniques can be used on their own, or in combination with the strokes usually used on the neck, head and face.

1 Settle your hands lightly around your partner's scalp for a few moments. Keeping your hands in the cupped position, lift them slowly away from the head as if they were drawing out the pain.

2 Cup your hands around the head again, placing your thumbs between the eyebrows. Apply gentle pressure with your thumbs for a count of five, then release.

3 Working from inner to outer edge, apply a press/release motion under the ridge of both eyebrows using the tips of your index fingers. Then use your thumb pads to press/release over the top of the cheekbones, working out from the nose to the edge of the temples.

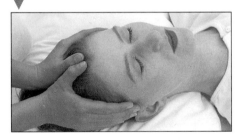

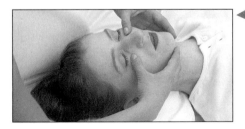

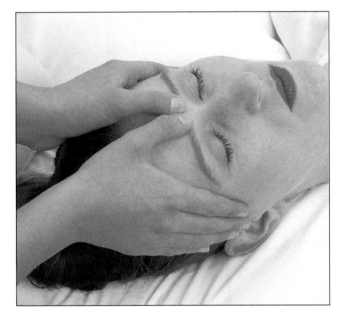

Recommended Oils

Where the specific cause of a headache is known the following essential oils may bring relief.

Hyperactivity, overwork: Marjoram

Anger, worry, hyperactivity: Chamomile

Sharp, piercing pain, lethargy, despondency: Peppermint, rosemary

Mild pain, lethargy: Lemon

Colds, sinusitis: Eucalyptus

Note: All essential oils should be blended with a vegetable carrier oil before use.

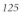

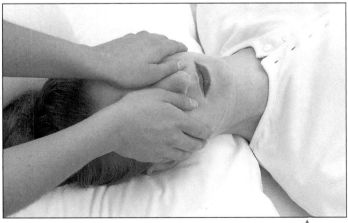

4 Briskly rub your hands together to create heat, then softly lay your slightly cupped palms over the eyes for a count of five to soothe and relax the eye muscles. Withdraw your hands slowly.

Easing Anxiety

Aromatherapy massage provides an excellent antidote to the symptoms of anxiety and stress. While the oils soothe and comfort, the strokes will return a sense of physical reality, helping to calm the anxiety. By restoring equilibrium, the massage and oils will assist in dealing more practically with the root causes of the problem.

A prolonged state of anxiety can deplete vital energy from the body, leading to a general state of nervousness and tension. This has a detrimental effect on the physical and emotional state of health.

Soothing Away Stress

A furrowed brow is a common sign of mental anxiety, as the facial muscles constrict under stress. Releasing tension from the brow, temples, jaw, and neck will certainly help to calm the mind. Focus on these areas while giving a soothing head, face, and neck massage to an anxious partner.

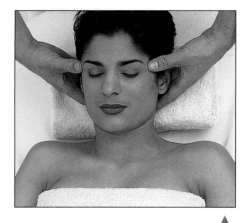

3 Placing your fingers around the head, use the thumb pads to stroke in soft, clockwise motions over the temples to ease mental stress.

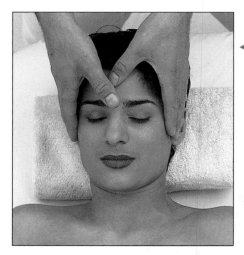

2 Using the palms and fingers, brush your hands soothingly in alternating motions from one side of the forehead to the other. With the fingers of your right hand pointing to the left temple, draw your hand lightly across the brow, before lifting off to let your left hand repeat the motion from the right temple.

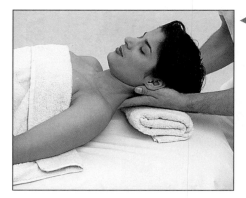

The Head and Neck

1 Muscles in the centre of the forehead tend to knit together with worry. Using your thumbs, stroke one after the other in short, firm slides, to ease the tension from the area that lies between, and directly above, the eyebrows.

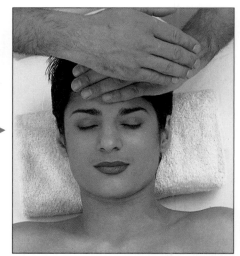

4 Releasing the neck and helping it to extend away from the shoulders will lengthen and loosen muscles that have constricted in this vital area. Place both hands, fingers pointing downwards, along each side of the top of the spine. Ask your partner to breathe deeply and relax her neck and head back into your hands. Pull your hands gently but firmly, with the fingertips slightly indented into the tissue, up the back of the neck and then out from under the head.

Recommended Oils

There are a number of essential oils suitable for relieving anxious feelings or anxiety attacks. Because these feelings are complex and can involve a wide range of physical symptoms, the range of oils that may be helpful is also broad.

The balancing effects of either lavender or geranium are useful, as are their relaxing qualities. Marjoram is also very relaxing, although the comforting, enveloping sensation of ylang ylang or the euphoric relaxing nature of clary sage may be preferable.

Pulsing the Joints

Passive movements to loosen and relax the joints of the body will help your partner to release tension locked into the musculature surrounding the major segments of the body, which will have contracted under anxious feelings. It is important to encourage your partner to give up the control of movement and weight of her limbs into your hands, thereby enabling her to trust you and free her tension. Gently rotate, wiggle, stretch, and rock the joints of the body in line with their natural movement. Encourage your partner to breathe into these areas to allow a greater sense of connection to her body. You can follow up these passive movements with massage on the arms, hands, legs, and feet to allow tension to be released from the body.

NOTE Never try to force someone into relaxing, and always respect their level of tension. If she is unable to let go of the weight and movement in her limbs during the passive movements, then simply continue with the massage.

Further Work

- A gentle foot massage will help bring your partner down to earth, and stabilize her emotions
- Calm, still, hands-on holds on the body will induce feelings of peace, helping the individual to deepen and relax their breathing
- The massage strokes for insomnia will work equally well for relieving symptoms of anxiety

The Passive Movements

The shoulders are one of the most affected areas of the body during a period of anxiety and tension, as they tend to tighten and rise, putting the whole posture under stress. These passive movements will help the shoulders to relax.

1 Keeping the elbow slightly flexed, lift the arm away from the body. To secure your hold, clasp the wrist and hand and slip your thumb between her thumb and index finger. Place your other hand supportively behind the shoulder. Encourage your partner to let you take the entire weight of her arm, and begin to rock it gently so that the movement travels up into the shoulder joint. Lift and lower the arm as you rock it to encourage a complete release of tension.

2 Lifting the arm vertically above the body, pull gently upwards to create an easy stretch in the joint before slowly releasing the traction. Then, with the elbow slightly flexed, bounce the arm gently up and down into the shoulder socket, and against the support of your hand.

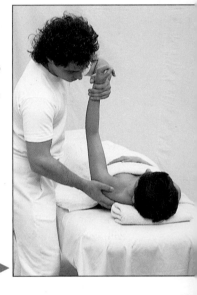

3 This gentle stretch in the legs releases tension from the hips and pelvis. Positioning yourself below your partner's feet, clasp the back of both ankles with your hands. Lean back in your own body to pull her legs towards you, and then slowly and easily release the traction.

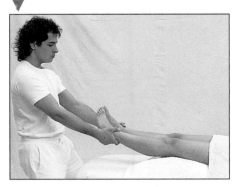

If the anxious feelings are causing a sense of alienation, adding sandalwood, rosewood, or frankincense to the chosen blend may help.

Some anxiety attacks centre directly on the belly, in which case neroli is the ideal choice.

If the anxious feelings prevent sleep, orange will help relax the body and promote sleep. Orange also has an uplifting aspect, which can raise the spirits as the anxious feelings pass away. Cypress can give a feeling of cleanliness once the experience has ended.

Strokes and Oils for Insomnia

Soothing, hypnotic strokes and sedative essential oils help to separate the activities of the day from the necessary period of sleep and rest at night, and enable the insomniac to break the vicious cycle of sleeplessness.

In cases of insomnia or bad dreams that lead to sleeplessness, it is important to reduce the intake of stimulating drinks such as tea and coffee, and to avoid eating late at night. It is also helpful to create a relaxing ritual to prepare for falling asleep. The suggested massage treatments, given here and for the treatment of anxiety, combined with a recommended blend of aromatherapy oils, will prove invaluable for this bed-time preparation.

A Gentle Wave

The following sequence of strokes washes over the limbs and extremities of the body in outward flowing motions, creating a gentle stream of movement that draws tension and anxiety away from the central core of the body. The soft, downward pulling strokes have a hypnotic and sedative effect, which will calm the emotions and quiet an over-active mind, thereby helping to induce relaxation and sleep.

As you apply the strokes, combine them with an awareness of your breath, drawing your hands down on the inhalation and pausing briefly on the exhalation. This almost imperceptible pause in the motion will create a lovely wave-like feeling, rather than a straight pulling effect. Rub a little oil into your hands and mould them to the body, letting them impart a steady softness, and always begin the sequence on any limb from above the major joint, such as the shoulder or hip, in order to draw tension away from the constricted area.

Take the stroke right out of the head, hands, or feet, and beyond the actual physical body, as if you are emptying it of the stress and worrying thoughts that may inhibit sleep. Each sequence should be performed up to five times on each part of the body. Begin by pulling your hands along the back of the neck and out of the head and hair, as shown in the soothing-away-stress programme for anxiety.

1 Place one hand over the top of the chest, and the other over the muscles on the back of the shoulder, so that the fingers point towards the centre of the body. As you breathe in, pull your hands steadily outwards to the edge of the shoulder and down to just below the joint. Pause briefly as you exhale, letting your hands rest and lightly cradle the top of the arm.

▼

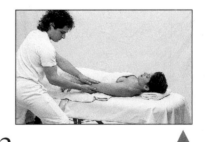

▲

2 Adjust your position so that you can continue the pulling motion down the length of the arm. As you breathe in, pull both hands down to just below the elbow joint. Relax as you breathe out, and then continue the slide down the forearm and below the wrist with your next inhalation.

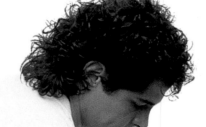

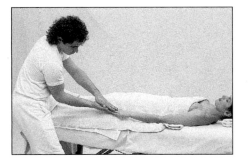

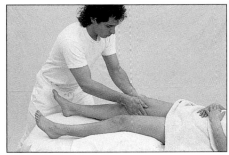

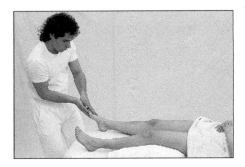

3 Draw your hands over both sides of your partner's hand and fingers, taking your stroke out beyond the body as the hand settles back on to the mattress. Repeat steps 1 to 3 on the other side of the body.

4 Begin the hip, leg, and foot sequence by laying both hands slightly above the pelvic girdle to cradle the side of the body. Pull both hands down over the hip socket as you inhale, separating them as they reach the thigh in order to hold each side of the leg: rest briefly as you exhale. With the next inhalation, draw your hands down the leg to just below the knee.

5 Continue this wave-like motion down the lower leg to just below the ankle, and then – sliding one hand under the foot, with the other on top of the foot – pull gently and steadily until your hands pass out over the toes. Repeat this sequence of strokes on the other side of the body.

Sedating Strokes on the Legs and Feet

Soft, soothing, downward flowing strokes over both legs will further enhance the calming and sedative effect of your massage.

1 Using the flat surface of both hands, ▶ softly stroke down the legs from the thighs until your hands pass over and out of the feet. Repeat the movement as many times as you like to allow your partner to relax.

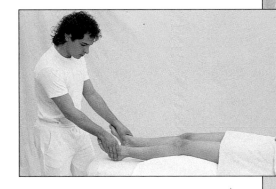

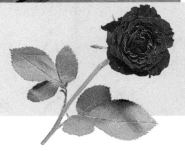

2 To increase the sedative effect of your strokes, complete these sequences with a still, calm hold of your hands over the front of both feet. This will draw the energy down the body, bringing a sense of balance and equilibrium.

Recommended Oils

All the relaxing, sedative oils are useful for insomnia: chamomile, clary sage, lavender, marjoram, mandarin, neroli, orange, rose, rosewood, and sandalwood. For sleeplessness brought about by bad dreams, try blending frankincense or lemon with one of the oils listed above. Ylang ylang can be very helpful for disturbed sleep following a nightmare.

Alleviating the Symptoms of Cold

While a cold will normally run its course, combining self-massage with aromatherapy treatment can bring considerable relief to the symptoms. Adding the recommended essential oils to a vaporizer or bowl of steaming water will enable you to inhale their remedial effects, helping to clear the head and soothe the throat and chest while boosting the immune system. After inhaling, apply some self-massage strokes to the relevant pressure points on the head, face, and feet to relieve blocked sinuses.

A cold can usually be treated at home with plenty of rest, which allows the immune system to fight off the viral infection. In the normal course of events a cold usually takes about a week to clear, but if the symptoms persist longer than this, or worsen, then it may be advisable to consult your doctor. Drink plenty of fluids and increase your intake of fruit and vegetables to help cleanse the body of mucus.

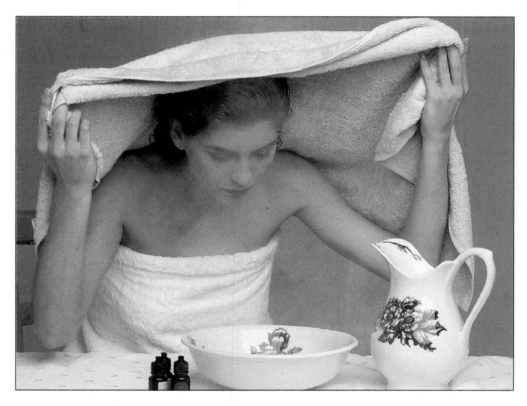

Inhaling With Essential Oils
Pour your blended oils into a bowl of hot water and, as they vaporize, inhale the steam as deeply as possible. The oils will begin to decongest blocked nasal passages and soothe the cold symptoms. If you hold a towel over your head this will delay the effects of evaporation. Be careful to place the bowl in a safe position.

Recommended Oils
A large number of essential oils can be comforting and helpful in relieving cold symptoms. Some of these are listed below. Tea tree, which acts as an antibiotic and antiseptic, is perhaps the most useful, while eucalyptus is invaluable for relieving a blocked nose and head. However, because most colds present a mixture of symptoms you should choose one oil for each symptom, and then add essential oil of tea tree to make an appropriate blend for your cold.

Self-massage
Enhance the remedial effects of the essential oils and steam by applying some self-massage and pressure on specific points to aid decongestion.

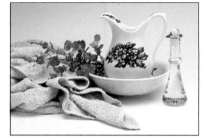

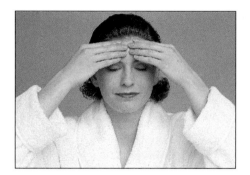

1 Massage all over your brow, starting from the centre and working out with small circular motions from your fingertips.

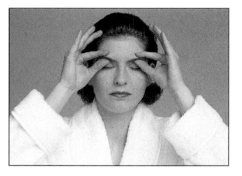

2 Release pressure from the sinus passages by pinching along the ridge of your eyebrows with your thumbs and index fingers, starting on the inside corners and working, step-by-step, to the outer edges.

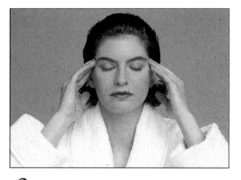

3 Stroke your temples with your fingertips, moving them counter-clockwise in circular motions, This will alleviate the stuffiness that can lead to headaches.

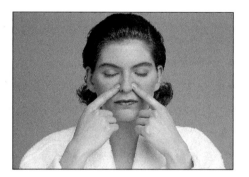

4 To relieve congested nasal passages, use your fingertips to press gently into each side of the outer rim of the nostrils at the edge of the cheekbones. Hold for a count of five and then slowly release the pressure.

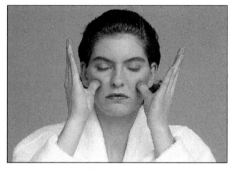

5 The small indentations beneath the ridge of the cheekbones indicate the location of some of the sinus passages. Apply thumb pressure slowly up into the hollows. Hold for a count of five and release. This will help clear the head.

Reflex Points for Clearing the Sinuses
Check your foot zone therapy chart to locate the reflex points corresponding to the sinus passages. Rest your lower leg over your knee and, supporting the foot with one hand, use the tip of your thumb to apply a slowly increasing pressure to the pads of the toes. Work from the big toe to the smallest toe.

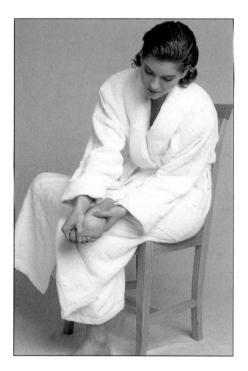

Cold in the early stages: Nutmeg
Runny colds: Ginger
Bronchitis: Cedarwood, eucalyptus, frankincense, neroli, orange, peppermint, rosemary, sandalwood
Other chest infections: Benzoin, cedarwood, ginger
Catarrh: Cypress (watery catarrh), frankincense, jasmine, lemon, black pepper, sandalwood
Congestion: Frankincense (chest), lemon, eucalyptus

Boosting the immune system: Bergamot, grapefruit, lavender, lemon, marjoram, rosewood
Warming: Jasmine, neroli, nutmeg
Uplifting: Bergamot, cedarwood, cypress
Stimulating the appetite: Ginger, peppermint, black pepper

All oils are to some extent antiseptic, and will assist in preventing the spread of infection.

Massage for Digestive Disorders

When stress is manifested physically in the abdominal area, massage and touch can bring the sense of safety and comfort needed to relax and relieve mild digestive disorders and abdominal discomfort.

Emotional tension can cause us to tighten our abdominal muscles and reduce our breathing in order to avoid the experience of painful or uncomfortable feelings. If we are unable to assimilate those emotions, or express them appropriately, they can manifest themselves as physical disorders, particularly playing havoc with the digestive system. Massage helps to deepen breathing, allowing the muscles to soften and expand, and to restore harmony and equilibrium.

All the strokes shown on the belly in The Whole Body Massage are suitable when stress is felt in the abdominal area. Reflexology, shiatsu, hands-on breathing techniques, and passive movements can also bring relief to simple digestive disorders.

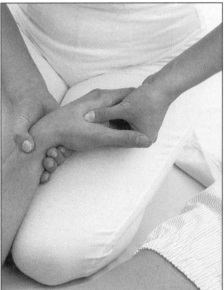

Reflexology for the Digestive System

Check the foot zone therapy chart on page 46 for the correct location of the reflex points for the liver, pancreas, stomach, small intestine, and colon. Press systematically on each of these points with the tip of your thumb for up to three seconds, while supporting the foot with your other hand. The pressure gradually eliminates toxic build-up in the reflex points corresponding to the digestive system. Repeat the treatment over several days until any tenderness in the foot zones has disappeared.

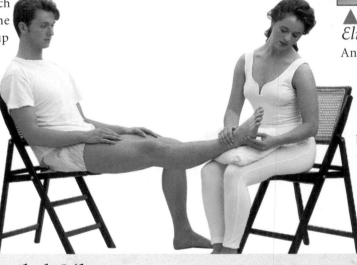

Elimination Point

An important shiatsu point for the release of intestinal congestion is the one found on the web of skin between the thumb and index finger. The exact location is indicated by its tenderness to pressure. This point is known as Large Intestine 4, or in Chinese terms as "the Great Eliminator". Press gently on this point for up to five seconds, then release the pressure gradually.

Recommended Oils

For specific digestive complaints the following essential oils and blends may be useful.

Constipation and pain: Three drops each of ginger, orange, bergamot, and clary sage

Sluggish digestion: Peppermint, black pepper, palmarosa, nutmeg

Indigestion, colic, flatulence: A drop of peppermint, three drops each of ginger, lemon, bergamot

Flatulence: Bergamot, black pepper, fennel, ginger, lemon, marjoram, neroli, nutmeg, peppermint, rosemary

Colicky pain: Bergamot, chamomile, clary sage, ginger, cypress, lemon, orange, peppermint, sandalwood

Constipation: Black pepper, fennel, ginger, marjoram, neroli, nutmeg, orange, peppermint, rose

Diarrhoea: Cypress, chamomile, ginger, lemon, orange, peppermint, black pepper

Holding and Breathing

Still, calm holds over the abdominal area will encourage deeper breathing, allowing the release of pent-up emotions and stress. The following holds will all help to promote relaxation and eliminate tension, enabling the digestive tract to function properly.

1 If your partner is under extreme stress and is experiencing abdominal discomfort, ask him to lie on his side with his knees drawn up slightly. Put pillows under his head and between his knees to create a feeling of security. Place one hand over the lower back and the other on the belly, and ask him to breathe slowly and deeply from the abdomen. When the abdominal muscles are relaxed, rub the belly with gentle clockwise strokes.

2 Ask your partner to lie on his back with his knees raised. Place one hand under the small of the back and ask him to drop the weight of his pelvis towards your hand. Place your other hand over the abdomen so that its warmth helps to dissolve constriction in the muscles. Then ask your partner to direct his breathing towards your hands and to imagine that each breath is helping the belly to expand and release tension. Then move your top hand to hold different parts of the abdomen.

3 Encourage deep but gentle breathing in the diaphragm and solar plexus region by placing one hand below the mid-back and the other over the top of the abdomen. This will encourage the release of tension that can lead to digestive problems. As the area relaxes, gently massage it with soft circular strokes of your palm.

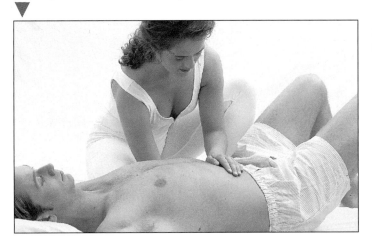

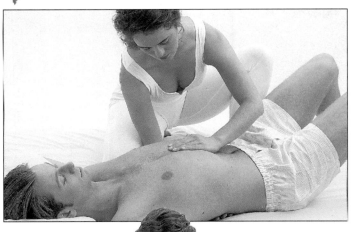

Relieving Abdominal Cramp

You can help to relieve tightness in your partner's belly by pushing his knees towards him. Ask your partner to bend his knees, keeping his feet on the mattress. Adjust your own posture so that you can lean your weight forward as you perform this passive movement. Slowly push the knees towards the trunk of the body, taking care not to force them beyond their natural point of resistance. Help to lower your partner's feet to the mattress, then repeat the movement twice more.

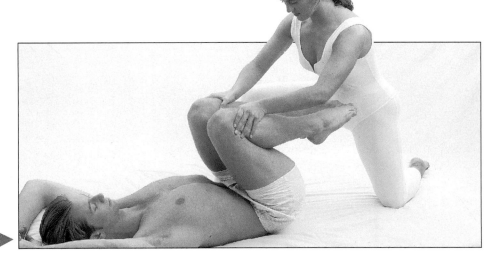

Improving Circulation

A healthy circulatory system is vital to the well-being of both mind and body. Massage, combined with a healthy diet and exercise, is an excellent way of boosting both blood and lymph circulation in order to promote health and vitality.

The circulatory system is divided into two parts: blood circulation that is pumped by the heart; and lymph fluid circulation that is moved by muscle action. The lymphatic system carries waste products to the lymph nodes, which act as filters to prevent harmful substances from entering the bloodstream, and is an important part of the body's immune defence system.

Poor circulation may be caused by hereditary factors, but it is also affected by a sedentary lifestyle, smoking, an unhealthy diet, or emotional stress and tension. A sluggish circulation will cause a depletion of vital nutrients in the body, leading to exhaustion, ill-health, and even depression as toxins build up and the elimination process is impeded.

Boosting and Draining

The signs of a sluggish circulation can be detected in pale, mottled, or blue-tinged skin, which is usually cold to the touch. The most common areas of poor circulation are the extremities of the body. Lift the limb and apply flowing strokes to boost and drain the blood supply on its return to the heart.

1 Cold arms, hands, and fingers indicate poor circulation. To assist the return of blood to the heart, raise your partner's forearm and clasp his hand with whichever of your hands is closest to his body. Wrap the other hand over the back of the wrist and drain firmly down the arm towards the elbow with a long steady stroke. Glide lightly around the elbow and back up to the wrist. Swap hands to repeat the movement on the inner forearm.

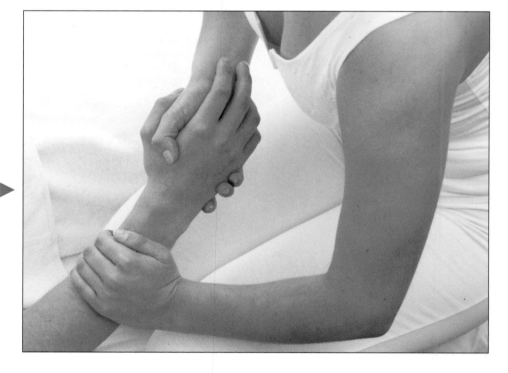

2 Help to increase vitality in the legs and feet by first applying the basic effleurage stroke from the ankle to the back of the knee, with the lower leg in a raised position. Wrap both hands over the back of the ankle, little fingers leading, and firmly stroke up the calf. This position also helps to drain excess water from around puffy ankles.

3 Deeper drainage strokes can be achieved by using your thumbs to stroke, in alternating short slides, from the ankle to just below the back of the knee. Repeat several times.

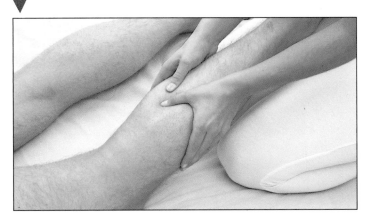

Warming Up

Hands and feet that are cold as a result of poor circulation can be warmed up by briskly rubbing them between both hands. The friction produces heat and stimulates the blood supply.

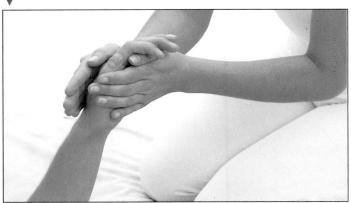

Stroking Towards Lymph Nodes

Lymphatic massage follows a specific procedure and requires the therapist to have a clear knowledge of the distribution of lymph vessels and nodes throughout the body. However, in a basic massage, gentle, upward effleurage strokes towards the major superficial lymph nodes – such as those in the back of the knee – can assist the lymphatic circulatory system to eliminate toxins from the body, particularly after kneading, friction, and deep tissue strokes.

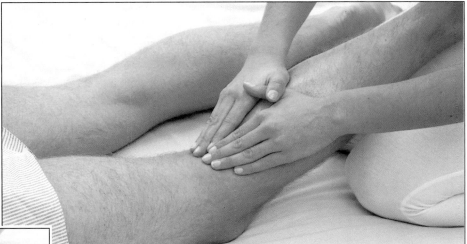

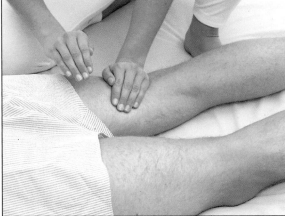

Benefiting the Skin

Pale, flaccid skin benefits from the stimulating effects of all percussion strokes. In particular, the suction effect of cupping draws the blood up towards the skin, bringing vital oxygen and nutrients to its peripheral nerve endings and underlying tissues.

Varicose Veins

The return of de-oxygenated blood to the heart from the lower half of the body is against the pull of gravity, and so the veins have valves in them that open and close to prevent back-flow. When a valve is damaged the veins become dilated, causing the condition known as varicose veins. This condition can be exacerbated by pregnancy, obesity, or prolonged standing. It is not advisable to massage directly above or below a varicose vein, but gentle upward-flowing effleurage over the sides of the leg, or away from the damaged vein, will ensure that the area is not neglected during a massage.

Recommended Oils

The following essential oils aid circulation: Benzoin, cedarwood, cypress, eucalyptus, grapefruit, geranium, lemon, mandarin, neroli, rose, rosemary.

To address the problem more fully, create a blend that includes a detoxifying oil from the list of oils recommended for cellulite and one of the general tonic and stimulant oils.

Convalescence and Recuperation

After an illness or injury the body is left in a vulnerable condition, and a period of convalescence is vital to give the immune system time to rebuild its defences. Massage helps to promote this important transition.

Gentle, hands-on holds are ideal for the first fragile stages of convalescence. The touch of your hands will comfort the body, stimulating the nerves that replenish the vital organs, and return the body to a normal resting state. As your partner recuperates, whole body massage will tone up the muscles, boosting circulation and increasing the body's overall vitality and sense of well-being.

Healing Holds

These soothing holds help to balance the nervous system and increase the body's energy levels. Start at the head, gently placing your hands over the forehead, temples and cheeks, then work methodically down both sides of the body to the feet.

1 Gently cup your left hand over your partner's temple and place your right hand over the heart area. This helps to encourage a sense of integration between mind and body.

2 Slowly withdraw your left hand and rest it on top of your right hand. Tune in to the heartbeat and the rise and fall of the breath.

3 Move to the side and rest one hand on your partner's chest and one over the solar plexus. This helps to decrease anxiety and encourages deeper breathing.

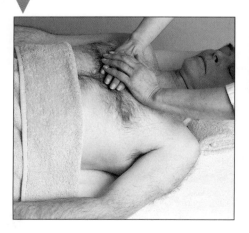

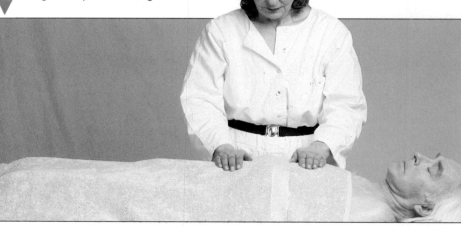

Clearing the Head

A prolonged period of inactivity can cause the shoulder and neck muscles to tense up, restricting the circulation which, in turn, leads to headaches. Relax the shoulder and neck area by kneading the shoulders, then follow this with a neck, head and face massage.

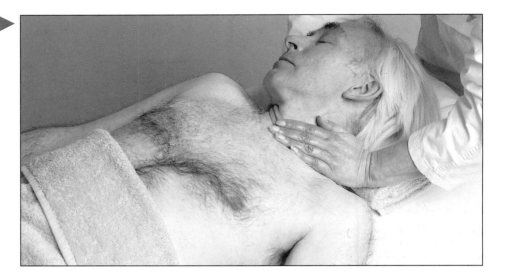

Getting Ready for Action

As your partner recuperates and becomes stronger, he will be eager to resume normal activities. When he has reached this stage in his convalescence, focus your massage on the feet and legs to boost a sluggish circulatory system, and massage the arms and hands to renew their strength and dexterity.

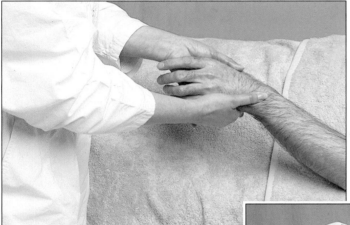

1 Massage the hands and fingers to release tension and increase flexibility.

2 Now massage the forearms, using draining strokes to help the circulation flow back to the heart. To loosen and warm the muscles, use one hand after the other in a fanning motion, working from the wrist towards the elbow.

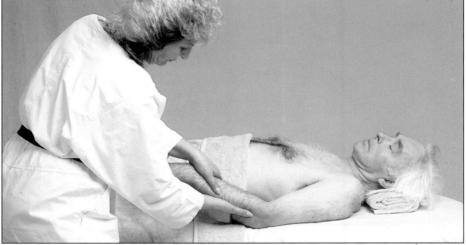

Recommended Oils

The period of convalescence is usually a time of physical and emotional fluctuation. The patient may experience bursts of energy, followed by fatigue when the spirits fall. The oils that are useful for convalescence include black pepper and orange to stimulate the appetite, which may still be lacking at this time. The stimulating quality of black pepper and tea tree may help overcome lethargy and also boost the immune system. Orange and nutmeg both have an uplifting and comforting nature, and are more gentle, and these oils may be all that are needed to get over the last part of an illness.

Most important, during this recovery period the immune system needs boosting. The oils to choose for this are bergamot, black pepper, rosewood, and tea tree. Mandarin is a pleasant, relaxing tonic oil, and clary sage is also very useful.

Cellulite and Detoxification Massage

Cellulite is detectable by the bumpy "orange peel" look of the skin on the fleshy areas of the body. It is caused by the accumulation of toxic deposits in the fatty tissues. Massage alone cannot rid the tissues of such deposits, but it can greatly assist the process.

Cellulite, which collects mostly on the hips, buttocks, and upper arms, is not specifically related to body weight and affects people of all sizes, especially women. It usually results from a sluggish circulation and poor elimination of toxins from the body, and in order to improve the condition it is necessary to use a combination of approaches. This includes a change of diet to cut down on the intake of toxins such as refined carbohydrates, caffeine, and alcohol. This should be combined with an increase in the daily intake of fresh vegetables and water. Regular exercise is also important, as it helps the lymphatic system rid the body of waste products.

The following massage programme, combined with the appropriate essential oils, should become part of a daily routine for six to eight weeks if you are to achieve a smooth and healthy skin. Mechanical massage instruments are also useful for this purpose.

Self-help

A quick self-massage programme to stimulate the circulation and elimination process from fleshy cellulite areas can be carried out several times a day, such as when dressing and undressing, or after taking a bath or shower. Squeeze and knead the thighs and buttocks, and follow up with percussion movements.

Hack, cup, and pummel the thighs briskly to tone the area and revitalize the blood circulation.

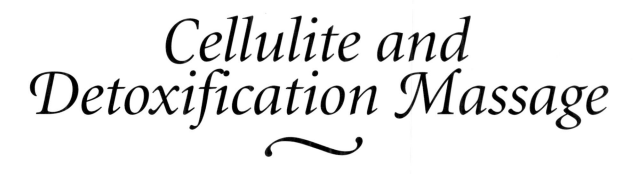

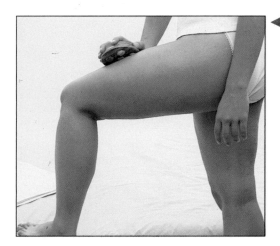

Hand-held massage instruments such as this wooden six-ball roller are ideal for making the circular pressure motions that help to smooth out cellulite spots on the thighs.

Recommended Oils

To stimulate and detoxify: Black pepper, eucalyptus, fennel
To stimulate circulation and prevent water retention: Geranium, lemon, grapefruit

Note: A useful blend would be three drops of lemon, two drops of geranium, two drops of fennel, and one drop of black pepper in 10 ml/2 tsp vegetable carrier oil.

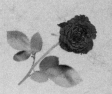

Cellulite Reduction Massage

If your partner is worried about cellulite, focus your attention on the problem areas of the thighs and buttocks during the massage. By using the correct sequence of basic massage strokes, you can soothe, tone, and stimulate the whole area, boosting the blood supply to the tissues and helping to increase the lymphatic drainage of waste products.

1 Soothe, warm, and relax the thigh muscles with upward flowing effleurage strokes such as integration and fanning motions. Repeat several times, always returning the stroke to the back of the knee by gliding your hands around and down the sides of the leg.

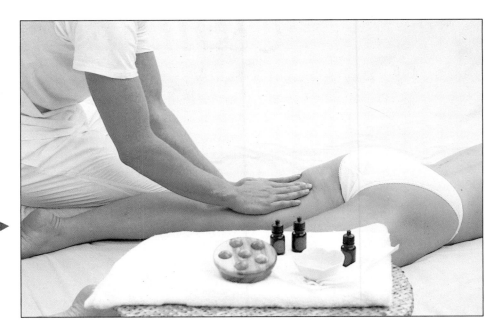

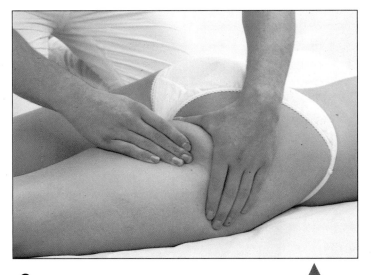

2 The lifting, squeezing, and wringing action of kneading strokes are ideal for enlivening the thigh and buttock muscles and helping the exchange of tissue fluids. Knead thoroughly over the whole area. Follow up with effleurage strokes to boost the circulation.

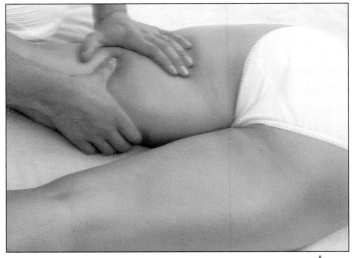

3 Deep friction strokes help to break up toxic deposits. Sink and rotate your thumb pad on one area at a time, using your other hand to push the tissue towards the stroke. Follow these strokes with fanning motions to aid the elimination process.

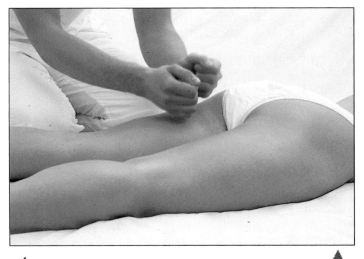

4 Pummelling, hacking, and cupping strokes are ideally suited to cellulite conditions. Briskly strike the thigh and buttocks, one hand following the other in rapid succession, flicking off the skin at the moment of contact.

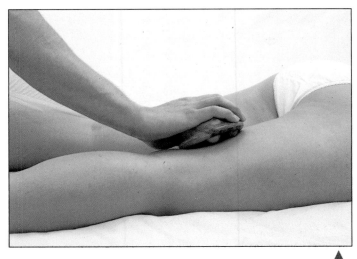

5 Soothe the thighs and buttocks with effleurage strokes. If you have a mechanical roller, use it to add to the benefits of your cellulite massage by moving it in circular motions over the flesh. This is particularly effective when the skin is oiled.

Baby Massage

All babies thrive on being cuddled, touched, and massaged, for skin-to-skin contact is essential to the nurturing of an infant, helping her to bond with her mother and father, and to develop emotional and physical health and self-esteem.

Massage and touch can become a natural part of play with a young baby, especially during and after bath time, or before she is dressed. No formal routine is needed, just gently stroke the baby's body and limbs, using effleurage circles and fanning motions.

Alternatively, softly squeeze, knead, and perform passive movements on the arms, legs, fingers, and toes. Your touch will comfort and soothe the baby, helping her to explore and discover the wonders of her body.

Soothing and Feathering

1 Hold your baby close to you, so she can feel the warmth of your body, the beat of your heart, and the rhythm of your breathing, enabling her to melt into you and be comforted by your presence.

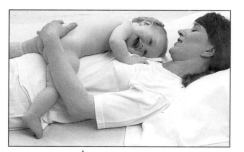

2 Babies love to lie against the softness of your body. Soothe her by placing one hand over the base of her spine, while gently stroking her head.

3 Running your fingertips up and down the baby's back will make her giggle with pleasure as the feather-like touches brush her delicate skin.

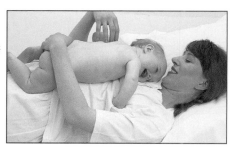

Recommended Oils for Babies and Young Children

It is both safe and beneficial to use essential oils with babies and young children, as long as you ensure that the dosage is correctly prepared and you exercise common sense when selecting the oils. As a precaution, avoid the very stimulating, strong-smelling oils, and choose instead from the following. All the oils listed are suitable for massage when applied in the recommended dosages.

Flexing and Wiggling

4 The baby will thoroughly enjoy a game of passive movements, where you move and gently flex the joints in her little arms and legs. Bend her knee towards her body and then straighten out her leg. Carry out the same action on the other leg. Repeat several times.

5 Babies never seem to lose interest in their fingers and toes; add to this fascination by wiggling and rotating the little joints one by one. ▶

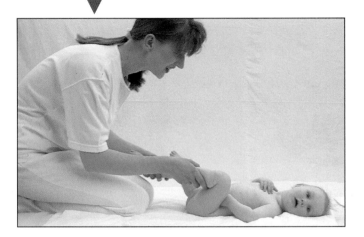

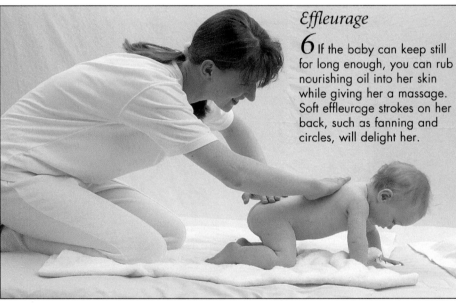

Effleurage

6 If the baby can keep still for long enough, you can rub nourishing oil into her skin while giving her a massage. Soft effleurage strokes on her back, such as fanning and circles, will delight her.

Kneading and Squeezing ▲

7 Chubby little arms and legs are made for gentle kneading and squeezing. Press the limbs softly between your thumb and fingers.

Newborn Infants

Recommended oils for specific conditions:
Fretfulness: Chamomile, geranium, lavender, mandarin
Nappy rash and skin irritation: Chamomile, lavender
Cradle cap: Eucalyptus (*Eucalyptus radiata*), geranium
Teething: Chamomile, lavender
Dosage: 1–3 drops of essential oil in 30 ml/2 tbsp vegetable carrier oil.

For Infants 2-6 Months of Age

All the above oils are effective with children in this age group, as well as mandarin and neroli. For sickness, peppermint may prove to be calming: put a drop of peppermint oil on a cotton wool ball and place at the foot of the baby's cot.
Caution: Avoid using peppermint on infants under 2 months of age. As an alternative, try spearmint.
Dosage: 3–5 drops of essential oil in 30 ml/2 tbsp of vegetable carrier oil.

For Infants 6-12 Months of Age

In addition to the oils suggested above, grapefruit, palmarosa, and tea tree can also be used. For hyperactive children, marjoram can be very helpful. However, as this problem is usually complex, you should always seek the advice of your family doctor as well.
Dosage: 3–5 drops of essential oil in 30 ml/2 tbsp of vegetable carrier oil.

For children of all ages, coughs and colds can be eased by using eucalyptus, lavender, and tea tree in a diffuser, in doses appropriate to the child's age.

Massage for the Elderly

Many elderly people live full and active lives, and aromatherapy massage provides a valuable contribution to the maintenance of their physical and emotional health. The contact of touch through the medium of massage is especially important for alleviating feelings of isolation, which may result from loneliness or bereavement.

Whole body massage is beneficial to older people, but if they are uncomfortable about undressing, then massage on the hands, feet, and face is equally helpful. Still, hands-on holds, to induce feelings of calm and peace, can be applied to the body while the person is fully clothed.

A condition commonly affecting the elderly is the onset of osteoarthritis, a degenerative disease of the joints caused by wear and tear. One or several joints of the body may be affected. Gentle massage with the recommended essential oils brings great relief. However, it is not advisable to massage over the joints if they are inflamed, swollen, or disintegrated. In these circumstances, still holds will allow the warmth of your hands to subtly comfort the affected area.

Still Hands-on Holds

Lay your hands gently around an arthritic or painful joint to allow the warmth and presence of the hands to penetrate the tissues, helping to increase circulation and reduce stiffness.

1 Focus your attention and breath into your hands before gently cradling the shoulder. This supportive hold will help the shoulder relax.

2 Osteoarthritis commonly affects the knee joints in older people. Cup the knee between your hands to bring it warmth and comfort.

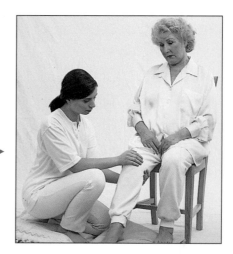

Recommended Oils

Using essential oils for the elderly presents no particular difficulties, yet it is advisable to bear in mind two general points. First, as we age our metabolism slows down, so that any chemical introduced into the body will remain there slightly longer. Second, because of this slower metabolic rate and a less physically active life, the whole system can become more toxic. This is particularly true for those people who must

Relaxing the Spine

The vertebrae at the top of the spine are another potential trouble spot with the progression of age. As flexibility is lost, mobility in the neck and head is reduced. Gentle massage will boost the blood supply to the surrounding tissues, helping the whole area to remain supple.

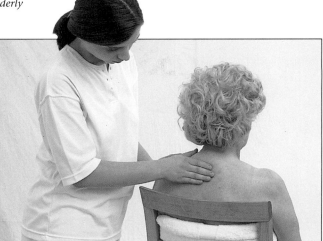

1 Soft, circular effleurage strokes over the top of the spine, at the base of the neck, and between the shoulder blades will ease away tension. While massaging with one hand, use the other hand to support the front of the body.

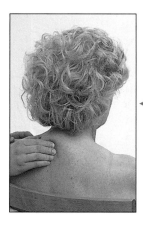

2 Excess tissue frequently builds up over stiff, tense areas, further prohibiting flexibility. Once the muscles are warmed with effleurage, sink into a deeper level of tissue with friction strokes. Use small circular motions from your fingertips to loosen and stretch the areas surrounding the top of the spine.

Staying Supple

Regular hand and foot baths with essential oils are an excellent preventive measure against stiff and aching joints at the extremities of the body. Massaging the hands and feet will also help to keep the wrists, fingers, ankles, and toes supple, giving the whole physical system an extra boost.

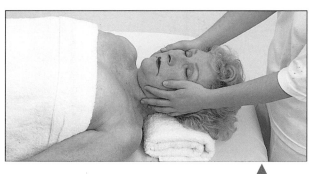

1 Support the wrist with your fingers, and apply circular and sliding strokes with your thumbs to ease away tension from its tiny bones.

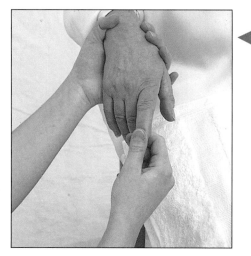

2 Many older people wish to pursue their hobbies, which may require dextrous hands and fingers. If the joints are not inflamed or in a degenerated condition, regular hand massage with gentle passive movements and stretching of the fingers will assist this continued flexibility. (For other strokes suitable for the hands, see the whole body massage programme.

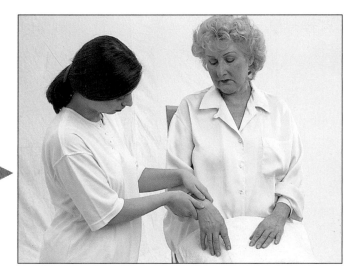

A Soothing Neck and Face Massage

A soothing neck and face massage is an excellent means of easing away physical and emotional tensions in elderly people. The loving contact of your hands will be especially comforting in times of loneliness, distress, and bereavement.

necessarily live a more sedentary life, or are in residential homes or hospitals.

With these points in mind, it is best to avoid the highly stimulating oils and make use of the gentle essential oils that have similar uses. A more dilute blend of the essential oil should perhaps also be considered. Oils that are particularly appropriate are frankincense, geranium, ginger, grapefruit, jasmine, juniper, lavender, marjoram, nutmeg, neroli, rosemary, and sandalwood.

For arthritis, try benzoin, black pepper, chamomile, cedarwood, eucalyptus, ginger, juniper, lemon, marjoram, and nutmeg.

For aches and pains, try ginger.

For grief and loneliness, choose from marjoram, rose, and nutmeg.

For constipation try fennel, ginger, marjoram, or black pepper.

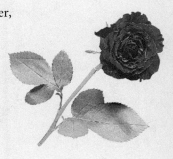

A Quick Massage

A quick 15-minute massage can work wonders in alleviating the day's tension from the body and mind. Focus your strokes on the head, neck, and shoulders, which are the main areas of tension. By letting your hands and oils bring relief to this part of the body, and the underlying stresses and strains, you can immediately restore a sense of well being.

The following strokes will relax and revitalize your partner in just a short amount of time. Ask him to straddle a chair so that you can easily reach his upper back, neck, and head. Remind him to keep his spine and neck lengthened throughout the massage so he can maintain a relaxed and open posture. Choose a blend of essential oils to help ease away muscular tension and restore vital energy. Start by placing your hands over both shoulders for some moments, to allow your partner time to relax and let go of tension. Then spread a little of your essential oil blend over the upper back, shoulders, and neck, using effleurage strokes to soften and warm the muscles.

1 Anchoring your fingers to the front of the shoulders, loosen the muscles across the top of the back by lifting and squeezing them between the heels and fingers of your hands, in an upward rolling, kneading motion.

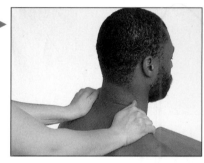

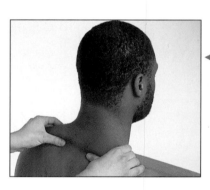

2 Keeping your fingers gently hooked to the front of the shoulders, deepen the kneading action on the shoulder muscles with circulating thumb-pressure strokes.

3 Once the shoulders have started to relax, begin to loosen the neck muscles. Use one hand to support your partner's forehead, then clasp the neck between the thumb and fingers of your other hand. Lift, squeeze, and release the muscles with a rotating action, moving up to just below the skull.

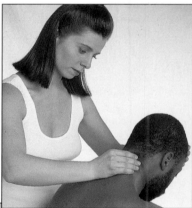

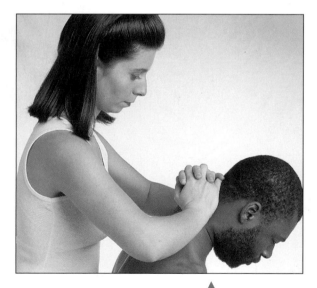

4 Clasp your fingers loosely together and cup the base of the neck beneath the heels of your hands. Sink the heels slightly into the tissue and slide them gently towards each other to lift and squeeze the muscles. Release the pressure slowly before gliding the heels in a circular motion to knead higher up the neck.

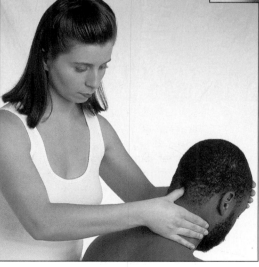

5 With the head leaning forward, use your thumb pad or fingertips to ease constricted areas under the base of the skull. Apply pressure slowly, in and upwards, just under the ridge of the bone, and rotate on one spot at a time.

6 Stimulate the scalp to loosen and increase circulation with fingertip rotations, as if you were shampooing the hair, but ensure that the pressure sinks into and moves the scalp. Hold the head securely between both hands to give it support.

7 Relieve tension in the head and neck with a lifting action. Place the heels of your hands securely on each side of the head, just above the ears. Gently squeeze the head and lift upwards with the pressure of your heels, then release slowly. Repeat the lift from behind and in front of the ears.

▼

8 Standing close to your partner, rest your forearms over the shoulders beside the nape of the neck. Ask him to inhale as you lean your weight down into your forearms, and to exhale as you release the pressure. Repeat twice before gradually moving out, step by step, to the edge of the shoulders.

▼

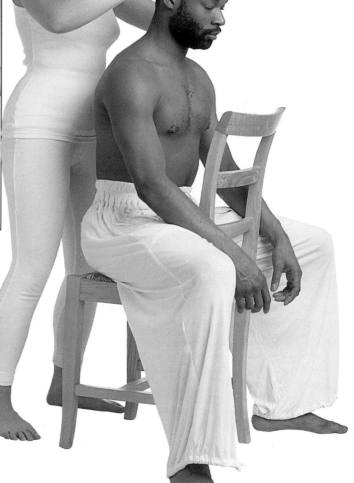

9 Apply a firm but relaxed stretch to the neck. Rest one forearm on the shoulder, and place the other hand over the same side of the head. Apply gentle pressure on both parts, so that the shoulder moves down and the head leans away to create a gentle traction through the neck. Ask your partner to let you know when the stretch has reached its natural point of resistance, and then release the pressure slowly. Repeat the movement on the other side of the body.

▼

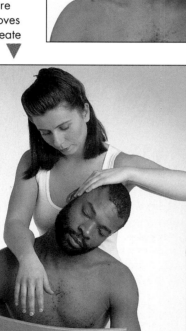

10 Invigorate the whole area with light hacking from the sides of your hands. Keeping your wrists loose, but the hands firm, hack briskly but gently over the scalp. Then hack more firmly across the top of the shoulders, taking care not to strike the spine.

▼

11 After the stimulating ▶ hacking, soothe the head, neck, and shoulders with these lovely overlapping strokes, using one hand after the other. Stroke from the forehead over the back of the head and then down to the base of the neck. Complete the session with a still hold, placing a hand over each shoulder for several moments before drawing away.

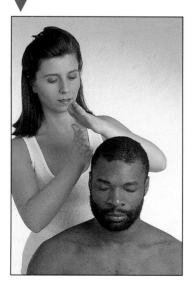

The Sensual Massage

One of the most wonderful ways for an intimate couple to relate to each other is through touch and massage. The skin is so highly sensitive that it is able to transmit and receive loving messages and feelings conveyed through the hands. Such messages and feelings nourish not only the physical body, but also the mind and emotions.

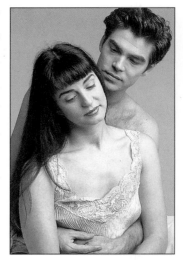

Massage can become an integral part of a relationship, a means of deep communication, a way to show how much you care for each other. Use the Whole Body Massage programme, and the recommended aromatherapy recipes to help one another relax after a stressful day, or to replenish vitality when you are tired. By carefully selecting your essential oils you can enhance the mood and beneficial effects of your massage.

Touch within a loving relationship has many dimensions. It can be therapeutic, playful, sensual, or intimate. It is a beautiful way to explore, refresh, and delight each other's bodies.

Languid Strokes

1 Having mixed your chosen blend of essential oils, spread it over the back of your partner's body with soothing, languid, and sensual strokes. Take time to allow the flowing movement of your hands to relax him physically and emotionally before applying your strokes.

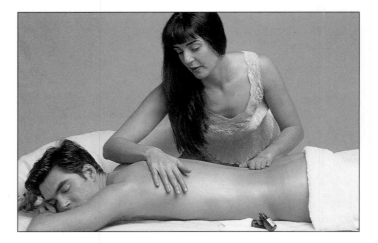

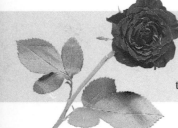

Recommended Oils

When choosing essential oils for sensual massage the most important consideration is personal taste. The massage will not be a pleasurable experience if the person giving or receiving it finds the blend of oils disagreeable. This is a time when both partners should allow an intuitive choice to guide them towards a blend of oils that they find most appealing.

Moulding into the Contours

2 As you ease tension from his back, let your hands become soft and pliable, so that they mould and encompass the shapes and curves of his body.

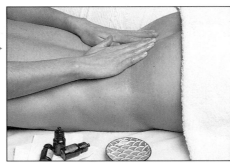

Kneading the Buttocks

3 Kneading on the buttocks not only brings a deep relief of tension to the lower back area, but can also create pleasurable and sensual feelings.

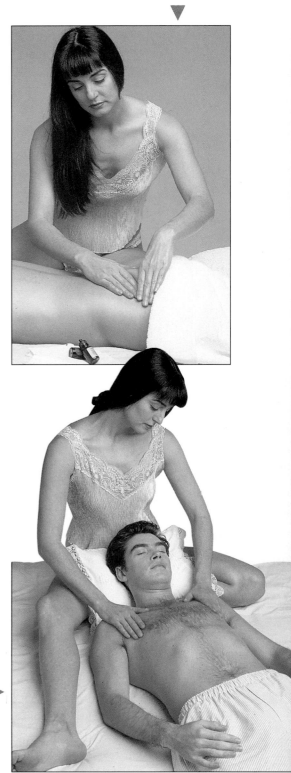

Massaging the Chest

Relaxing the chest and rib cage with massage helps your partner to release tensions and breathe more fully. This will enable him to become more open and more able to connect with his feelings. Begin the chest massage with the opening integration movement, and then add strokes from the whole body programme. Sit or kneel comfortably behind your partner so that his head is supported in your lap. Spread the oil over his ribcage, increasing the amount used if he has a lot of hair on his chest.

1 Place both hands flat over the top of the breastbone so that your fingers point down the body. Stroke gently and steadily down to its base.

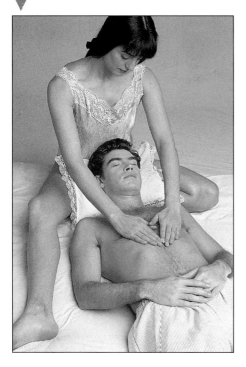

2 Without breaking the flow of motion, fan both hands out over the lower ribs, towards the sides of his body, so that your fingers slip slightly below the back. Moulding your hands to his rib cage, pull them up towards the edge of his armpits.

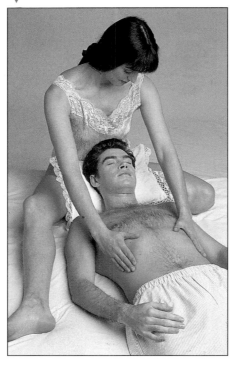

3 Flex your wrists, gliding both hands into the body and out towards the edge of the shoulders, increasing the pressure slightly to open and stretch the top of the chest. Slip both hands softly around the shoulders and slide them lightly back over the pectoral muscles, towards the breast bone. Repeat this lovely integration stroke several times.

There are, however, a few oils that seem to have a universal appeal: jasmine, rose, rosewood, sandalwood, and ylang ylang. These oils are the embodiment of luxury, and are indeed some of the most precious and therefore the most expensive to buy.

They have a warming and enveloping quality, freeing the mind of the mundane and opening it to the exotic and romantic.

To spice and stimulation to your chosen blend, add either black pepper or frankincense

Caressing

Soft caressing is profoundly relaxing, especially on the face and jaw. Tenderly stroke one hand after the other along the sides of the face. A gentle face massage is one of the most loving gifts you can bestow on your partner.

◄

Soothing the Brow

Use the combination of strokes described ▶ in Focus on the Face, focusing on the brow to soothe away the day's anxieties and to restore a sense of equilibrium.

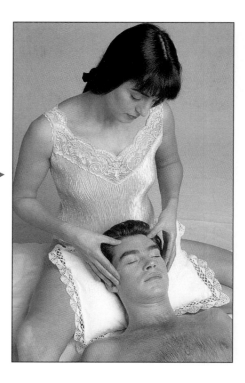

Soft and Flowing

A sensual massage can be made up entirely of soft, flowing effleurage strokes, using the flat of the hands to soothe the skin and relax the nervous system, while at the same time bringing tactile joy to the senses. This overlapping stroke, using the palms of the hands, creates the sensation of many hands caressing the body. It feels particularly wonderful on the legs and arms. One hand follows the other in short, tender brushes to the limb, with the leading hand lifting off the skin to loop over the following hand, ready to repeat the stroke.

▶

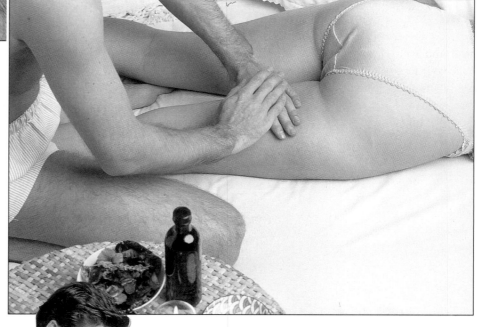

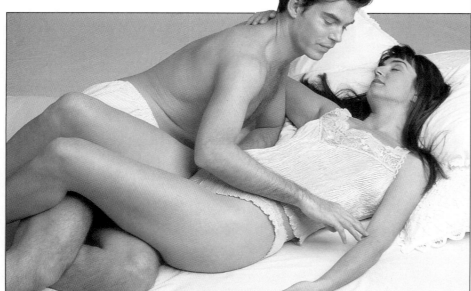

Feather Touches

Delicate feather touches are playful and deliciously arousing to the nerve senses, bringing the skin alive with shivers of pleasure. Soft skin areas, such as the undersides of the arms, the inner thighs, and the nape of the neck, are most receptive to these teasing strokes.

1 Using only the barest minimum of touch, slowly trail your fingertips down the highly sensitive skin on the underside ◄ of the arm.

2 Many people love having their necks rubbed and stroked, which is pleasurable and soothing. Using one hand after the other, stroke the fingers down the nape of her neck in overlapping motions.

▼

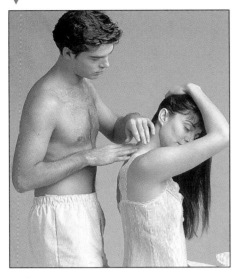

Head Strokes

Stroking, combing, and massaging the head and hair induce feelings of calm. Rake your fingers through her hair, then gently massage the scalp with circular motions from your fingertips. ▶

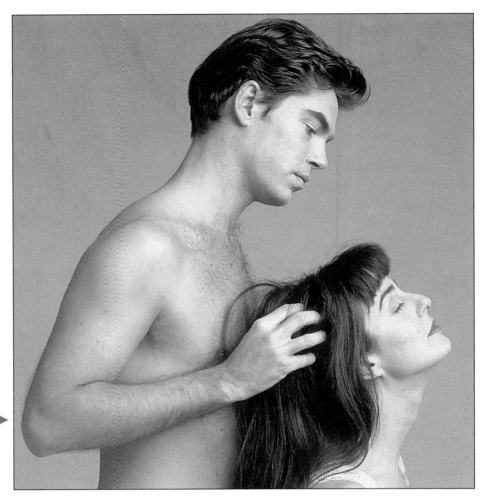

Moments of Intimacy

The close and intimate moments within a relationship open up precious feelings of vulnerability and love. Moments of still, quiet touching and eye contact will deepen your bond.

Energy and Auric Massage

Knowledge of the body's auric and energy vibrations has always existed in spiritual and healing practices, but has been largely ignored by modern medicine and science. Today, healers, psychics, body workers, and massage therapists are again tuning into the subtle body energy when working the health of the whole person.

There is an electro-magnetic energy field known as the aura that surrounds all living things in both the animal and plant kingdom. The word "aura" derives from the Sanskrit for "air", and the same word in Latin means "breeze". Both words suggest that the aura is a subtle but constantly moving energy field.

The influence of the energy field on our health and well being is a fascinating area to explore with massage and aromatherapy. The aromatherapy massage brings to the aura the benefits of healing and balance, thereby helping to prevent the physical body from manifesting symptoms of ill-health and emotional disturbance.

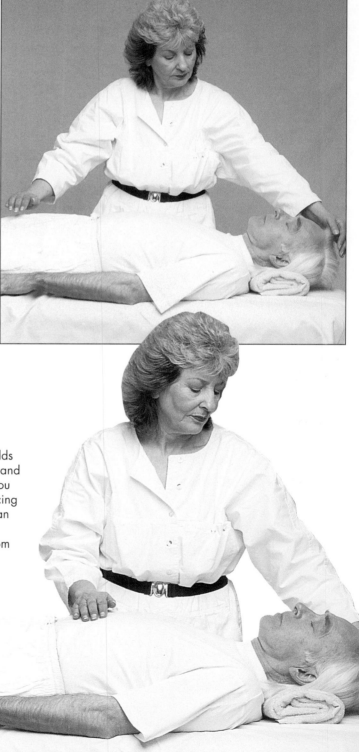

Preparation for Energy and Auric Massage

Assemble the appropriate essential oils with some vegetable carrier oil or unscented moisturizer. Lay the person down comfortably, making certain they feel warm and safe. It is not necessary for them to undress. Take time to become still and meditative within yourself by bringing your whole attention to your own body and breathing. This will increase the sensitivity in your hands, helping them to tune in to subtle energy vibrations.

Balancing Body Energy with Healing Holds

1 Begin the programme of auric massage with a session of healing holds to bring a sense of unity to the body, and to return equilibrium to the mind. If you are doing the holds for energy balancing as a complete session by itself, you can put the recommended oils in an aromatherapy burner to infuse the room with their healing fragrance.

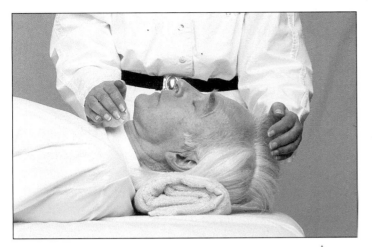

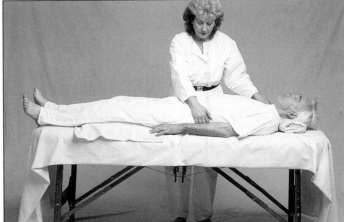

2 Raise your hands to shoulder level and let them drift down towards the body, with great sensitivity and awareness, to find the edge of the person's aura. This is felt as a tangible but subtle vibration. Softly enter this energy field, letting your hands come to rest, without weight, over the body. Tune in deeply through your hands to the person's essential energy, with the intention of restoring harmony to the whole being. Hold gently until your intuition tells you to move your hands to connect and balance other parts of the body.

3 This polarity hold brings a sense of integration and balance to both sides of the body. When standing on the left side of the body, place your left hand over his right shoulder, and the right hand over his left hip. Imagine a current of energy passing between your hands.

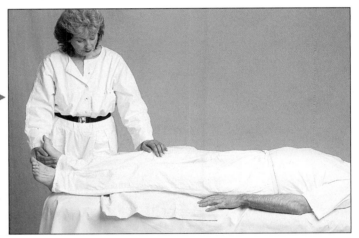

4 Healing holds on the legs and feet can help to earth the physical body, bringing an inner stability to the emotions. Start with a hip and foot hold to connect the whole leg. Then, when you are ready, place your right hand over the knee, keeping the left hand on the hip. Finally, place your left hand over the knee while cupping the right hand beneath the sole of the foot.

Clearing the Aura

When the person becomes calm through the loving touch of the healing holds, you can begin the auric massage. Take the blended oils and spread a small amount into the palms of your hands. Alternatively, add one drop of the oil to a small quantity of moisturizer and rub it into your hands. Now stroke over the aura in smooth, slow, rhythmic strokes towards the feet, working down the body and then over the limbs, one at a time. Do this three times, working over the aura's spiritual, emotional, and physical levels. Start by clearing the spiritual plane (45-60 cm/18-24 in above the body); then move lower down on to the emotional level (15-20 cm/6-8 in above the body); and finally, on to the physical level (5-7.5 cm/2-3 in above the body).

Complete your session by letting your hands hover over the belly and heart, before settling softly on to the body.

The Chakra Energy Levels

The centres of energy, known as "chakras", relate to the endocrine glands and so provide a bridge between the subtle and physical anatomy of the body. Their function is to transform energy from one level to another. The most important seven chakras form a line from the base of the spine to just above the head. In Eastern tradition, each chakra has a vibrating sound and a colour that relates to it. All seven chakras represent a different aspect of our physical, emotional and spiritual life, and have a positive and negative electrical charge. Although they operate independently of one another, they are also interrelated. Auric massage with essential oils can restore the balance between them.

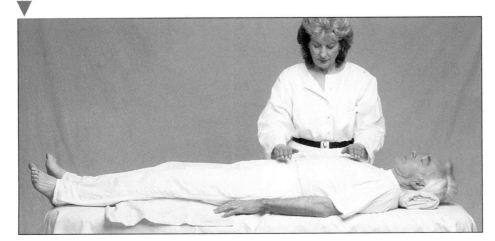

Chakra Balancing

By trusting your intuition, and moving your hands sensitively above the body in an auric massage, it is possible to detect subtle variations in the relationship of one chakra to another. Stress affecting a specific area of life may manifest in a related chakra, leaving that part vulnerable to disease. This can be felt as an overcharge of vibration or holes in the aura, which could represent potential ill-health. Harmony can be restored by using the essential oils related to the disturbed chakra, and applying auric healing holds to balance it with the other chakras.

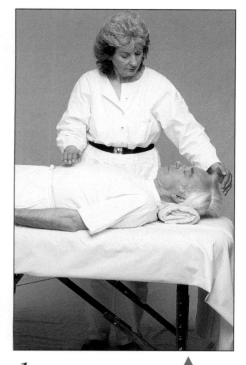

1 Restore calm to the solar plexus chakra by balancing it with the crown chakra. If the auric vibration feels dense or overcharged, softly sweep your hand over the area and away from the body, to help disperse the excess energy.

2 The throat chakra is the centre of communication. When someone is experiencing difficulties with self-expression, help to clear and recharge the energy on an auric level by gently undulating your hand above the throat.

The Seven Chakras

- The base chakra: Associated with the colour red and the adrenal glands. Connection to basic life survival, stamina and physical drive, the basic constitution, and elimination. Essential oils: Frankincense, black pepper, clary sage
- The belly chakra: Associated with the colour orange and the reproductive gland. Sense of yourself, relationships with others, concrete activity, ability to put ideas into action, fertility. Essential oils: Chamomile, fennel, marjoram, orange, peppermint, rose, sandalwood
- The solar plexus chakra: Associated with the colour yellow and the pancreas and spleen. Decision making, activity in the world, intellect. Essential oils: Frankincense, fennel, juniper, lavender, peppermint, neroli, rosemary, rosewood
- The heart chakra: Associated with the colours green or pink, and the thymus gland. Vulnerability, hopes and dreams, self-esteem, empathy, spiritual purpose. Essential oils: Benzoin, bergamot, geranium, mandarin, peppermint, rose, sandalwood, ylang ylang
- The throat chakra: Associated with the colour sky blue. Self-expression, inner growth, the place of synthesis between inner vision and outward expression in any form. Essential oils: Chamomile, clary sage, sandalwood
- The brow chakra: Associated with the colour indigo and the pituitary gland. Personal ethics, morality, and spiritual law, perception of the arts, perception of inner vision. Essential oils: Benzoin, clary sage, jasmine, juniper, orange, rosemary
- The crown chakra: Associated with the colour violet and the pineal gland. Spiritual control of physical plane, the point of connection between spiritual and physical life. Essential oil: Cedarwood, cypress, eucalyptus, frankincense, juniper, lavender, mandarin, neroli, rose, rosewood, sandalwood

Note: Some oils help re-balance the upper and lower chakras in a general way: try jasmine, lavender, or sandalwood

Protecting the Aura

You can use visualization techniques in conjunction with essential oils and auric massage to bring an energetic safety and protection to a friend at a time when he may feel particularly sensitive and vulnerable. Imagine that you are gently sealing the aura from harsh external forces with a layer of pink light. Rub the blended oils into your hands, and then send the intention of goodwill and protection into your hands as you draw them over the aura from the crown to the base of the body.

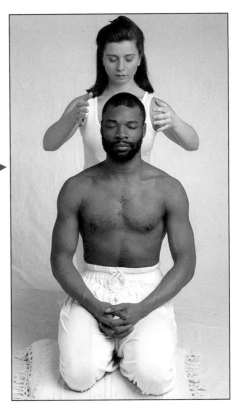

1 Focusing your total attention into your hands, visualize spreading the seal of pink light over the aura, starting from the crown of the head. ▶

◀ *2* Slowly draw your hands down over each side of the body to gently protect each chakra.

3 Complete this aura protection massage with a balancing hold, letting your hands hover at a distance over the base of the spine and the head. When you feel ready, let your hands drift away from the body and sit silently with your friend for some moments.
▼

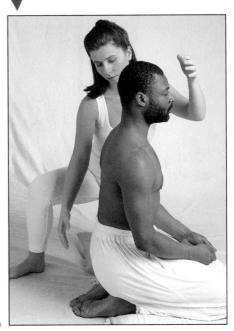

Completing Auric Work

When massaging the aura, your hands can feel overcharged and heavy with static energy. Release this down to the earth by shaking your hands gently towards the ground, or by placing them on wood. Consciously let go of the session when it is over and wash your hands in cold water. As a further cleansing, drink a glass of water and offer one to your friend.

Essential Oils for Common Ailments

This chart provides a ready reference to those essential oils that are suitable for use in the home, and some of the more common complaints and disorders they may be used to treat.

	acne	arthritis	athletes foot	bad breath	boils, blisters,	brittle nails	broken veins	bronchitis, chest infections	bruises	burns	chilblains	cold sores	cystitis, urinary infections	dandruff	dermatitis	earache	eczema	'flu
BENZOIN		■						■			■		■					■
BERGAMOT	■			■				■				■	■				■	■
BLACK PEPPER		■																■
CEDARWOOD	■	■						■					■					
CHAMOMILE	■	■								■	■		■	■		■		
CLARY SAGE	■				■													
CYPRESS								■					■					
EUCALYPTUS		■						■										
FENNEL									■									
FRANKINCENSE								■									■	
GERANIUM	■									■	■		■				■	
GINGER	■	■							■									■
GRAPEFRUIT	■																	
JASMINE																		
JUNIPER	■												■	■	■		■	
LAVENDER										■						■		
LEMON	■	■			■	■					■	■						
MANDARIN																		
MARJORAM		■						■	■		■							
NEROLI							■											
NUTMEG		■																
ORANGE								■										■
PALMAROSA	■												■		■			
PEPPERMINT				■				■								■		
ROSE							■										■	
ROSEMARY	■	■						■						■	■		■	
ROSEWOOD	■																	
SANDALWOOD	■							■					■				■	
TEA TREE	■		■					■		■		■				■		■
YLANG YLANG																		

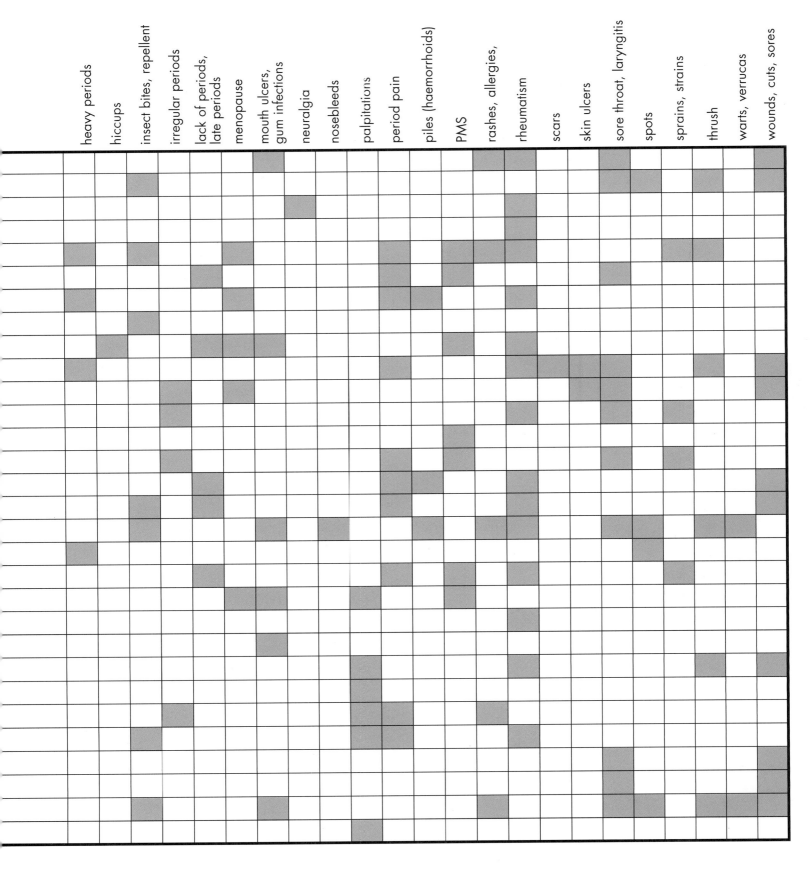

Useful Addresses

Massage
For information about courses

The International Therapy
Examination Council Ltd
James House
Oakelbrook Mill
Newent, Gloucestershire
GL18 1HD

The Massage Training
Institute
24 Brunswick Square
Hove BN 13 1 EH
Tel: 0273-20758

Training Centres

The Academy of On-site
Massage
14 Brunswick Square
Hove BN13 1EH
Tel: 9273-20758

London College of Massage
5 Newman Passage
London W1P 3PF
Tel: 071-323-3574

Clare Maxwell-Hudson
PO Box 457, London NW2 4BR

The School of Holistic
Massage
c/o Nitya Lacroix
75 Dresden Road
London N19 3BG
Tel: 071-253-4994

General Information

The Institue of
Complementary Medicine
Unit 4
Tavern Quay
London SE16
Tel: 071-237-5165

Aromatherapy
*For information about courses,
and essential oils*

International Society of
Professional Aromatherapists
The Hinckley and District
Hospital
The Annex
Mount Road, Hinckley
Leicestershire LE10 1AG
Tel: 0455 637987

Index

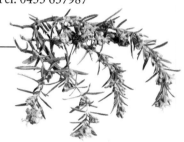

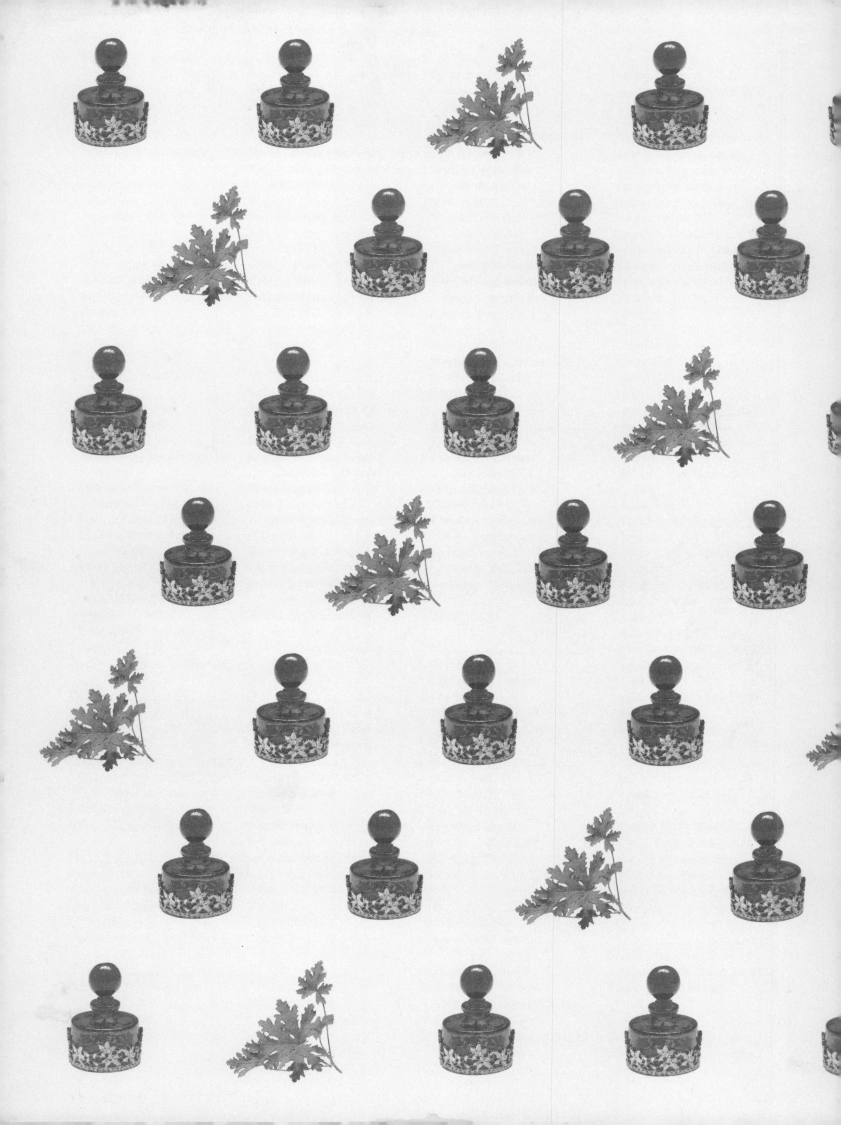

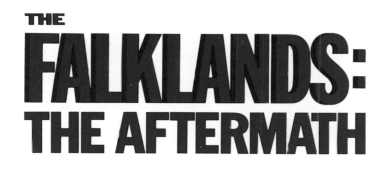

THE
FALKLANDS:
THE AFTERMATH

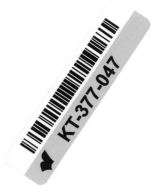

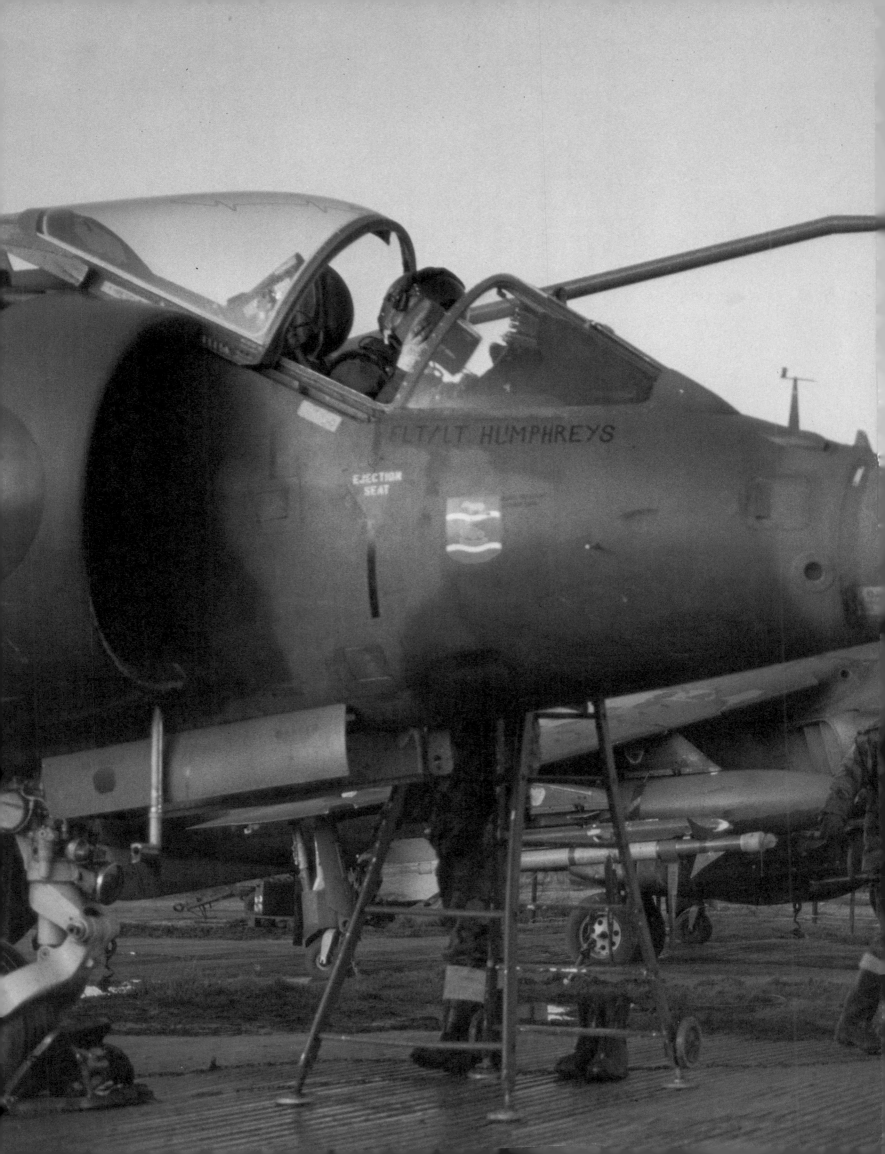

THE
FALKLANDS:
THE AFTERMATH

Marshall Cavendish

Published by Marshall
Cavendish Books Limited
58 Old Compton St, London
W1V 5PA

Edited and designed by
Grub Street, London

© Marshall Cavendish
Limited 1984

Printed in Italy
ISBN 0 86307 202

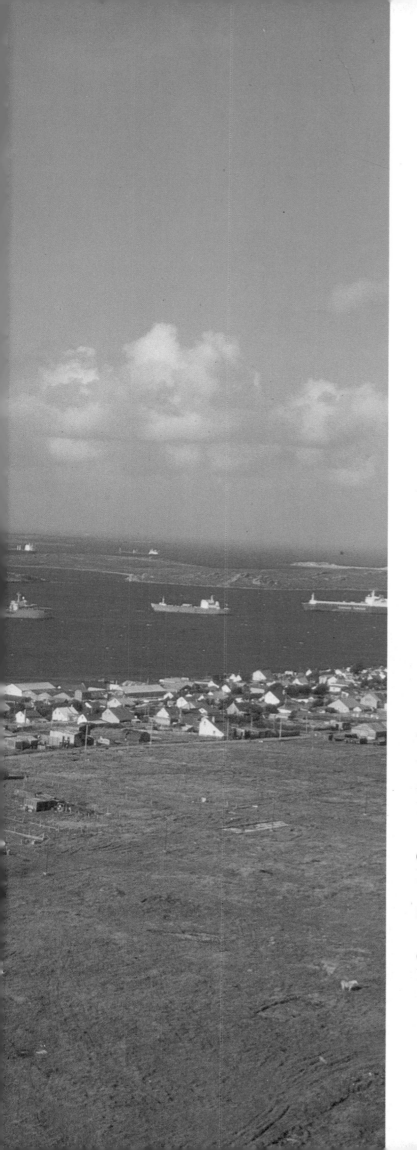

CONTENTS

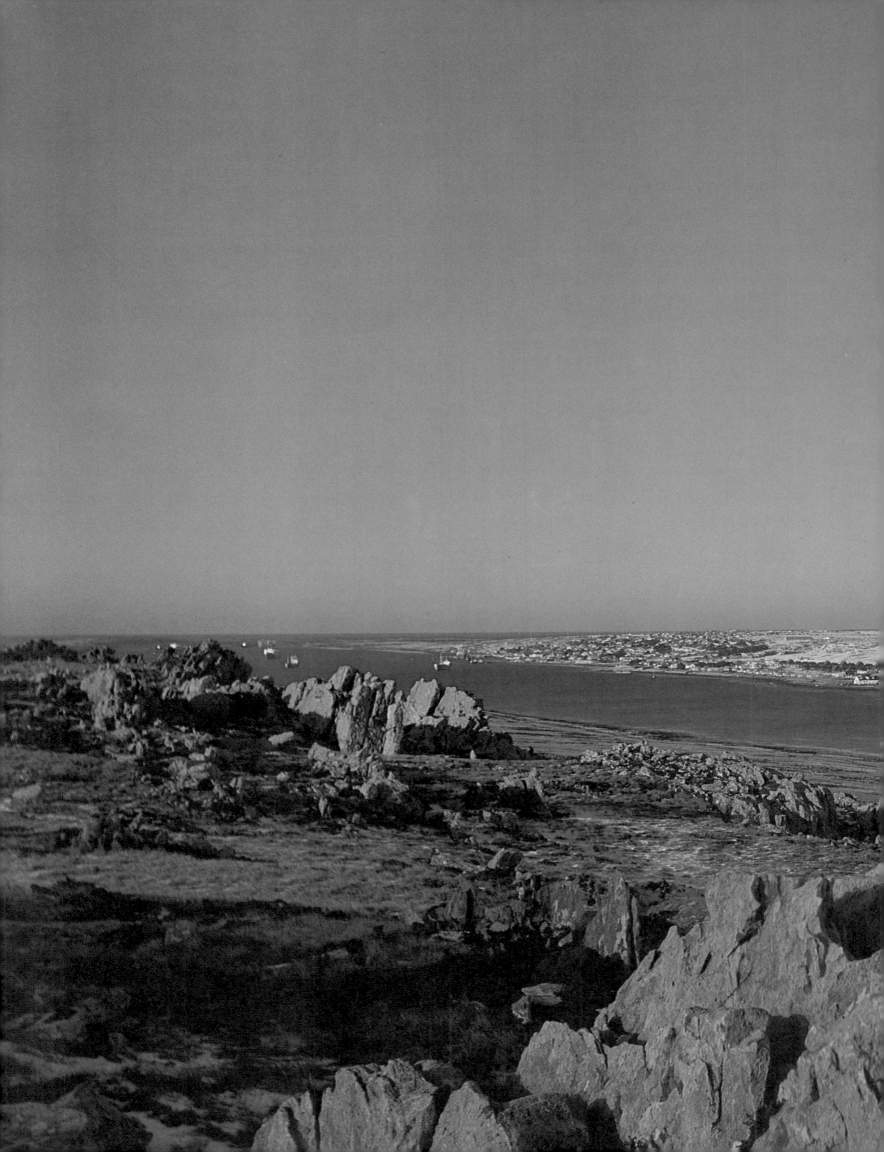

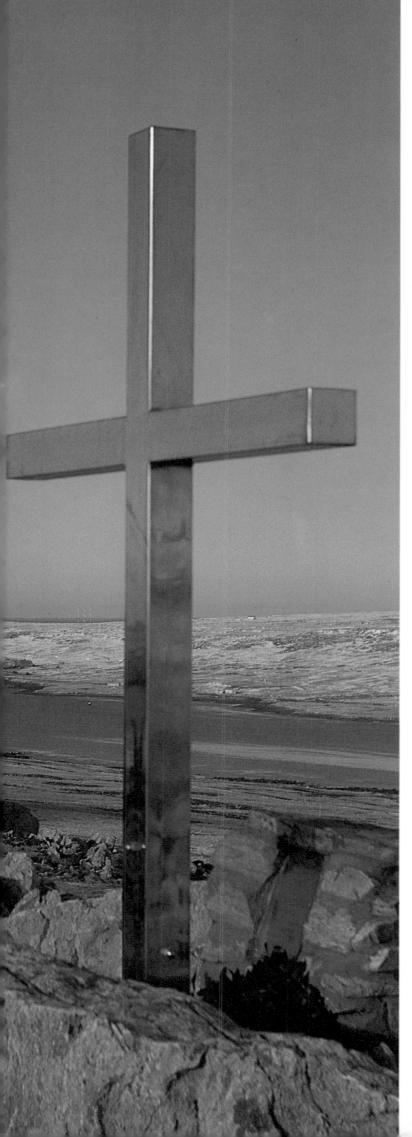

INTRODUCTION

The Falklands War, bravely fought and won, left large and costly question marks behind it. For those who followed the course of the original conflict, here is the equally fascinating account of the events that followed in the year after the decisive military victory of June 1982.
It was a year of intense and testing military activity. In these pages we tell the story of the race against time and weather by the British armed forces to secure Fortress Falklands, and the steps taken by Argentina to rebuild her shattered arsenal. It was a year of huge decisions, committing millions of pounds to vast construction projects.
And for those who had fought the war, it was a time of personal and painful adjustments. We are privileged to have been able to interview many of the fighting men concerned.
The Falklands : The Aftermath is a companion to *The Falklands War*. We are proud to present it to complete the story of a conflict that cannot be forgotten.

Peter Way
Consultant Editor

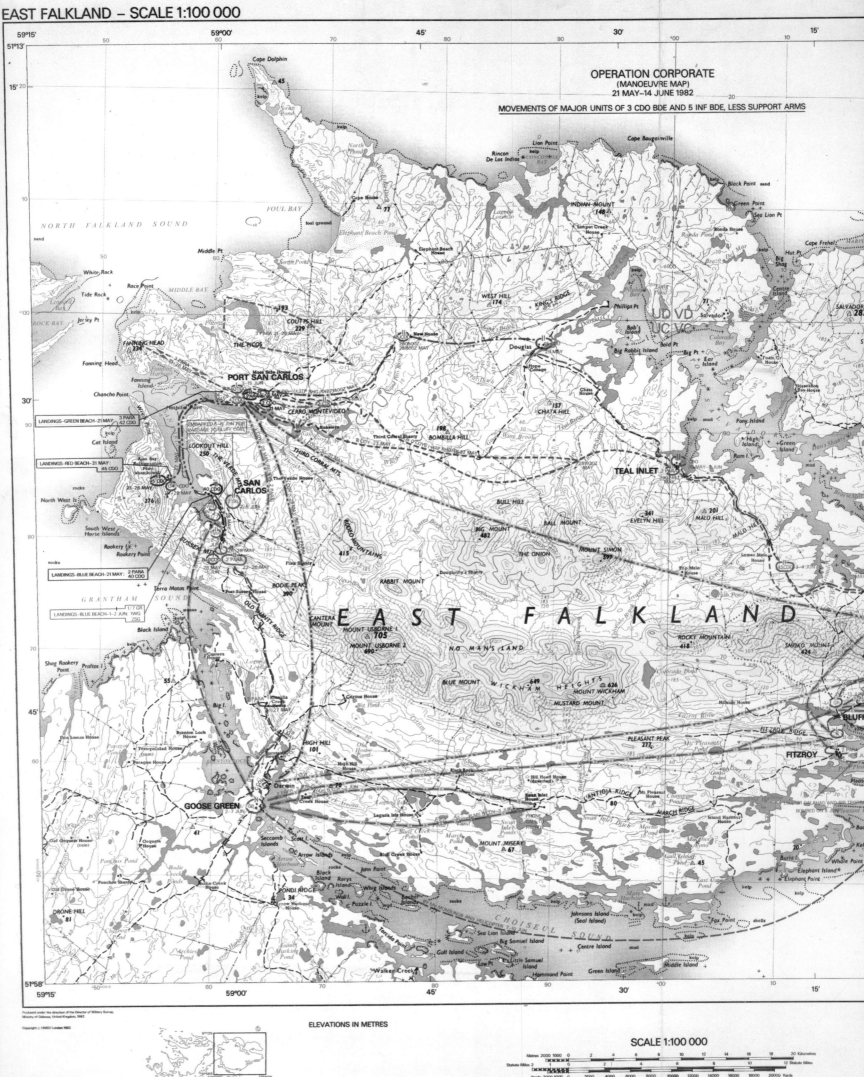

EAST FALKLAND – SCALE 1:100 000

OPERATION CORPORATE
(MANOEUVRE MAP)
21 MAY–14 JUNE 1982
MOVEMENTS OF MAJOR UNITS OF 3 CDO BDE AND 5 INF BDE, LESS SUPPORT ARMS

NORTH FALKLAND SOUND

MIDDLE BAY

FOUL BAY

E A S T   F A L K L A N D

GRANTHAM SOUND

CHOISEUL SOUND

LANDINGS–GREEN BEACH–21 MAY: 3 PARA 42 CDO

LANDINGS–RED BEACH–21 MAY: 45 CDO

LANDINGS–BLUE BEACH–21 MAY: 2 PARA 40 CDO

LANDINGS–BLUE BEACH–1–2 JUN

PORT SAN CARLOS

SAN CARLOS

GOOSE GREEN

DARWIN

TEAL INLET

BLUFF

FITZROY

Cape Dolphin

FANNING HEAD

ELEVATIONS IN METRES

SCALE 1:100 000

SERIES GSGS 5465A
EDITION 1-GSGS

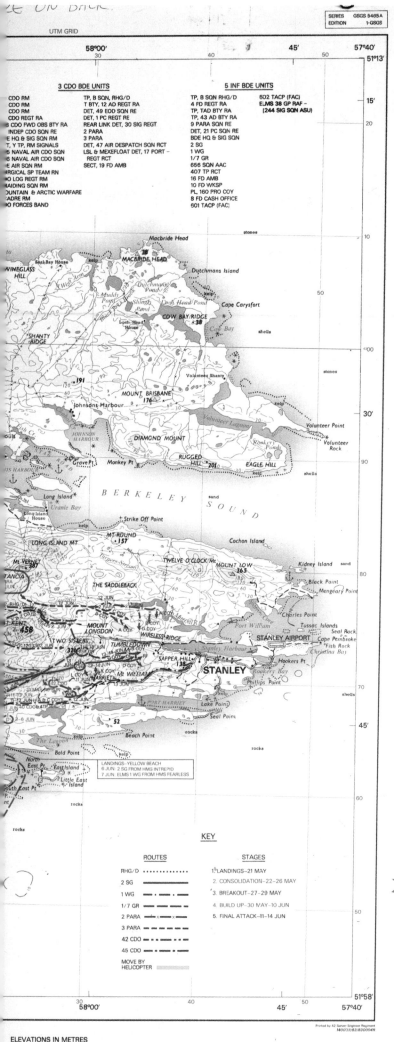

SERIES GSGS 5465A
EDITION 1-GSGS

UTM GRID

3 CDO BDE UNITS	5 INF BDE UNITS	
CDO RM	TP, B SQN RHG/D	602 TACP (FAC)
CDO RM	4 FD REGT RA	ELMS 38 GP RAF –
CDO RM	TP, TAD BTY RA	(244 SIG SQN ASU)
CDO REGT RA	TP, 43 AD BTY RA	
3 CDO FWD OBS BTY RA	9 PARA SQN RE	
INDEP CDO SQN RE	DET, 21 PC SQN RE	
E HQ & SIG SQN RM	BDE HQ & SIG SQN	
T, Y TP, RM SIGNALS	2 SG	
5 NAVAL AIR CDO SQN	1 WG	
6 NAVAL AIR CDO SQN	1/7 GR	
E AIR SQN RM	656 SQN AAC	
RGICAL SP TEAM RN	407 TP RCT	
O LOG REGT RM	16 FD AMB	
AIDING SQN RM	10 FD WKSP	
OUNTAIN & ARCTIC WARFARE	PL 160 PRO COY	
ADRE RM	8 FD CASH OFFICE	
O FORCES BAND	601 TACP (FAC)	

3 CDO BDE UNITS second column:
CDO RM — TP, B SQN, RHG/D
CDO RM — T BTY, 12 AD REGT RA
CDO RM — DET, 49 EOD SQN RE
CDO REGT RA — DET, 1 PC REGT RE
3 CDO FWD OBS BTY RA — REAR LINK DET, 30 SIG REGT
INDEP CDO SQN RE — 2 PARA
E HQ & SIG SQN RM — 3 PARA
T, Y TP, RM SIGNALS — DET, 47 AIR DESPATCH SQN RCT
5 NAVAL AIR CDO SQN — LSL & MEXEFLOAT DET, 17 PORT –
6 NAVAL AIR CDO SQN — REGT RCT
E AIR SQN RM — SECT, 19 FD AMB

KEY

ROUTES		STAGES
RHG/D	••••••••••	1. LANDINGS–21 MAY
2 SG	————	2. CONSOLIDATION–22-26 MAY
1 WG	—·—·—·—	3. BREAKOUT–27-29 MAY
1/7 GR	—··—··—··	4. BUILD UP–30 MAY-10 JUN
2 PARA	—x—x—x—	5. FINAL ATTACK–11-14 JUN
3 PARA	— — — —	
42 CDO	—·— ·— ·—	
45 CDO	— — — —	
MOVE BY HELICOPTER	▬▬▬	

LANDINGS–YELLOW BEACH
6 JUN: 2 SG FROM HMS INTREPID
7 JUN: ELMS 1 WG FROM HMS FEARLESS

ELEVATIONS IN METRES

Chapter 1
THE WAR IN PERSPECTIVE

The Falklands War is now history. Specific events can be recognized as turning points of the conflict. Argentine motives and the British choice of targets during Operation Corporate (the combined services strategy to free the islands) are better understood in the aftermath. As each arm of the forces reflects and counts its losses, certain important conclusions can now be drawn.

A map showing the disposition and movements of the major British land forces on East Falkland, from the San Carlos landings to the Argentine surrender.

Printed by 42 Sarver Engineer Regiment

9

In retrospect, a key decision of the war was that of the Argentine invaders to film and photograph the surrender of Naval Party 8901. If the British public had not been confronted on TV and in the Press by the young, tired Royal Marines, their faces smeared with camouflage cream and their hands raised in surrender, the national hurt would not perhaps have been so great. Without that impetus of anger, hurt pride and patriotism, the political acceptability of using the Task Force would have been very questionable. As it was, the politicians were actually following the national feeling demonstrated by the sendoff given to the ships as they left for the South Atlantic.

However it is worth examining the reason that Royal Marines were on the islands and why they went into action against the Argentine special forces and marines who had landed.

Naval Party 8901 had been sent to the Falklands after incursions by Argentine nationalist individuals and groups. They were adequate for the job of rounding up these eccentrics, but everyone agreed that the Royal Marines remained only a 'trip wire' if Argentina planned a full-scale invasion.

The fire fight around Government House and the brief but effective armour ambush sprung on an Argentine marine LVTP7 armoured amphibious troop carrier could have been the beginning of a longer guerrilla action on the island.

In fact the Governor, vested with the 1939 emergency powers which made him commander-in-chief, decided on surrender, fearing that the small port would be destroyed in the fighting. It was the prag-

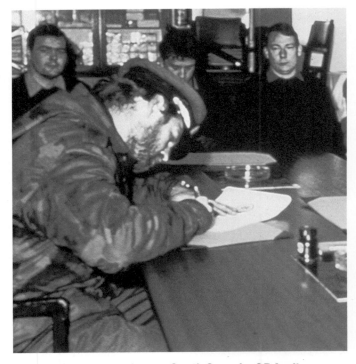

Torturer Astiz surrenders on South Georgia, 25 April.

matic decision of a wise public servant, but it left a very bitter taste in the mouths of the Royal Marines who were to make up 3 Commando Bde. The short and highly successful fight at South Georgia with the destruction of one, and almost certainly a second helicopter as well as the unique distinction of an 84mm anti-tank weapon causing severe damage to the frigate *Granville* did something to redress the sense of grievance.

If the surrender of NP 8901 shaped the war, then the triumph remains the assembly and despatch of the Task Force. Over a Bank Holiday, ships and men were readied and sent to sea. The comparatively leisurely progress south allowed valuable training and anti-submarine drills as well as combat air patrols.

The liberation of South Georgia on 25 April perpetuated the idea that this would be a war with no real casualties. The British had no accurate idea of how many had died in the Argentine invasions, and the death of one Argentine seaman aboard the submarine *Sante Fe* was regarded as a small price for the victory. There was moreover the success of capturing Lt Cmdr Alfredo Astiz, who the French and Swedish governments were keen to interview about the disappearance of various people.

The sinking of the Argentine cruiser *General Belgrano* on 2 May, the day after the first air attacks on Stanley, catapulted the war to a new level. However British casualties were still only from accidents and minor wounds from Argentine air attacks on the Task Force.

The loss of the Type 42 destroyer *Sheffield* to an air-launched Exocet missile brought home the reality

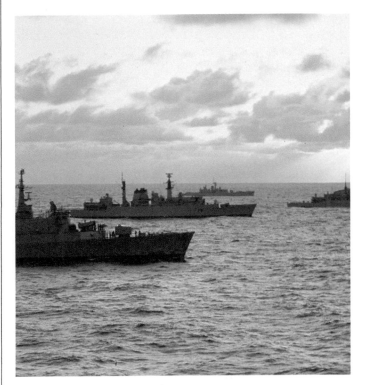

Task Force heads south, 5 April.

of the war to the British public. The servicemen had realized that losses were inevitable and in their planning for the landings at San Carlos personnel at Northwood, the UK HQ of Operation Corporate had steeled themselves for the loss of a major vessel like *Canberra* or even a carrier.

The use of Vulcan bombers, the naval bombardments and the Total Exclusion Zone around the Falklands were an indication that ruthlessness in war is not the preserve of a few traditionally belligerent nations. In effect Northwood and the planners in the Task Force were told to get on with the job, and their advice was accepted by the war cabinet.

How good news was manufactured

The only indication of political pressure was the way that 'good news' was sent soon after bad. Following the loss of the *Sheffield*, the SAS raided Pebble Island on 14 May. This small community on the northern tip of West Falkland had an airstrip with some Pucará counter-insurgency fighter bombers as well as transports. The main target was a suspected radar site which would have given the Argentine garrison warning of any naval operations in the Falkland Sound (the water between the two islands). The SAS raid was a model of well-coordinated, aggressive special forces action. Long after the campaign and the raid were over a veteran of Pebble Island recalled it with some satisfaction and added 'I really don't know why we did it'.

The raid destroyed aircraft and also established the state of morale and leadership on the island. The landings at San Carlos escalated the war. Though

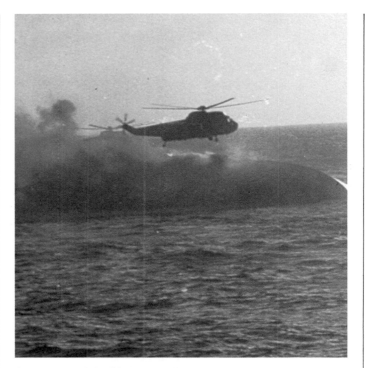

Coventry sunk by Skyhawks, 25 May.

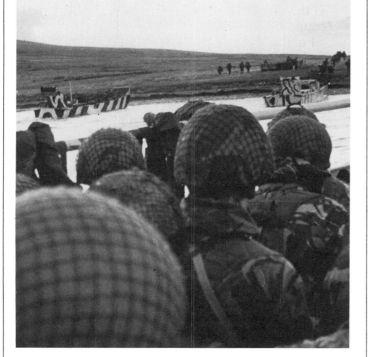

Troops go ashore at San Carlos, 20 May.

there were no British casualties (the beach and coast had been checked by Special Forces who had been ashore on the islands for nearly a month), the naval and air war became savage.

In retrospect, the Argentine Air Force (FAA) should blame not the men of the Royal Navy and the Rapier crews ashore, but their own armourers and intelligence officers. If the air attacks had been launched against the troop transports and logistic ships this would not only have caused heavier casualties among the soldiers and marines (as Bluff Cove was later to show), but the destruction of logistic ships with their loads of ammunition would have caused terrible devastation.

The FAA Mirage and A4 Skyhawk pilots went for the 'grey ships' as ordered and did not press attacks on white *Canberra* or blue *Norland*. On a few occasions they put bombs either through ships, or into them, but the low level at which these attacks were delivered meant that the fuses lacked time in free flight for the bombs to arm. They arrived on target as so many thousands of pounds of dangerous high explosive, and not the devastating explosions that wrecked ships like *Ardent, Antelope* and *Coventry*.

For the men on the ground, watching the air attacks on the 'gun line' of ships in San Carlos and the Falklands Sound was a moving and awesome experience.

Following the loss of *Coventry* and *Atlantic Conveyor*, the latter hit by Exocet missiles, there was a renewed need for 'good news'. It came from Goose Green and Darwin.

The night-and-day action fought by 2 Para not

only reflected the aggression and skill of the soldiers, but highly flexible command. This flexibility allowed the second in command to take control after the death of Colonel 'H' Jones (who won a posthumous VC) and so to win the battle. It also revealed that the leadership and values of the Argentine officers differed dramatically from their British counterparts. The concept of honour and a sense of manly dignity had an important part in their conduct — even, as one British officer observed, if honour meant a good fight in which the conscripts died but the officers surrendered with dignity.

To the north, 3 Para and 45 Commando had set off to march to Douglas and the Teal Inlet. The epic yomp or tab was across a grim mix of soggy peat and rock and boulder-strewn country. Hard going, but worse when carrying up to 100lb. Simple physical fitness, combined with leadership at all levels, saw the paras and commandos through their march.

While the paras and commandos were on their way, men of the SAS had landed on Mount Kent. Inserted at night by helicopter pilots using passive night goggles (night-vision equipment), they had been patrolling on the high ground and found that it was very lightly held. It appeared that General Menendez had taken men off the mountain to reinforce the garrison at Goose Green — swelling it to nearly two battalions.

Mount Kent is the key to the perimeter of interlocked crags and high ground that cover the western approaches to Stanley; a prize worth seizing. On the night of 31 May, elements of 42 Commando were

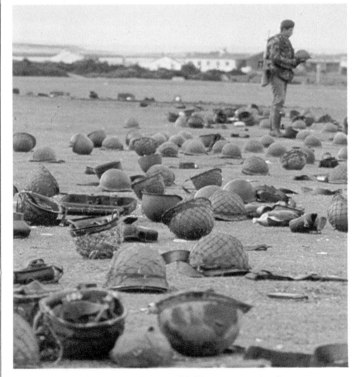

Argentines quit Goose Green, 21 May.

landed on it and began to secure it with all haste.

The following day, 5 Brigade landed at San Carlos. They had been transported south by the liner *QE2* and then cross decked at South Georgia to *Canberra*, 'the great white whale'. Now the Commander-in-Chief Land Forces Falklands, General JJ Moore was on the island to take the pressure off Brigadier Julian Thompson commanding 3rd Brigade.

On 2 June, Brigadier Tony Wilson of 5 Bde sent 2 Para eastwards to Fitzroy which had been left unguarded by the Argentine forces. Their heli-lift by the surviving Chinook from *Atlantic Conveyor* might have been a master stroke of initiative, but nearly ended in disaster when they were just saved from being shelled by their own guns. The Chinook should have been at Goose Green, but so far east observers took it for an Argentine machine.

The Scots Guards and Welsh Guards were transported around the coast from San Carlos, though the tough little Gurkhas of 1st Battalion, 7th Gurkha Rifles marched to Goose Green. On the second lift the RFA *Sir Galahad* and *Sir Tristram* were attacked and wrecked by FAA A4 Skyhawks and 51 men were killed. These were the heaviest losses to be suffered by British forces since the Korean War.

Information policy at the MoD in Whitehall allowed ministers to make evasive replies to questions about the severity of the losses. After the war it was said that this was for operational reasons, and certainly the Argentine press were convinced that losses were much greater and that therefore British plans for further attacks towards Stanley would be disrupted. Like many of the casualty reports, however, it did cause concern among the next of kin of men in the 1st Battalion Welsh Guards.

To compensate, the Welsh Guards received two companies from 40 Commando who had been dug in around the Brigade Maintenance Area (BMA) at San Carlos. The unhappy 40 Commando who had landed with their comrades from 42 and 45, as well as 2 and 3 Para, saw very little action. They were retained at San Carlos because there was always the threat that the Argentine garrison on West Falkland would attempt a raid on the BMA. The Argentine garrison did make one small attempt but this was quickly rounded up by the Gurkhas.

The Harriers had attacked coastal shipping as well as the airfield at Fox Bay. The RAF Harrier reinforcements which flew from the UK to the South Atlantic, with inflight refueling, was one of the epic logistic operations similar to that which kept mail and crucial supplies flowing, as well as allowing four Vulcan attacks on targets around Stanley.

Though derided for a lack of accuracy, the Vulcan attacks which put 21 1000lb bombs on or near the runway had a dramatic effect on the morale of the men billeted in the area. The use of the controversial

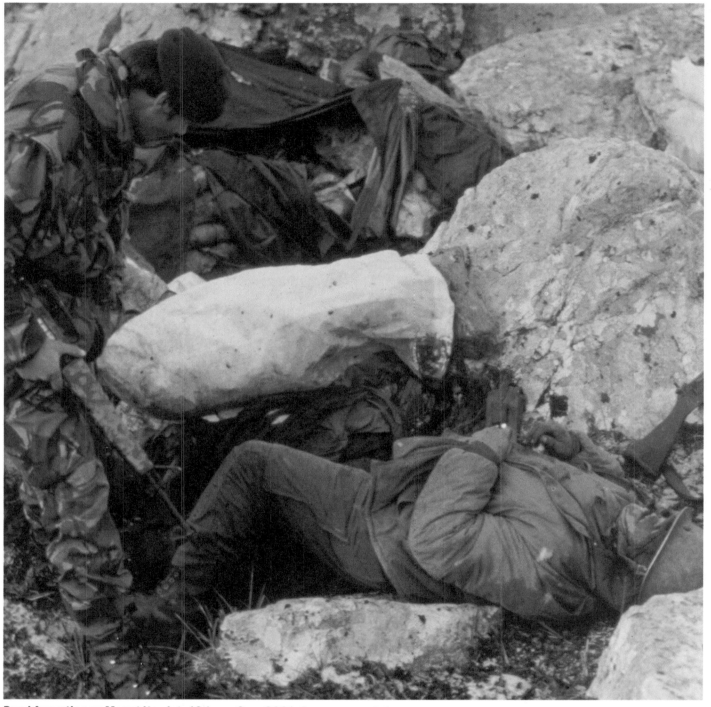

Dead Argentine on Mount Harriet, 12 June. Over 300 prisoners were taken.

cluster bombs by Harriers, bombs which spread destructive shrapnel over a wide area, were another indication that the war was being waged with a strong service influence and few political constraints.

Argentine air activity was not at an end after the Bluff Cove attacks. A nightly shuttle by C130s between Stanley and the mainland continued, allowing them to move men and equipment into the area and evacuate wounded. Their A4s also made an attack on 3rd Brigade HQ, which may have been located by the radio direction-finding equipment that they had bought from the UK before the conflict.

Air activity was not confined to fighter ground-attack work. The Sea Harriers on Combat Air Patrol (CAP) were able to intercept the Argentine Mirage, Dagger and A4s as they made their way towards the Falklands. With their excellent all-aspect AIM-9L Sidewinder missiles, they ran up 16 confirmed kills and one probable, and four downed by 30mm cannon fire and two probables — a total of 23 kills.

Four Argentine aircraft were meanwhile destroyed on the day of Bluff Cove, whilst 3 and 5 Bde were preparing for their night attacks. The first of these was on 11 June with the assaults on Mount Longdon, Mount Harriet and Two Sisters.

On Two Sisters, 45 Commando fought a grim action with a reinforced company of the Argentine 4th Infantry Regiment. The latter were armed with 0.50in heavy machine guns well dug in. The position was taken with four dead and eight wounded. On Mount Harriet, 42 Cdo sent one company through the minefields to the south, advancing upon the position by the least-expected route. The attack brought revenge for Juliet Company — a composite company including men from NP 8901. They took their objective at the price of one man dead and 13 wounded. On Longdon, 3 Para fought a savage action against 7th Infantry Regiment that cost them 14 dead and 35 wounded. A survivor from the regiment recalled the attack with awe as it was pressed against their well-dug positions. During this action Sergeant Ian McKay won a posthumous VC.

There was a delay of one day, and then action resumed with ammunition brought forward for the 105mm light guns of which 3 and 5 Brigade had fired some 3000 rounds — excluding the naval-gunfire support which had cost HMS *Glamorgan* 13 men when she was hit by a land-launched Exocet while supporting 45 Commando.

The guns received over 400 rounds each for the attack and during the second night attack they fired 2400 rounds.

The night attacks of the 13 and 14 June began with a diversionary action by the Scots Guards which went up a track to the south of Tumbledown. It worked, since this was the axis that the Argentine troops most expected an attack to come from.

The Scots Guards and Tumbledown

The Scots Guards had a hard fight for Tumbledown which did not end until dawn. This delay prevented the Gurkhas from getting onto Mount William before the fighting had almost ended. The men of 2 Para, profiting from the experience of Goose Green, had worked out what they were proud to call an 'all-arms battle'. They had naval-gunfire support, the guns of a troop from the Blues and Royals, fire from the 105mm light guns of the Royal Artillery plus the mortars of 3 Para. With this level of support and well-planned and implemented attack, all went well on Wireless Ridge.

The Welsh Guards advanced from the south but became entangled in a minefield where two of the Royal Marines attached from 40 Cdo lost feet on mines. At first light the Welsh Guardsmen were helilifted to attack Sapper Hill, but by then the fighting was almost over.

While 2 Para were knocking on the door of Puerto

ONE WHO WAS THERE
Private Ian Davis

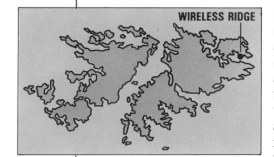

WIRELESS RIDGE

He looks fine at first sight. His left upper arm and shoulder are covered and bandaged, and he sits very still in the chair, and you notice that a couple of fingers are missing from his right hand. He speaks very calmly, very matter-of-factly all the time, and in the same voice informs you that the left arm is due to be taken off on 9 August.

Private Ian Davis of 2 Para joined the army at 16 and is now 24. Why did he join the Paras? 'One reason, because my old man was in the Royal Corps of Transport, and I didn't want to follow him because I was supposed to be the rebel of the family.' All his childhood was spent with an army background, living in married quarters. He wanted to be a soldier too. 'I used to play truant from school, and just go on Salisbury Plain, and watch the soldiers over there.'

Ian Davis spent six months patrolling the Falls Road in Belfast in 1976. Between 1979 and 1981 he did his second Northern Ireland tour, two years this time, mainly in Armagh. When the Falkland crisis blew up he was on embarkation leave for Belize, where the 2nd Battalion was due to carry out a six-month stint. 'I can remember seeing the Falklands on TV, and I knew that 3 Para were going, and I was sick as a dog because I knew that we were going to Belize. I joined the army to be a soldier and fight, and that's what I wanted to do. So when I got a telegram a couple of days later I was really pleased.'

Ian Davis first came under close fire just after Camilla Creek on the way to Goose Green. 'To come under fire — to me it seemed as though I was back in Brecon (on exercises), until somebody got hit. The first bloke that was hit was my mate. He got caught by a machine gun. He was the advanced platoon, and I being one of the medics, we stayed up on the echelon. Then we went forward as they started to take casualties. He was the first one we got to.'

He worked through Goose Green and then beyond. On 14 June they reached Wireless Ridge on the way to Stanley. 'As we got to the top we lay in a gully. One of the platoons went forward, and then someone called for a medic. I ran across, and was just about to treat the bloke, and the One Five Five dropped in on us. That's a 155mm cannon, the biggest

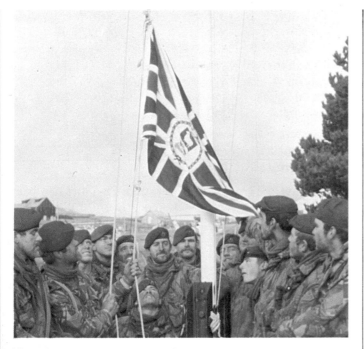

Victorious troops restore the flag at Stanley.

Argentina (the new Argentine name for the port), negotiations began to bring about the surrender.

These were the outcome of a radio link established by the British and which assisted the quick implementation of surrender negotiations. Using a satellite radio link the team, which was finally headed by General Moore, were also able to talk to Whitehall as the talks were in progress. Once again the Government did not impose any political pressure and the two generals were able to sign the simple surrender document.

The Falklands War had begun because President Leopoldo Galtieri had thought that recapturing the Malvinas would give his unpopular government a new lease of popularity. For a short time it worked but then the bubble burst.

The British reaction was not only unpredictable to Dr Costa Mendez, the Argentine Foreign Minister, but it also seemed excessive. It should however be seen in a wider context — to fight for 1800 people, on a windy, wet island at the other side of the world — is not a very convincing *causus belli*. The war was fought over principles. An attack had been made not only on British servicemen, but also on the British citizens who had become the unwilling captives of a government with a very dubious record on human rights. If the withdrawal of the Ice Protection vessel *Endurance* had been seen as a signal of weakening British will by the Argentine government, what would the world have made of the surrender of the islands? Fear of setting a precedent must have been a central consideration when the decision to sail was taken.

one they had on the islands. It dropped about ten metres away. We were out in the open, so . . . It took away the shoulder, the arm, the bone, two fingers — shrapnel smashed my shoulder-blade. The bloke who was next to me — he died. I was awake all the time. I had to keep awake. I had to treat myself. I was the only medic with the company. I knew that if I'd gone to sleep I wouldn't have woken up, because I would have bled to death. I lost six pints on the way to Fitzroy. They pumped as much blood into me as they could, but they couldn't give me anaesthetics.'

Pte Davis spent the best part of the following month on the hospital ship *Uganda*. While he was there he rang up his fiancee, a Belfast girl, telling her he was injured, but not daring to tell her the extent of the damage. From *Uganda* he was taken in the survey ship *Hydra* to Montevideo, flying from there to Ascension Island, and thence to Brize Norton. He arrived back in the UK exactly a month after he was blown up, on 14 July.

The long series of treatments began, in hospital in Woolwich. Now his fiancee had to know how badly he had been hurt. He actually tried to put her off the idea of marriage, telling her how difficult life could be, not wanting her to go through with it from pity. He need not have worried. She stuck with him, and they were married on 31 October 1982. The hospital treatment continued at Woolwich, but he wanted to be back with the regiment, and left hospital in January 1983. The couple got married quarters at Aldershot. Treatment alternated with sick leave. Pte Davis began to come to terms with the idea that his army career was all but over. There was nothing more that the surgeons could do for his left arm. The damage was too great, and could not be rebuilt. Like many others coming back from the Falklands he suffered from bouts of depression, and would go out deliberately to get drunk, to blot everything out. Yet even after learning that he would have to lose the arm, his single-mindedness began to pull him through. 'I've got no regrets about it. I joined the army to do that sort of thing, and when it came I was really happy. It was the only way I could prove to myself that I had learned what I was taught.'

Ian Davis seems to have spent his life proving himself to himself. Once he knew the army was over for him he began to replan his life. Having decided that there could be a future in computer programming, he went out and bought himself a computer and began to teach himself how to use it. His resilience is almost frightening. He claims that the loss of the arm does not really bother him. He has little time for the Falklands as a cause, reserving his respect for his dead friends. He believes all the medals should have gone to them.

THE LAND LESSONS

In December 1982 the British Government published a White Paper, *The Falklands Campaign: The Lessons*. It had been awaited with interest by defence commentators and experts, who in some instances had been guilty of irresponsible guesses about weapons, equipment and organizations.

The returning servicemen, Royal Marines and Paratroopers as well as Guardsmen and Gurkhas, would agree with at least one of its conclusions. 'We have learned a great deal from the Falklands Campaign. Many of the lessons are not new but they are no less important for that'. One veteran of the Korean War in conversation with the gunners of 29 Commando Regiment asked them what they had learned and received the simple reply 'To dig'. 'Yes,' he answered 'I learned that in Korea'.

The Falklands were a proving ground for several pieces of equipment and weapons that had been developed by the British and never tested in action. The most notable were the Rapier and Blowpipe SAM systems, the Scorpion and Scimitar from the CVRT (Combat Vehicle Reconnaissance Tracked) family, and the CET (Combat Engineer Tractor). Though they never encountered the Argentine AML90 armoured cars, they did valuable work at the close of the campaign in action against fixed positions. Their second-generation night sights did not 'bloom out' when used in an environment with ordinary white light and so the AFVs were able to see and fire when flares and tracer were lighting up the darkness. The AFVs of the Blues and Royals in action on Wireless Ridge employed their main armament against positions and then as the defenders attempted to withdraw engaged them with GPMG (General Purpose Machine Gun) fire.

They had shown beforehand that the vehicles could travel over not only the rough rocky going of the Falklands, but more importantly over the very soft ground on the island. In one case, a vehicle commander had jumped down from the turret and sunk up to his knees in the soft ground — the armoured vehicle, however, due to its well-designed tracks and weight distribution had not penetrated the surface turf. It was a pity that the cross-country properties were not fully appreciated until the end of the campaign and the CVRTs were not sent over Sussex mountain to support 2nd Parachute Regiment at Goose Green and Darwin.

Taking a day or so to settle in at San Carlos, Rapier was the greatest air-defence land success. One of the problems of the system was that the crews had not been able to go ashore at Ascension to test their equipment. It had been stowed near the ship's engines where it suffered from vibration and heat. Once in action, however, it claimed 14 confirmed kills and six

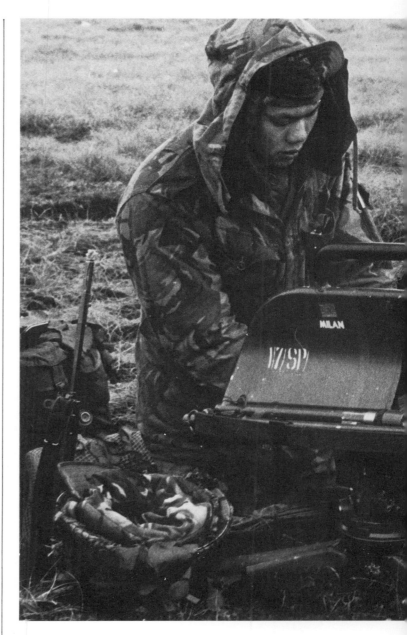

Above: Gurkhas consider Milan anti-tank system.
Right: Rapier battery of 9 Btn 12 Air Defence Rgt RA.

probables. Even Blowpipe, which was used by both the British and Argentine forces, had nine kills and two probables in British hands. The White Paper was at pains to dismiss the French claims that their Roland SAM was effective — in fact it destroyed only one of the five Harriers lost in action.

More significant was the effect of the Argentine radar-directed Oerlikon twin 35mm AA guns which destroyed three Harriers. Close-range AA fire was an important factor in local defence — the sight of tracer fire coming up at a pilot is more likely to put him off his bombing or rocket run, than the impersonal audial warning that radar is tracking him prior to a missile launch, or even that a missile has been launched. The men of 3rd and 5th Brigade found that GPMG and tracer fire not only put pilots off, but it even

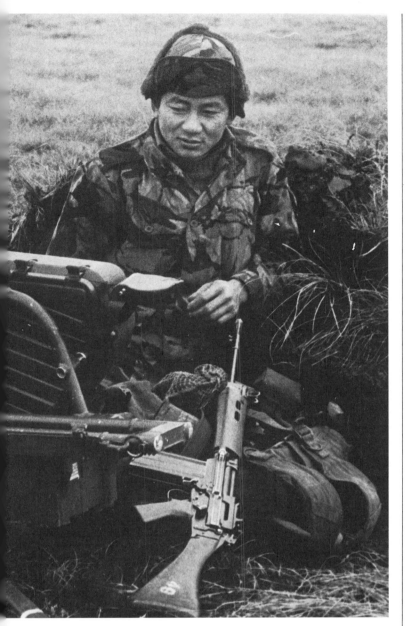

occasionally brought their aircraft down in flames.

Some units went south equipped with the M79 grenade launcher. This weapon, developed by the US Army for Vietnam, proved to be invaluable in action against fixed positions. Other weapons that were used for 'bunker busting' included the Milan anti-tank missile, which was described as extravagant by some commentators — the missiles cost about £8000 at a conservative estimate. At Goose Green, 2nd Parachute Regiment watched an Argentine soldier run from one bunker as a Milan streaked towards it, and then have to make the same hasty exit from another as it in turn became a target.

The 66mm one-shot anti-tank rocket was also used to good effect, along with the heavier 84mm. The feeling was that although the 66mm was excellent and two could be easily carried by one man, the 84mm was bulky and heavy in the assault.

Soldiers who saw the effect of the 5.56mm round fired from the M16 or Armalite were not impressed when they compared its effect with that of the 7.62mm round from the Self-Loading Rifle (SLR). The bigger rifle round would knock over a man with its greater kinetic energy. One Royal Marine recalled a fire fight in which his Argentine enemy had taken three hits with 5.56mm rounds and was only obliged to surrender because the third round had clipped his forehead and blood from the wound was blinding him.

The automatic fire of the GPMG was invaluable in the assault, and the Royal Marines and 2nd Parachute Regiment were lucky to have either an extra LMG (Bren Light Machine Gun) or GPMG in each section which doubled their firepower. One Argentine survivor recalled the sight of tracer fire hitting a machine gun position; the incoming fire resembled a fan as individual GPMG gunners located the target and engaged it from their positions.

Light guns in fierce action

The 105mm Light Gun developed by the Royal Ordnance factories was also tested in action. It fires a 35.4lb shell to a maximum range of 10.56 miles, and so outranges the Argentine Italian-made Oto Melara 105mm Pack howitzers with a range of 7 miles. However, the Argentine French 105mm guns could reach targets 13.6 miles away and fired a 95lb shell. The gunners were well served by their observers who were well forward, locating targets in the Argentine-held areas of the island.

In the interviews after the surrender the Argentine officers said that the naval bombardment kept their men awake and caused some destruction, but it was the fire from the Royal Artillery 105mm light guns which was most destructive of life and equipment.

A less-publicised area of Operation Sutton (the codename for the Falklands land battle) was the

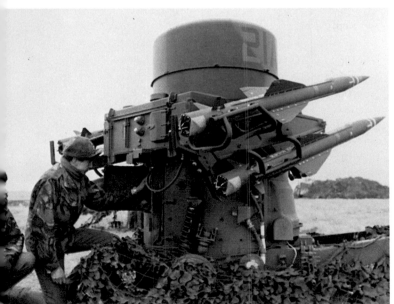

ONE WHO WAS THERE
Private Steven Hood

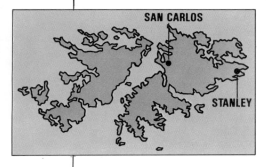

Private Stephen Hood joined the Parachute Regiment when he was 16 years old, as a junior soldier. He went into the Second Battalion when he was 17 and a half. He is now 24 years old. He joined the army 'to get away from home, basically'. He enjoys the army sometimes, but says there have been a lot of hassles. As to the regiment, he states simply that he loves it.

Before the Falklands his previous active service had been a two-year stint in Northern Ireland. Like the rest of 2 Para, Pte Hood learned that he was going to the Falklands about three weeks before they went. They had all thought that they were going to Belize, but Belize was postponed at the last moment. Stephen Hood had been medically downgraded with burst-eardrum problems, but he was determined to go out with his battalion, saw a specialist and insisted that he was going. The doctor passed him, and he travelled out with most of the rest of 2 Para on *Norland*.

Pte Hood had had medical training and went to the Falklands as a full medic. 'To tell you the truth, I thought we'd get as far as Gibraltar and turn back. I thought it'd be a three-weeks' cruise. Of course, I'd just got married, five months before. My wife dropped a child about four days before I left. A girl.' The marriage was not to survive the Falklands campaign.

Stephen Hood lives in barracks in Aldershot. His wife and their baby daughter live in the town. 'I'm separated now. It's because of the Falklands we're separated. A lot of guys out in Belize now — they're separated. When I came back I was a little bit mental there, you see. I lost one good friend, a Scots lad. I saw him. It was alright there at the time, because it was war. I was prepared to die, so were the rest. That was our job. When I came back, of course, I was a different man. My wife, she had missed me and all of this, and she'd had post-natal depression. The marriage just fell apart. She was always crying. When I was out in the Falklands I'd get letters, I'd get bad letters from her. Of course, she was depressed. And then, when I came back, it didn't click. We couldn't get on again. It just fell apart.'

They were together until Christmas 1982, and then she left him. They have an arrangement, and he gets to see his daughter. Barracks life has been slack in the year since getting back from the South Atlantic. He has had some leave, and gone on some exercises. His thoughts return again and again to the Falklands. What had left the greatest impression on him? 'The fact that you had to go and kill somebody, and that person you're going to kill is trying to kill you. Then you see your mates get killed, and you've got to pick them up and carry them away. That's probably just me, the way I feel. I enjoyed it, don't get me wrong, but I didn't at the same time...'

Time and again he returns to the subject of his dead friend. 'My friend died, and I keep going out to see his grave. He's buried in Aldershot, although he comes from Glasgow. And I always go and see his grave, and I can't get that out of my system. I had other mates who were killed as well. I knew them all.'

Stephen Hood suffered another burst eardrum at Goose Green while under Argentine shelling, but he found that even in the most stressful conditions his medical training won through. From San Carlos Bay to Goose Green to Darwin, Wireless Ridge, and finally Stanley he carried on working, treating the injured, administering drugs and intravenous drips, getting the wounded back to safety. 'You're all psyched up to go, and you've got a job to do, and you do it...'

How the lessons of the war saved a life

Back in Aldershot, just over a year after returning from the Falklands, his training came in useful again. Stephen Hood stumbled across a head-on collision which had just occurred. A 15-year-old boy had been severely injured and was bleeding badly from abdominal wounds. Passers-by were making ineffectual attempts to help. As Hood said, he went 'straight into the Falklands bit'. He took charge, located the bleeding, applied the necessary pressure at the right place to stem the flow, and kept the boy comfortable until the ambulance arrived. The medical training had taken over, and he indubitably saved the boy's life.

In 1986, Pte Hood will be 27 years old and will have completed his nine-year engagement in the Second Battalion of the Parachute Regiment. He says he would like to sign on again, though only if he can stay in the regiment. He can no more see himself 'wearing a black beret' than being a civilian. However he believes that the authorities are keeping an especially close eye on men who have been to the Falklands, and getting rid of them if there's any sign of trouble. He would like to continue training as a medic. He has experienced more of life and death than most of us manage in half a lifetime. Yet, he complains, the authorities still treat them, he and those who went with him, as little boys. His final comment on the Falklands: 'I'm glad I went... but I wish I hadn't.'

admirable support given by the Logistic Regiment of 3 Brigade. Later they took on some of the responsibility for 5 Brigade. However in the White Paper, 5 Bde, which has now been tasked for out of area operations will be improved. 'The combat arms units were already in being and include two parachute battalions (2 Para, 3 Para), an infantry battalion and engineer support. To these we have just added an armoured reconnaissance regiment and in the course of next year we will add an artillery regiment, an Army Air Corps squadron and certain logistic support units. RAF Hercules transport aircraft are currently earmarked for the brigade and the fitting of station-keeping equipment to a number of Hercules aircraft in 1985 will give the brigade an assault-parachute capability.'

The gulf between theory and action

In effect these improvements to 5 Brigade will make it airmobile and so parallel the amphibious capability of 3 Brigade, giving even greater flexibility for out-of-area operations.

Organization and equipment are worthless unless they are linked to well-trained and motivated men. The Royal Marines and paras in 3 Brigade and the men of 5 Brigade gave different and at times slightly conflicting comments on leadership. The democratic style of the paras and marines was contrasted with the more formalized approach adopted by the Guards and Gurkhas. The value of basic physical fitness, competent weapon handling and the cohesion and strength that come from units that have worked together for years was on the other hand amply demonstrated. The ability to patrol and work at night, and to do so in small section strength units is a reflection of the responsibility that Northern Ireland has placed on the young corporal and junior leader.

Though patrols might gather valuable intelligence, it was important that this was widely disseminated. The excellent special forces who were ashore before the landings at San Carlos had communications that allowed them to talk directly to 10 Downing Street and Northwood, via Hereford. But the information had to find its way to the soldiers and marines who were about to attack the next hill the following night on their way to Stanley. Sometimes it failed to do so.

It was also interesting that some of the *ad hoc* prisoner interviews yielded information that was passed to Brigade but to the men who had conducted the interviews it seemed to become lost in the Brigade intelligence cell — and so thereafter battlefield intelligence went direct to the neighbouring battalions who could make immediate use of it.

In contrast to the 'higher world' of military intelligence, the men on the ground relearned one important lesson about the final phase of an attack. In theory, the re-organization phase when the sergeant, or CSM (Company Sergeant Major) assesses the ammunition needs of his unit and the casualties suffered and prisoners taken, is a time for the Directing Staff to have a quick discussion before the next attack. The reality in action was very different and 2nd Parachute Regiment (who fought two actions; Goose Green and Wireless Ridge) took the precaution to ask a large number of men from their B Echelon (the cooks, clerks and storemen) to bring ammunition forward and casualties to the rear.

In effect, reorganization is the critical moment in an attack; a time to regain control and command after the violence and confusion of the assault and maintain the momentum of the action.

Ultimately the land battle was won by the men who had an uncomplicated aim — to remove the Argentine garrison from the island. They knew that the best way to do this was to reach Stanley. Selection and maintenance of the aim is the first principle of war, and in the Falklands it was again proved true.

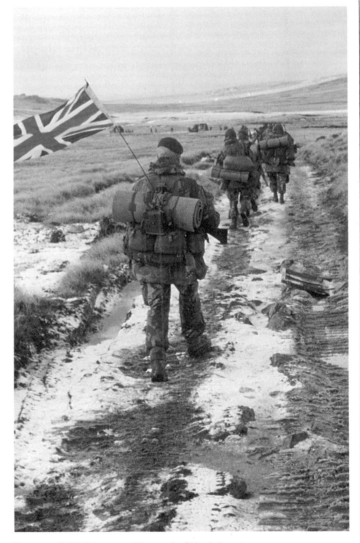

Troops of 45 Cdo near the end of their long yomp.

THE NAVAL LESSONS

The naval lessons of the Falklands were numerous. In the first place, territory must still be physically occupied if a decisive conclusion to a war is to be achieved and so the British had little option but to expel the Argentine forces from the islands. The RN had no hope of maintaining a blockade for it had neither numbers of ships nor a handy base.

The sinking of the cruiser *General Belgrano* has been claimed to prove that nuclear submarines succeeded in imposing a blockade. But the fact is that the only way in which the submarine *Conqueror* could prevent the Argentine cruiser from entering the Total Exclusion Zone was to torpedo her — in other words, the submarine could not affect the outcome until the British Government took the momentous decision to step up the level of conflict.

The use of elderly Mk8 torpedoes to sink *General Belgrano* highlighted the desperate urgency of getting new torpedoes into service. The Mk24 Mod O Tigerfish is not a totally successful weapon, and the more effective Mod 1 variant only started coming into service in 1982. Neither of these Mods is ideal for attacking surface ships, as they have small warheads, whereas the next generation, the 21in Spearfish, has a much heavier warhead.

Submarines did, however, play an extremely important part in the conflict, not least by 'inserting' clandestine groups of SBS and SAS to reconnoitre landing beaches, sabotage airfields and generally provide much-needed intelligence. Apart from *General Belgrano*, no serious targets presented them-

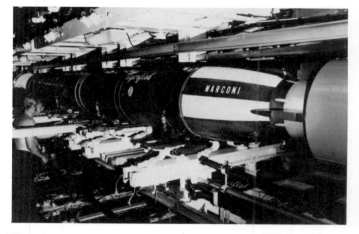

Tigerfish torpedo on a C-class nuclear submarine.

selves in the Total Exclusion Zone. There have been suggestions that a submarine was in position and able to torpedo the carrier *Vienticinco de Mayo* on 2 May, and that permission was refused. The *Armada Republica Argentina* played no further part in the fighting, probably because Admiral Anaya wished to preserve it as a 'fleet in being' or a pawn in the inter-service wrangle which was bound to follow the collapse of the junta's hopes for a bloodless conquest of the Falklands.

The British faced two massive problems in choosing to fight in the Falklands. The first was the sheer size of the logistic support needed; by the end of the campaign nearly 700,000 tons of fuel had been sent south, along with 100,000 tons of freight. The second was the small number of aircraft, both fixed-wing and rotary-wing; any shortcomings in air

Type 23 — The new generation

On the drawing board before the Falklands War, the Type 23 or *Daring* class of frigates has been modified to take the RN's experiences there into account (particularly in regard to fire hazards). This 'new wave' design will replace the destroyers and frigates sunk in the conflict. A new surveillance radar is to be installed — Plessey's Type 996. Other Falklands losses will be made good by new Type 22 ships (silhouette), two of which will be called *Sheffield* and *Coventry*.

defence must take account of the fact that only 28 Sea Harriers were faced by at least three times their number of Skyhawks and Mirages.

The logistic problem was solved by rapid mobilization of merchant shipping, but the smallness of the *Hermes* and *Invincible* air groups meant inevitably that on occasions the Argentine airstrikes were able to penetrate the outer layer of the Task Force's air defence. What was remarkable was that they did not do so more often, for the British interceptors were deprived of any form of airborne early warning radar. This, as much as any other factor, accounted for the losses of the destroyers *Sheffield* and *Coventry*, the frigates *Ardent* and *Antelope*, and possibly the SS *Atlantic Conveyor*.

The second layer of Task Force defence was the medium-range Sea Dart surface-to-air missile, and the Argentine Air Force and Navy pilots have since made no secret of their respect for this weapon. The Argentine Navy owned the missile and so had ample opportunity to exercise against the two British destroyers also armed with it. The need to avoid the lethal 'missile box' over San Carlos Water did, of course, have the effect of forcing the attackers to fly so low that their bombs could not arm themselves, but that in turn exposed the weakness of the third British layer of defence.

Since the 1960s the RN had relied almost solely on the Sea Cat missile for close-range defence against air attack, and had not put any faith in rapid-firing guns. The Sea Cat missile remains reliable and accurate but the optical and blindfire control systems used to control it date from an earlier age, and simply cannot cope with fast-crossing targets. The replace-ment, Sea Wolf, is a lethal system intended to cope with sea-skimming missiles as well as high-speed air targets. It has been slow in coming into service, and only two Sea Wolf frigates were in the Falklands. Neither of these, *Brilliant* and *Broadsword* were able to test the system against Exocet missiles but it proved very successful against Mirages and Skyhawks in close combat. The new Type 23 frigate will have the lightweight version or even a vertically launched variant, and studies are in hand to retrofit it to the Type 42 destroyers.

Startling facts about Sea Dart

When used correctly the Sea Dart system demonstrated amazing low-level performance, shooting down at least two Skyhawks at a height of 50ft — officially an impossibility. The main problem with Sea Dart turned out to be manual injection of firing data from the surveillance radar to the Type 909 tracker radar; at least one operator was found to inject data incorrectly 50 per cent of the time because of stress, and there was also an understandable temptation to fire the missile outside its 'performance envelope'. In other words, the tracker radar locked-on at anything up to 100 miles, whereas the missile was only effective at 25 miles.

One of the biggest fears before the Falklands was that ships would exhaust their stock of missiles too quickly, but during the whole Falklands operation *Invincible* and the destroyers fired only about 24 Sea Darts — little more than the magazine-capacity of one Type 42 destroyer. Of these, only 12 were 'valid engagements' (ie, fired correctly) and eight of those destroyed their targets.

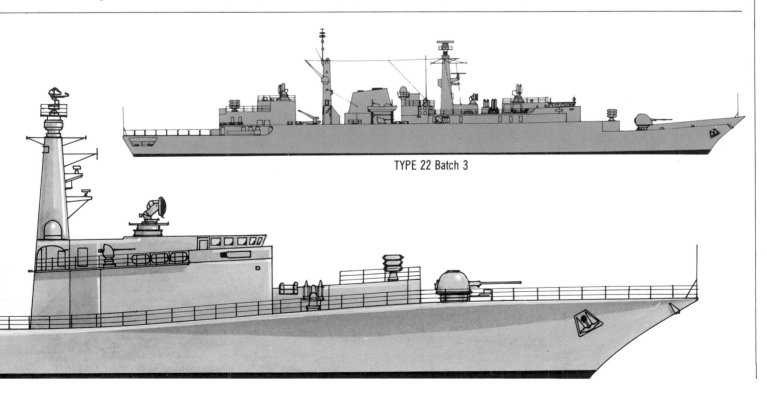

TYPE 22 Batch 3

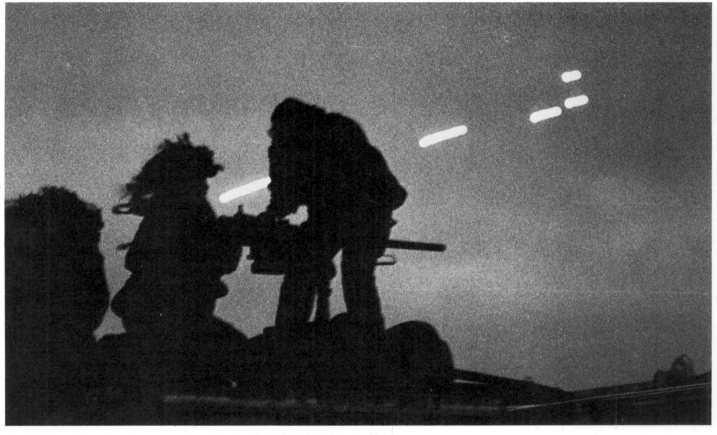

Rapid-firing close-range guns are back in fashion after San Carlos Water.

The lack of close-range guns to fire at aircraft which had broken inside the missile screen was keenly felt. Rapid-firing guns had gone out of fashion in NATO circles but the bitter air-sea battles in San Carlos Water showed that they still have a role to play. Type 42 destroyers were hurriedly armed with modern twin 30mm and single 20mm guns, and even 30-year-old twin 20mm from scrapped minesweepers were bolted onto decks of frigates and Royal Fleet Auxiliary ships. Five of the US Navy's 20mm 'Gatling', the Phalanx, were hurriedly imported, one for training and two each for the carriers *Invincible* and *Illustrious*, but the RN is now evaluating other gun-systems for future ships.

The 'black art' of electronic warfare is only vaguely understood outside service circles, and it would be impossible in the space of this article to explain what could or could not have been done to save HMS *Sheffield*. Out of six Exocets fired (five air-launched and one ground-launched) only two hit the targets they were aimed at. What had been missing from *Sheffield*'s defences was an active jammer, and energetic measures by British electronics firms resulted in jamming equipment becoming available before the end of hostilities. There was also a fear that the standard defence against missiles, the firing of clouds of 'chaff' or metallic strips, could not put up sufficient chaff to hide a large warship from the missile's radar 'seeker'. To generate more chaff the US Navy's Super-RBOC Mk36 chaff-launcher was hurriedly installed, and it is believed to be standard for future ships.

The use of aluminium in the superstructures of Type 21 frigates, *Ardent* and *Antelope* did not contribute in any way to their loss, and as it was not used in the Type 42 design it had nothing to do with the loss of the two destroyers. However all classes of British warships clearly had too much inflammable material aboard.

Two areas in which everything functioned much better than expected were maintenance of equipment and main propulsion. Many experts in and out of the Navy felt that computers and radars would rapidly go out of action and would be impossible to repair at sea, but this was not the case. Some of the radars such as the Type 965 and Type 909 are by no means modern in design, but even they were kept running. The RN only made its switch from steam turbines to gas turbines in 1967 when there was no proof that gas turbines would be able to cope with long periods of high-speed running. In practice both the older steam-driven ships and the new gas turbine frigates and destroyers performed magnificently. Perhaps the most significant miscalculation made by the junta was Admiral Anaya's belief that the Task Force would break down long before it reached the Falklands.

THE AIR LESSONS

After more than a year sifting through combat reports, the British Ministry of Defence considers that there were no remarkable new discoveries in the Falklands air war. Most of the lessons were old lessons relearned. Operation Corporate was entirely unexpected, and unlike the kind of conflict for which the RAF and Fleet Air Arm had spent a generation equipping and training.

Since 1968 Britain has confined itself to the NATO European context. It makes the occasional training flight to Gibraltar or Cyprus, and participates in exercises as far north as Norway. Tactical aircraft are sent by Britain to Red Flag meetings in the western USA: but the Falklands invasion was the kind of scenario that RAF Staff College graduates study in detailed appreciations which are promptly filed away before they have the slightest influence on official policy, planning or procurement.

It is a fact that the RAF only buys or builds new aeroplanes when the need is desperate. The air staffs write ORs (Operational Requirements) calling for new aeroplanes and other equipment, but no action is taken. HM Treasury has a vested interest in sanctioning very minimal defence expenditure, and major programmes, urgently needed and technically successful, are often cancelled midway at the stroke of a pen. It is against this background, therefore, that the notion of learning anything from the Falklands campaign must be judged.

For example, once more it will be noted that strike aircraft ought to have been properly equipped with ECM jammers and payload dispensers. They ought to have been equipped with self-defence missiles, and the pilots practised in their use. Helicopters of all kinds ought to have received their full kit of electronic support measures, all-weather and night-flying avionics and the latest navaids. Where appropriate, weapon-aiming sights and sensors ought to have been provided, along with armour over vital items. More than a dozen types of weapon and other externally carried loads could have been installed and fired from several types of aircraft to check compatibility. But it is very doubtful whether anything will be done to rectify the situation.

Harrier's fatal weakness exposed

The case of the Harrier is instructive. First developed for RAF use, in 1965–67, it was intended from the start to use the AIM-9B Sidewinder as a self-defence missile and to carry an as yet unspecified kit of active electronic warfare (EW) devices to improve its chances of survival in hostile airspace. As early as June 1967, development-batch Harriers had flown with AIM-9B Sidewinders, but on 2 April 1982 not one RAF Harrier

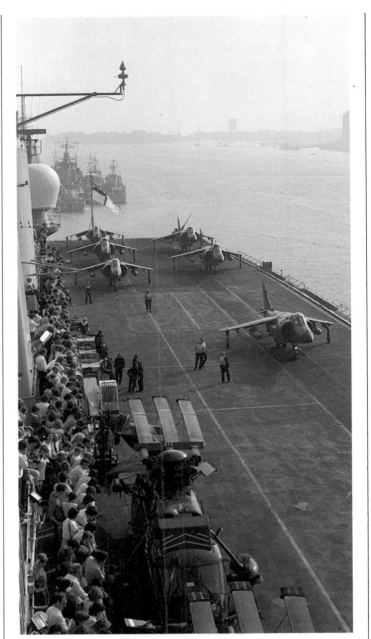

Sea Harriers aboard *Invincible* as the carrier docks at Portsmouth, back from the Falklands.

had provision for firing such a missile and not one Harrier pilot had any experience of it, unless he had previously served with a Phantom squadron. Though the ARI.18223 radar-warning receiver was fitted, no Harrier had any active ECM equipment at all. There was no provision for even a single bundle of chaff, though every Harrier squadron commander over the years must have written an official minute noting the fact.

The same kind of story can be told about every RAF and RN aircraft involved in Operation Corporate. As a result, the second quarter of 1982 saw fantastic activity by British industry and various technical shops in the fighting services — Navy, Army and RAF — to make good the lethargy and shortcomings

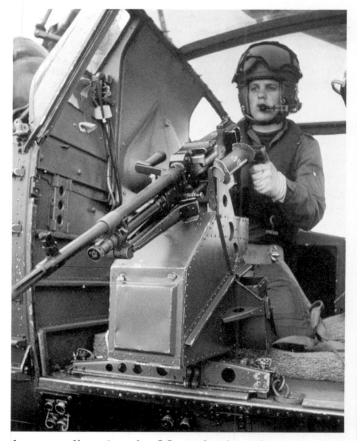

of previous decades. Amazing things were accomplished. The Harrier was in a matter of days cleared to fire Fleet Air Arm 2in rockets from the large 36-round pod, because of the suddenly realized inability of the Matra pod with 68mm SNEB rockets to function reliably in the strong electromagnetic environment aboard ships. It was also cleared to carry and fire Sidewinders in a single installation, and later, together with the Sea Harrier, to fire the new AIM-9L long-span Sidewinder (which had not previously been used by the RAF).

Working around the clock, British Aerospace revised a scheme prepared for the US Marines for a twin Sidewinder launcher and managed to install a suitably strengthened unit on trials aircraft which made use of existing wiring. It carries the pair of missiles slightly tilted, with the fins inclined inwards towards each other, but all four missiles fire perfectly, though in the case of the Sea Harrier, the head-up display weapon-aiming computer software needed to be reprogrammed to allow the Blue Fox radar to cue all four homing heads on to their targets. British Aerospace again made up for lost time in fitting long-range ferry tanks and an internal chaff/flare dispenser to the Harrier and Sea Harrier. The dispenser is very neat and was fitted immediately behind the speed brake, firing downwards from the rear fuselage. These urgently needed improvements, as well as an as yet undisclosed model of ECM jammer pod, were sent to the Task Force and put into action.

The basic techniques for operating short take-off, vertical landing aircraft at sea had been refined over the preceding decade. Many foreign observers had expressed surprise that the British vectored-thrust machines performed not only as advertized but set new records. The lessons here were learned not by the participants but by the rest of the world, who saw

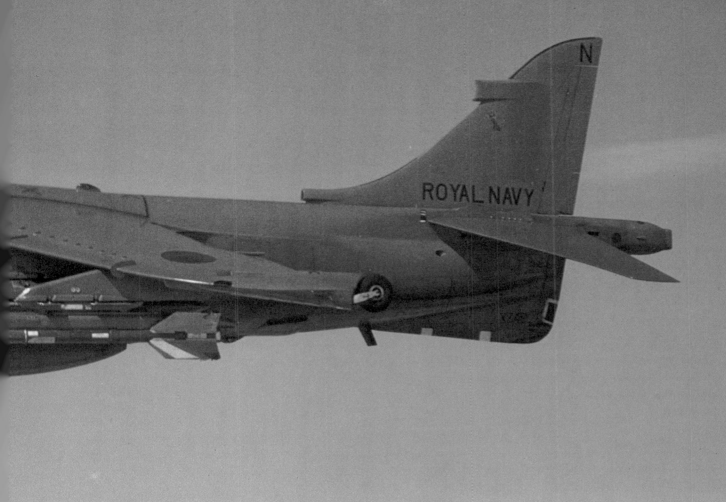

Air divisions of all three services had their successes. The Harrier's rugged and versatile character (above) proved a major asset to both the RN and RAF. Helicopters also played an important part. Left: An air gunner of 3 Cdo Bde Air Sqn mans a 7.62mm GPMG in his Westland Scout AH1. Helicopters have a key role in hit-and-run commando raids.

---

for the first time what had previously been dismissed as mere sales talk. Thanks to the rugged simplicity of the Harrier and Sea Harrier, these aircraft stood up to blizzards, Force 10 gales and conditions that would have halted operations by every other fixed-wing aircraft (including the most lavishly equipped machines carried on the giant US carriers). Yet despite the foul weather, six sorties a day was a fair average for each Sea Harrier, with 2376 sorties flown in 2675.5 hours during the actual fighting. Over 99 per cent of all planned sorties left on time. In the case of HMS *Invincible*, her Sea Harriers lost just one combat mission.

Early warning *was* available

Much has been made of the total lack of airborne early warning, so that radar detection of hostile aircraft took place just before their arrival over the ships. Combined with poor performance by the ship surveillance radars, this presented serious problems. It need not have happened. Thanks to Westland Helicopters and EMI, a Sea King HAS.2 was urgently fitted with the outstanding Searchwater surveillance radar in a pivoted kettledrum radar dome (or radome) on the right side,

and flight testing began on 23 July 1982. The first two Sea King HAS.2 (AEW) helicopters entered service with 824 Sqn aboard *Illustrious* as early as 2 August 1982, with six more following. Thorn-EMI had proposed exactly this same modification more than two years previously. Again, if the excellent BAe Nimrod AEW.3 had been developed to the planned time-scale, reaching No 8 Sqn RAF in March 1982, then with a tanker-support effort a high-flying radar could have watched over the entire TEZ (Total Exclusion Zone) throughout daylight hours.

The long list of things that urgently had to be done to the Gazelles of the Army and RM Commando Brigade Air Squadrons resembled that for the much larger fixed-wing machines. The chief items were: fit armour plate; install launchers for flares; install launcher pods for 68mm SNEB rockets (chiefly to provide smokescreens); install radio altimeter; install IFF (identification friend or foe) transponder compatible with Task Force interrogators; and modify the main-rotor blades so that two could be folded back for transport by sea. At least the Commando Brigade Gazelles also had upswept engine tailpipes, to provide protection against heat-seeking missiles, and GPMG installations to provide heads-down covering fire.

In World War 2, Britain had eight months of the Phoney War to prepare for battle. In the Falklands campaign there was almost exactly a month between the invasion of the islands and the final collapse of the diplomatic attempts to find a peaceful settlement. Next time there may be no such welcome period in which to rectify shortcomings.

ONE WHO WAS THERE
Tim Miller

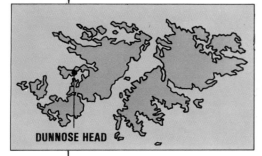

DUNNOSE HEAD

'The RAF bombed us on 23rd of May, at ten to nine to be precise. We were just sitting down having a cup of coffee, waiting for the BBC news to find out what was going on.' Tim Miller laughs out loud as he recounts this story, though he lost the sight of one eye in the Harrier strike at Dunnose Head on West Falkland.

He explains how it all happened: 'We weren't actually occupied by the Argentines there, but there was an unfortunate intelligence muddle up, and the Task Force got hold of the idea that the Argentines were there, and were using the grass airstrip at the settlement alongside the buildings for resupplying their garrison. Apparently what was happening was that the Task Force thought that they'd knocked Stanley airport out with the Vulcan raids, and they were picking up on their radar screens the Hercules coming out at night from Argentina, and then they were losing them off the West Falklands, off the radar screens, and so they thought, ah-ha, you know, there they are, landing on the West Falklands. Got the maps out. Farm on the West Falklands with a good hard air-strip on the west side, facing Argentina, Dunnose Head. So they got the idea they were going in there, and then the stuff was being distributed by light aircraft and helicopters.'

'Of course, what the Argentines were doing, first-class pilots that they are, they were literally hugging the grass bogs at night all the way into Stanley, and landing on the partly damaged runway. So unfortunately they sent in an airstrike to knock out the airstrip at Dunnose Head. They sent in some RAF Harriers. They knew we were there, but they thought there were some Argentines there as well, and because the farm was right alongside the airstrip, they pretty-well obliterated the farm as well, and caught us in the middle of it. There were eight of us there: Jimmy Foster and his wife, he's a farm manager, and their family, three kids, myself, and another single chap and his girlfriend. We'd heard jets before. We thought, ah, whose is it this time, ours or theirs? Rushed outside the door. Whoomph! I lost the sight of this eye, through shrapnel, and I got a piece in the wrist as well. My friend's girlfriend got a couple of little splinter cuts in her backside, that was all. We bandaged them up in a few minutes' Tim recalls.

In fact the little group at Dunnose Head, who never met an Argentine face-to-face in the whole course of the war, had already told *Hermes* by radio that there were no Argentines there. 'The *Hermes* had been trying to get hold of the Argentines to relay the first surrender call, and they couldn't get hold of any by radio. We heard them broadcasting and answered the *Hermes*, and we taped the surrender message. We told them that there were no Argentines at Dunnose Head. Obviously it didn't get to the right bloke, or else they didn't believe us. Eventually, later on that day, we managed to get hold of the Argentine garrison at Fox Bay by radio and pass the message on to them. I'll always remember the answer. The answer came back from the garrison commander at Fox Bay: "You tell British commander, kiss my asshole! Goodbye!" But by that time the *Hermes* had disappeared, and we weren't able to pass it on to Sandy Woodward.'

There was not much of the farm left, and they were afraid of a follow-up strike, so the little group trekked off across country to Hill Cove, on the north of the West Falklands, a large unoccupied farm which now housed 60 or 70 Falklanders, from Stanley and Fox Bay. After contacting San Carlos by radio and letting the Task Force know what had happened, Tim Miller was eventually picked up by a Special Boat Service unit and taken to a hospital ship at San Carlos. It was just two days before the end of the war. There was nothing the surgeons could do for his eye by now, and after a couple of days Tim got back to the farm at Dunnose Head and started the long cleaning and reconstruction process.

'First of all it was a case of clearing up the mess, in which we were helped by the forces. We had a troop of Gurkhas with us for a while, and the RAF. They felt a bit guilty about it, so they sent a crew out too, including the pilot who did it, who's going to be the best man at my wedding. It wasn't his fault. He was told to go and flatten Dunnose Head, which he did. He didn't know there were only eight Falklanders there and not 800 Argentines. And then after the cleaning-up session, we then had a squadron of Gurkha engineers a couple of months later, came out to bring a lot of building material, and spent about a month putting things to rights again, and getting the farm into a workable condition.'

'They patched up one of the houses using salvageable material, so we had reasonable accommodation for the summer. And then last summer took place as normal in temporary conditions, with, of course, servicemen to-ing and fro-ing — there's no army presence out there, but we get lots of visits, which we appreciate, from the navy. They ring up and ask if they can put a party ashore. We enjoy their company and they seem to enjoy ours. We're able to give them fresh meat and vegetables and what have you, and they bring some goodies ashore off the ship, and they bring mail and collect mail, that sort of thing.'

Tim Miller does not go to Stanley often, though he went more than usual in the year after the war, mainly for medical check-ups. He prefers to stay out in the camp, fishing for sea-trout, and reading books from the Stanley library which circulates them out to the camp settlements. In February he went into Stanley for the 150th anniversary festivities, travelling across country by horse and boat, and taking part in the horse races.

When the relatives of the servicemen who had died went out to the islands in April Tim Miller went to meet them as the Dunnose Head representative. He had a particular reason for going, as he had been communicating by letter with a Bolton couple whose son had died on HMS *Glamorgan*. After the service at San Carlos he went into Stanley with them and escorted them around the town for the day. In May he went to England. After attending the state opening of Parliament he attended a luncheon and talked to the ambassador of a major Latin American country. The ambassador told Tim Miller that there could be no realistic solution to the Falklands problem. However he did not think that the Falklands could continue as a colony, as this would be unacceptable to Third World countries. The ambassador suggested that the best solution for the Falklanders, and one which would get Third World support, would be some form of independence. And although that might take several years to build up towards, it would be a good idea to start proclaiming the intention at the earliest possible opportunity.

Tim Miller believes that the population of the Falklands needs to build up to at least 10,000 within fifteen years. He himself, in partnership with one of his brothers, at the end of the year after the war was attempting to purchase one of the sections of the Packe Brothers' holding on West Falkland, a 24,000-acre farm with 6000 sheep. In August 1983 he married a Manchester girl, a nurse — with the Harrier pilot as best man.

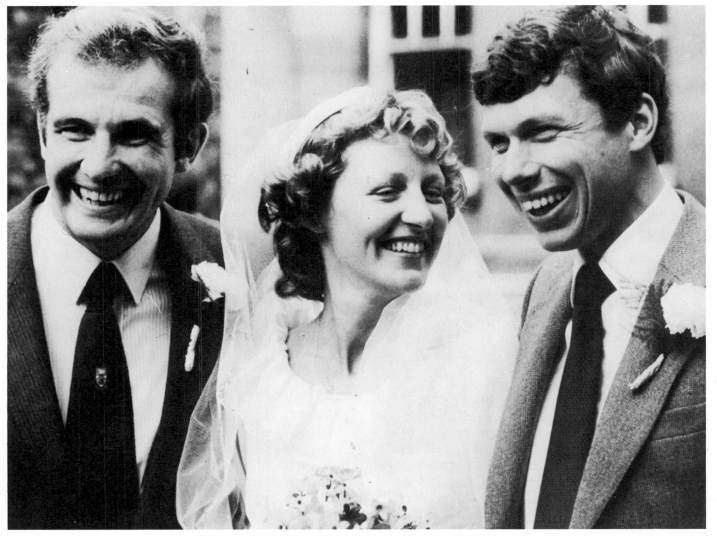

Tim Miller (left) marries Elaine Hodd, his penfriend. Flt Lt Mark Hare, who bombed Dunnose Head, is best man.

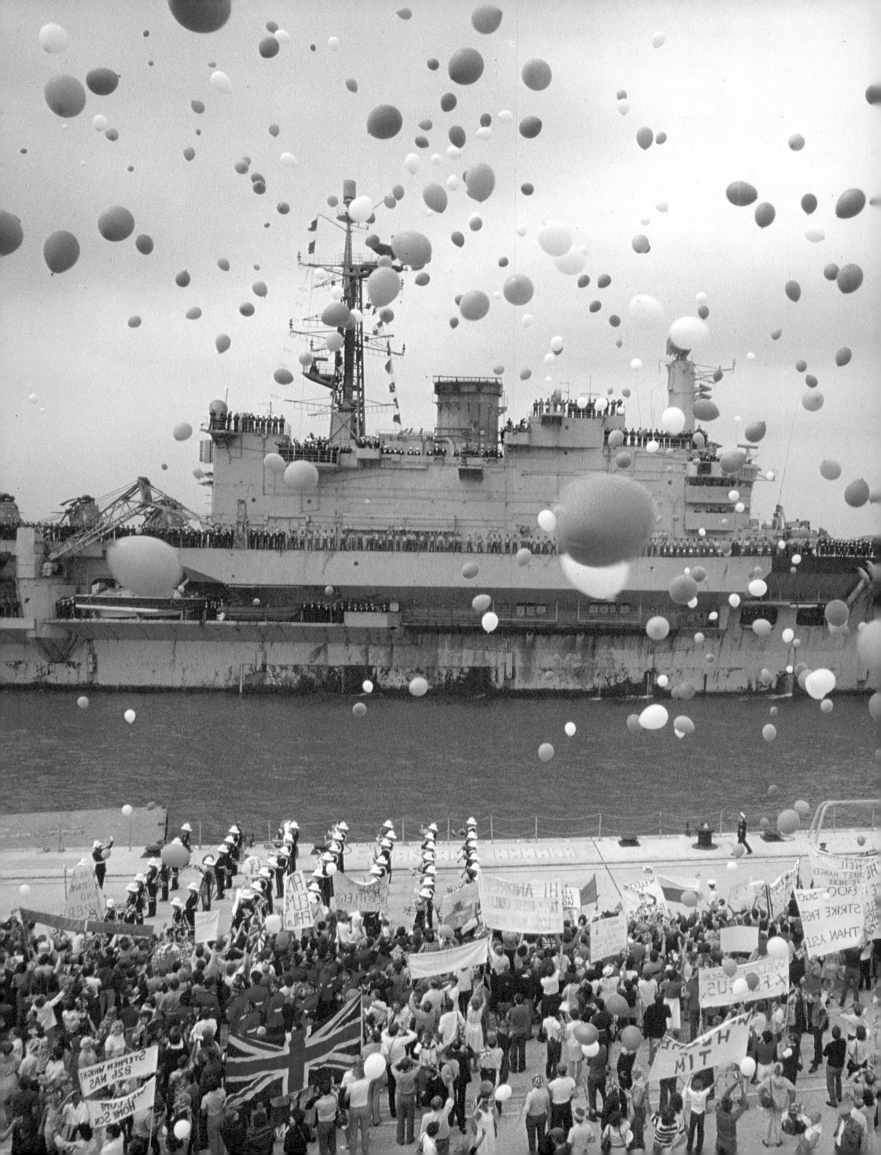

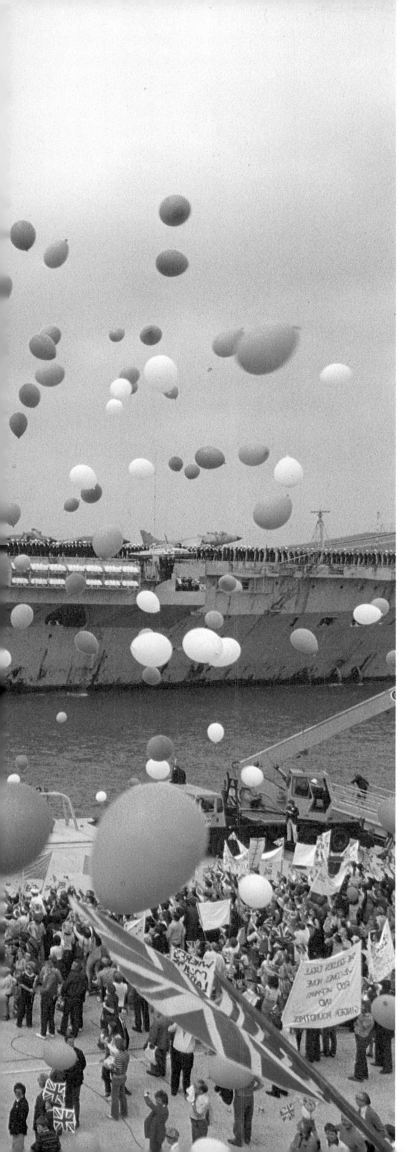

Chapter 2
BACK HOME

Among the most vivid memories of the Falklands War is the welcome given to the returning vessels. The story does not end with the streamers and balloons, however. Damaged ships need overhauling, refitting and updating. As the Royal Navy resumes its important NATO role, the significance of its recent experiences begins to emerge.

A jubilant greeting for the mercifully intact flagship *Hermes*. Her 28 Harriers were a mainstay of Task Force defences.

29

Nobody who saw the luxury liner *Canberra*, 'the great white whale', return to Southampton on 11 July, 1982 will forget the scenes of enthusiasm. Thousands of people and a flotilla of small boats turned out to meet the rust-streaked liner as she moved slowly up Southampton Water. Shortly after the Argentine surrender on 14 June she had embarked most of the Royal Marines of 3 Commando Brigade, and it was perhaps because she was 'bringing the boys home' that she got an even more rapturous reception than the liner *QE2* the month before.

In fact the first ship home from the Falklands was the destroyer HMS *Glasgow*, which had limped back to Portsmouth on 19 June, with the hole made by an unexploded bomb clearly visible just above the water-line. She had been hurriedly repaired in the South Atlantic by the repair ship *Stena Seaspread* but could not begin the 8000-mile haul back home until another air defence destroyer could relieve her. A week later another badly damaged ship, the frigate *Argonaut* arrived at Devonport, showing the scars of two bomb hits. Over the next four weeks the remainder of the damaged ships came in: the DLGs *Antrim* and *Glamorgan* and the frigates *Arrow, Brilliant, Broadsword, Plymouth* and *Yarmouth*.

With the new support carrier *Illustrious* heading south to join her sister *Invincible* it was also possible to relieve the flagship *Hermes*, which returned a week after the assault ship *Intrepid* on 21 July, exactly a month after the surrender. Although every ship returned to a vociferous welcome from relatives and members of the public, the battered-looking *Hermes* triggered off the same sort of emotions as *Canberra*. Her hard-worked air group of Sea Harriers and Sea King helicopters had already flown off to return to their home base at Yeovilton in Somerset, but the flag-wavers and topless girls in yachts knew and cared little for such details. Over a thousand officers and men were waiting to see their wives, girlfriends and children, who had waved goodbye to them three-and-a-half months before.

While officers and men forgot their cares in a period of shore leave, the dockyards took the ships in hand for the repairs which they so clearly needed. The destroyers and frigates were given extra light anti-aircraft guns, as well as new electronic countermeasures gear, rushed into service to cope with the threat from anti-ship missiles. The destroyers *Birmingham* and *Southampton* had already been given a hurried refit before leaving for the Falklands on 18 June, with the frigate *Rhyl*, but the dockyards were able to accept the additional burden of damage repairs with the same efficiency which they had displayed from the start.

To give one example, the destroyer *Exeter*, having been in action in San Carlos Water in May, returned to the UK and was then refitted with additional single

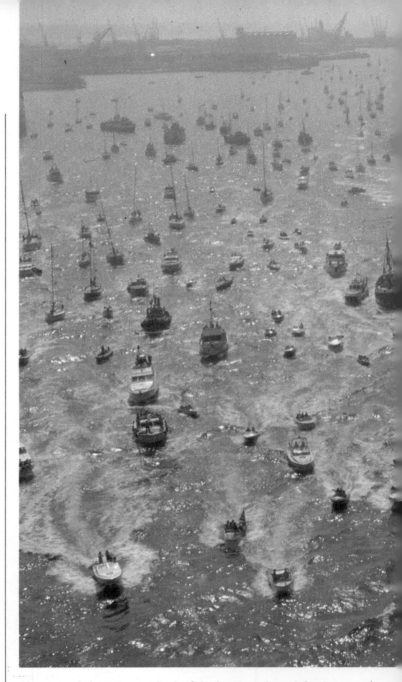

Men crowd almost every inch of deckspace aboard *Canberra* — which served as a troop and hospital ship — to respond to the welcoming armada (above). And, at right, in dry dock later at Southampton. After the war she needed a new boiler, among other things.

20mm Oerlikon guns and two pairs of 30mm guns amidships, as well as a new type of electronic jammer and American Super-RBOC chaff launchers. So rapid was the turnaround that she was running trials in October, and on her way back to the Falklands a month later. Early in 1983 TV viewers saw her captain, Hugh Balfour, demonstrating the firepower of his ship off Port Stanley, with tracers carving a pattern against the afterglow of a magnificent sunset.

Another example was the DLG *Antrim*, which had been damaged by an unexploded bomb on 21 May. It entered one of the missile-loading hatches and bounced off the deckhead before coming to rest. In spite of this damage, and holes from 20mm cannon shells fired by a strafing aircraft, she did not return to Portsmouth until 17 July. After a hurried refit, trials

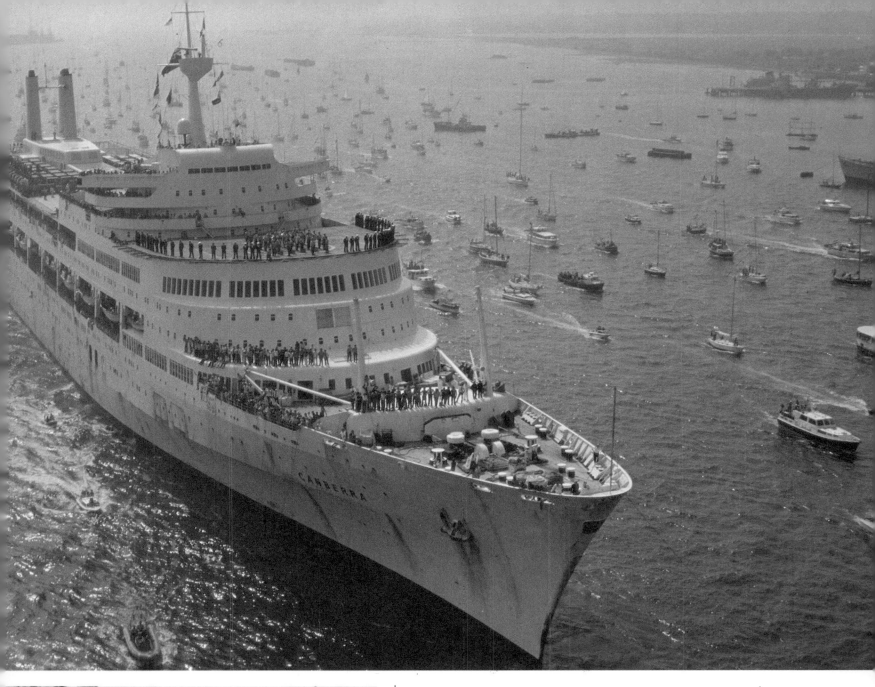

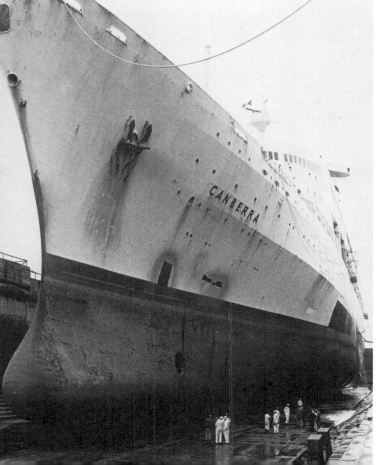

and work-up at the Portland training base, she too was on her way back to the Falklands on 8 November.

Born again: *QE2*, *Canberra* and *Uganda*

The naval dockyards had been responsible for converting the merchant ships 'STUFT' (or Ships Taken Up From Trade), but the responsibility for converting them back to civilian use rested with their owners. In fact, for most of them this involved little change apart from returning naval-communications equipment, particularly the satellite-communications terminals fitted back in April. A few ships had been given guns, and several had been fitted with helicopter platforms, and this meant a measure of repair work to replace fittings cut off during the hasty conversions. The two liners *Canberra* and *QE2*, with two and three helicopter decks respectively, required extensive refits before they could return to the passenger trade. The *QE2* finally returned to the North Atlantic trade on 14 August, transformed by a new colour-scheme. The educational cruise liner *Uganda*, which had

QE2 — Before and after

When *QE2* was requisitioned for service in the Falklands episode, the public imagination was fired. Luxury liner turns troop ship; what seemed at first like a pulp novelist's fiction was soon palpable fact. To the world's astonishment, *QE2* became the temporary home of Task Force troops who grew familiar with the liner's refurnished interior. *QE2* was

deliberately kept outside the war zone during the fighting, unlike her sister ship *Canberra* stationed in San Carlos Water. Both liners needed extensive refitting on their return to the UK. Since her return to the UK in 1982, £11 million has been spent on refurbishing her, including the installation of a new club lido and health spa. By November 1984 the figure will be £13 million. One of her four turbines was replaced after her Falklands sojourn. Today she is back sailing a variety of passenger routes all over the world.

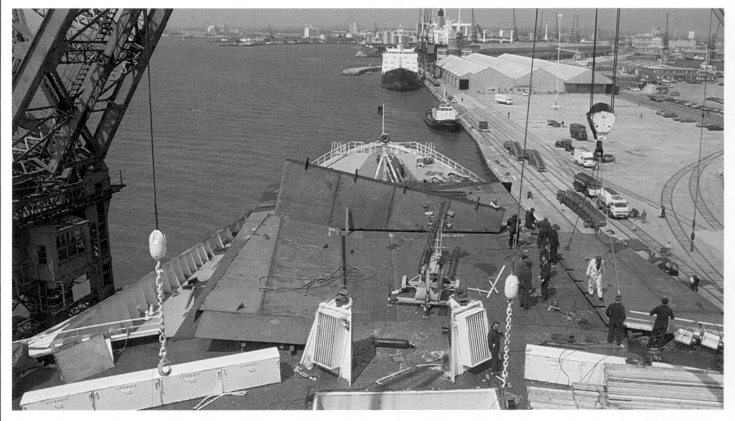

Above: Men at work on a wartime helicopter deck, which had to be removed. Many other tasks preceded her return to the trade.

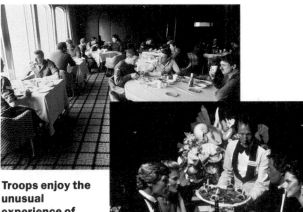

Troops enjoy the unusual experience of dining aboard *QE2*. Like *Canberra*, whose floor was damaged by boots, *QE2* endured wear and tear. The lower photo is of a luxury restaurant aboard *QE2*, from the current brochure.

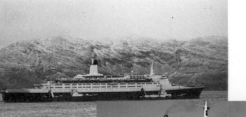

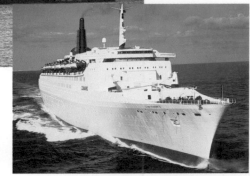

In South Georgia and (right) after her refit and new livery for the passenger trade. The 67,000-ton liner carried 3000 men to war and brought as many troops home as could be spared. She was fitted with an extra deck of light-alloy passenger accommodation.

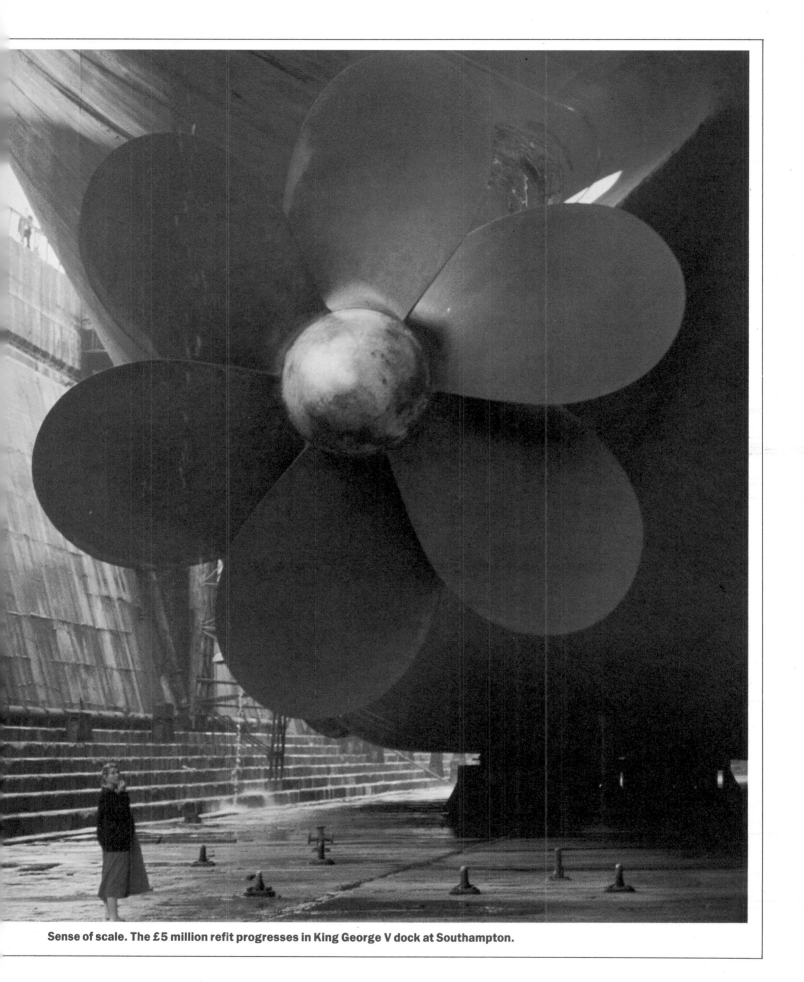

Sense of scale. The £5 million refit progresses in King George V dock at Southampton.

served as a hospital ship, left Southampton on 11 August, only two days after her return from the South Atlantic. She was bound for a repair yard at North Shields on the Tyne, and like the larger liners, had to have a helicopter flight deck removed.

The new support carrier HMS *Illustrious* was rushed to completion in June, and left before the end of the month. Three weeks later, after a fast run south, she met her sister *Invincible* and received two Sea Harriers from 809 Naval Air Squadron to join the other eight already embarked.

Although *Invincible* did not return to Portsmouth until 17 September, with the DLG *Bristol* and a fleet auxiliary, the welcome was on the same scale as that given to *Hermes* and other ships. To add to the sense of occasion Her Majesty the Queen visited the ship on the morning of her arrival, to greet her son Prince Andrew, who had flown a Sea King helicopter during the conflict. In spite of thick mist covering Spithead, an armada of small boats put out to surround the ships anchored in line abreast.

For the ships and men left behind in the Falklands there was little respite. The mere fact that the Argentine junta refused to admit any formal end to hostilities prevented the British forces from lowering their guard. Apart from any deliberate attack on the Falklands there was always the risk of a single kamikaze-style act of self immolation, and ships were ordered to be on constant alert.

The first ship into Port Stanley on 15 June was the trawler minesweeper *Pict*, one of five North Sea trawlers requisitioned but manned by Royal Naval personnel. With *Junella* and *Cordella*, *Pict* began to

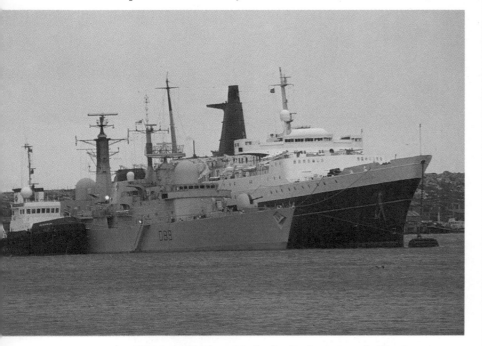

HMS *Cardiff*, the guided-missile destroyer, in Stanley harbour. Her blue anti-fouling streak is distinctive. She is flanked by *Rangatira* and a tug, *Irishman*.

sweep the outer harbour. From captured documents it was known that two fields of moored mines had been laid, so it was essential to clear the anchorage in advance and free it for shipping. When the remaining pair of trawlers, *Northella* and *Farnella*, arrived from South Georgia, there were five sweepers available and within a day or two numerous mines were cleared. By the beginning of July the last mines had been swept, using team sweeps in pairs to cut the mooring wires. Although the Argentines were known to have sophisticated mines those swept were locally manufactured copies of German World War 2 mines, and a sample of this type is now on display at HMS *Vernon*, the RN's mine warfare headquarters.

Underwater mines

The risk of further bottom-laid 'influence' mines actuated by hull-magnetism or propeller-noise could not be ignored, and at the beginning of July the five trawlers were relieved by the RN's latest mine-countermeasures vessels, HMS *Brecon* and HMS *Ledbury*. Using their high-frequency sonars these two ships 'hunted' for ground mines by scanning the sea-bed, and in the process located several wrecks, but no mines. They were able to handle the disposal of several tons of unsafe Argentine ordnance; the explosives were dumped on the seabed and the MCMV's PAP-104 remote-controlled disposal vehicle laid a demolition charge alongside. The sonar conditions were difficult, but the whole sweeping job was completed in five weeks, well inside the time allowed.

HMS *Junella* won the dubious honour of taking a specimen mine back to Portsmouth for examination. One of the 'floaters' was selected, and after it had been towed ashore by a Gemini inflatable dinghy, was defuzed on the beach by an explosives expert. Then the sinister horned sphere was hoisted onto *Junella*'s stern, to begin its 8000-mile journey back to HMS *Vernon*. As it was still packed with high explosive it had to be protected from the tropical heat by a covering of mattresses soaked in seawater. No patient in an intensive care unit could have received better attention!

The guided-missile destroyer *Cardiff* was among the ships which entered Port Stanley, and to the unholy joy of her boarding party they found the small coastguard patrol boat *Islas Malvinas* lying in the harbour. She was captured with no resistance, and after inspection was declared fit for duty. Honouring a tradition which goes back to the 18th century or earlier, she was soon recommissioned as a tender to HMS *Cardiff*, and to commemorate that connection was named HMS *Tiger Bay*, after the Cardiff water-front area.

Another ship captured was the naval transport *Bahia Buen Suceso*, one of two 3100-ton cargo and personnel carriers built in Canada in 1948–50. She

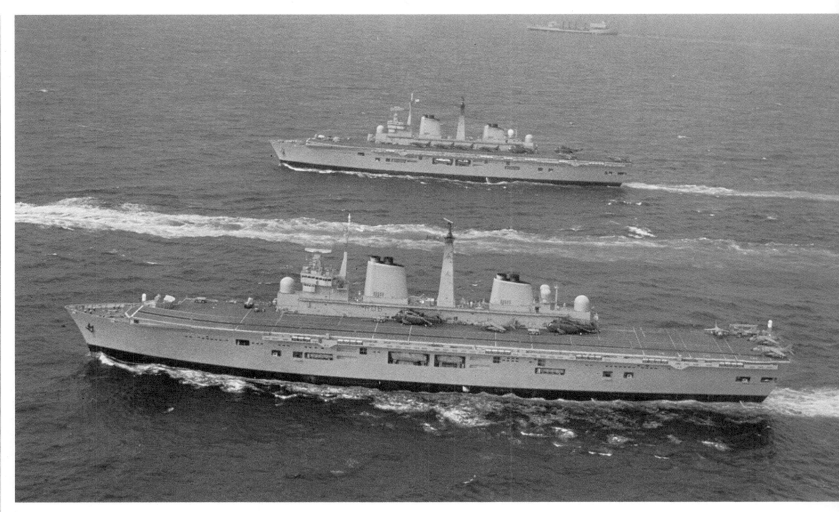

Support carrier *Illustrious* takes over from *Invincible* in the South Atlantic.

had taken part in the original operations to land a party of scrap dealers on South Georgia, the incident which had triggered off the Falklands War. She bore a charmed life, for on 16 May she had been attacked with 30mm cannon fire from two Sea Harriers and was run ashore in Falkland Sound. While still aground and abandoned by her crew, she was attacked with Sea Skua missiles fired by a helicopter, but her crew later reboarded her and finding that she was not seriously damaged, got her afloat again and reached Port Stanley.

The duty of defending the Falklands against any renewed Argentine air attacks rested on the Sea Harriers of the carriers *Hermes* and *Invincible* and the Harriers of the RAF based ashore. The plan was to replace the Sea Harriers and Harriers with Phantom high-performance interceptors. Before that could happen the runway at Port Stanley Airport had to be cleared of wrecked Argentine aircraft, the craters filled in, and the runway extended. *Hermes* and her air group of 28 Sea Harriers and Sea Kings staged a 'victory flypast' on 3 July before leaving for home two days later but *Invincible* and her ten Sea Harriers remained on station.

Invincible's commanding officer, Captain Jeremy Black admitted afterwards that this period was in many ways the most taxing of the entire South Atlantic deployment. The war was over, the men wanted to get home and see their families, but the tension remained. Each day the Combat Air Patrol waited for the 'Yellow Alert' or 'Red Alert' which they had come to know so well for 14 weeks. The ship's Type 1022 radar and similar radars in the escorting destroyers would give better warning of a low-level attack than the older Type 965 and radars in the destroyers which had been sunk, but there was still no form of airborne early warning radar to enable the Sea Harriers to have sufficient time to get into the best attacking position.

The problem of airborne early warning was finally solved, for in the last week of July *Illustrious* arrived. Included among her air group were two AEW Sea King helicopters, hurriedly converted to carry a long-range Searchwater radar. The two carriers exercised together, and some key personnel from the electronics, missile-defence and electronic warfare departments (as well as two Sea Harriers) were transferred from *Invincible* to her sister before she finally headed northwards on 29 July. The exchange of personnel was necessary to ensure that *Illustrious* did not meet trouble with a totally inexperienced ship's company.

Supporting stars of the Task Force : LSLs and others

The most melancholy task was to dispose of the burnt-out hulk of the Logistic Landing Ship *Sir Galahad*, which had been bombed at Bluff Cove on 8 June. With her sister *Sir Tristram*, not so badly damaged, she had been towed to Port Stanley after the surrender. She was too badly damaged to risk the long haul back home, and so on 24 June, after a particularly poignant memorial service held by the Welsh Guards, she was towed out to deep water and torpedoed by a nuclear submarine, believed to be *Conqueror*, the same boat which had sunk the cruiser *General Belgrano*. The moment was marred by the failure of the first torpedo to detonate, but eventually the battered logistic landing ship (LSL) went to the bottom.

Sir Tristram remained in Port Stanley, for accommodation was at such a premium that her troop decks could house a number of troops. Finally in May 1983 a commercial salvage ship, *Danlifter* arrived, to get her out of the water where experts could examine the bottom plating. At the time it had been thought that she might remain as part of the Port Stanley scene, but eventually *Sir Tristram* started her 'piggy-back' ride back to England, where she will presumably be rebuilt and put back into service.

The loss of two LSLs had left the Navy very badly off for logistic support, so early in 1983 two roll-on/roll-off ferries were chartered. They are the Norwegian *Grey Master*, which has become Royal Fleet Auxiliary *Sir Caradoc*, and *Lakespan Ontario*, which has become RFA *Sir Lamorak*. There was also an urgent need for a troop transport, and plans were announced to purchase a Danish passenger and vehicle ferry, SS *England*. The deal was later cancelled when Ministry of Defence experts reported unfavourably on her subdivision. As a replacement the British Rail Sealink ferry *St Edmund* was selected — a fitting choice as she had already been chartered for Operation Corporate. Under the name HMS *Keren* she was refitted on the Tyne, but did not sail as there was a dispute between the ferry crews and the owners.

Feeling that the dispute did not involve them, in April the Royal Navy took the high-handed action of marching a naval crew aboard, dressed in civilian clothes. The action of taking *Keren* to sea was regarded as strike breaking, and for a while tempers among the National Union of Seamen ran high, but eventually both sides compromised, and *Keren* returned to Newcastle, and got her civilian crew back again.

Elsewhere on the high seas, *Invincible*'s engineers reported on her way back that two of the four gas generators for her Olympus gas turbines had reached their limit of 5000 running hours. Although the machinery had given no trouble it was decided to test the capability that was designed into the ship, to permit her to change two gas generators. Although this exercise was possible, it should in theory have been done in a calm anchorage, with a repair ship alongside to lift out the defective generator. Instead the engine-room complement changed the two gas generators *at sea* within 48 hours, including stops for rough weather. Although done only as a test and not as a genuine emergency, it was an indication of how well the Task Force ships' machinery had performed throughout the campaign.

Once the RAF Phantoms were operational at Port Stanley and a new surveillance radar system was installed the Royal Navy could withdraw *Illustrious* and she returned to Portsmouth on 8 December. The air defence of the Falklands since then has been the responsibility of the RAF, but a number of ships remain, to provide cover against any attack on shipping, either from Argentine surface forces or submarines. There have been several probing flights around the edge of the Total Exclusion Zone, clearly by Argentines air-testing the British reactions. There has, however, been no serious attempt to renew hostilities. Even the much-publicised attempt to take a shipload of Argentine widows and relatives to the Falklands came to nothing, as the Argentine authorities refused to allow the visit.

The tiddlers of the Task Force were the offshore patrol vessels *Dumbarton Castle* and *Leeds Castle*. Displacing only 1200 tons and designed to patrol North Sea fishing grounds and oilfields, these ships earned the nickname of 'the Wells Fargo of the South Atlantic'. From 29 April, when they sailed for the South Atlantic, they performed a vital service as despatch vessels. At Ascension they helped to transfer loads from ship-to-ship, and then carried vital stores and mail to the Task Force. They made themselves indispensable, and did not leave the South Atlantic until the end of July. When HMS *Leeds Castle* arrived at Ascension on 1 August, homeward bound at last, she had steamed 26,944 miles (the equivalent of circumnavigating the world) at an average speed of 16 knots.

For the RN and Royal Fleet Auxiliary, as much as the Merchant Navy, there was an understandable desire to get back to the normal routine of exercises and training. The main role of the RN is to support NATO, and to maintain the British contribution several older escorts had been brought forward from the Reserve during the campaign. Ships which returned from the South Atlantic all needed some time in a dockyard to remedy defects and to replenish vital spares. In October 1982 HMS *Fearless*, under the

Sir Tristram — The ship that came back from the dead

RFA *Sir Tristram* was hit by rockets and 20mm cannon shells at Bluff Cove in the same attack which destroyed LSL *Sir Galahad*. She was lifted 'piggyback' by the salvage ship *Danlifter* (at bottom) and carried all the way to the Tyne. She arrived in the Tees on 13 June and will be examined with a view to rebuilding.

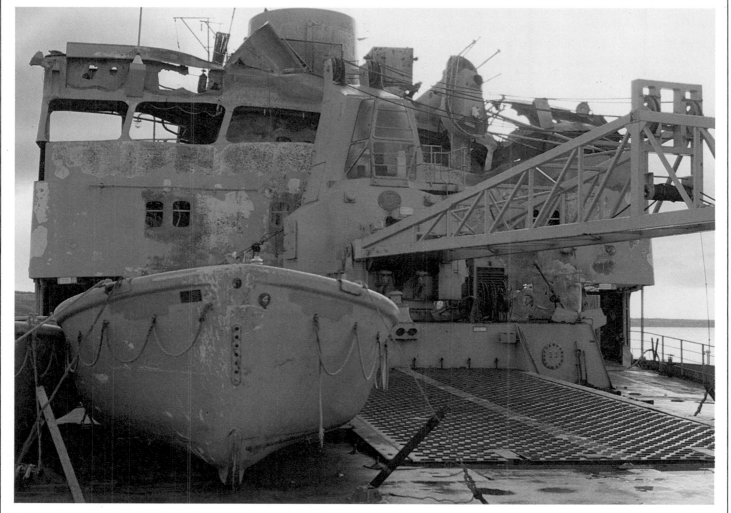

Sir Tristram's aluminium superstructure was burnt out by the fires which followed the attack.

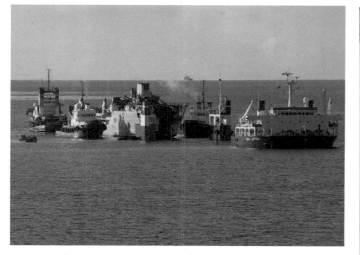

Danlifter does her stuff. The submersible barge gets ready to take her damaged charge on board.

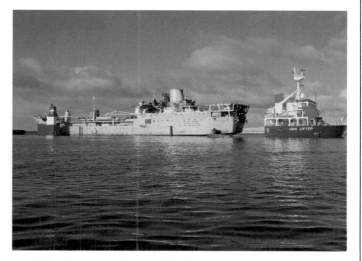

Danlifter then resurfaces with *Sir Tristram* in place.

same Captain Jeremy Larken who had been in the thick of the San Carlos landings, took part in the big NATO exercise 'Northern Wedding'.

This involved a large-scale landing on the coast of Jutland, in Denmark. The presence of the British assault ship and the same Royal Marines who had returned from the Falklands inevitably meant that the American and European journalists concentrated on the lessons of the Falklands operation, rather than the lessons of the current exercise. The US admiral on board the flagship *Mount Whitney* tried to explain that the long-term planning for 'Northern Wedding' actually *pre-dated* the Falklands affair, and that the real fear at Supreme Allied Commander Atlantic's HQ had been that the Royal Navy would no longer be able to provide its quota of ships. However he did add the wry comment that the chief lesson to emerge from the Falklands was that deterrence had failed — a comment that no British admiral would have been allowed to make.

In other exercises since then, particularly 'Spring Train', the Royal Navy has been putting into practice many of the procedures introduced during the fighting and afterwards. The all-important question of fire-fighting is now given a much higher priority than before, and during an exercise petty officers carry small smoke generators. They look innocent enough; small canisters with two yellow wires protruding from the top. Only when a torch battery links the two wires does it start to discharge dense clouds of smoke. On the frigate HMS *Alacrity* I watched a petty officer with a malicious grin on his face set one of these pyro-technic devices off next to the wheelhouse. He then opened a door into the superstructure to make sure that the smoke drifted inwards, and shouted 'Fire' at the top of his voice.

Even more impressive was the response; within a minute firefighters had appeared, each wearing breathing apparatus. As the PO observed, things have tightened up a lot since May 1982, and as many as ten smoke canisters had been set off in the engine room without warning, to simulate the sort of fires which had gutted the destroyer *Sheffield* and the frigate *Ardent*. It is noticeable that the number of sets of breathing apparatus has increased; before the Falklands the allowance for a frigate was only five, grossly inadequate for sustained firefighting. To make matters worse they were not easily rechargeable.

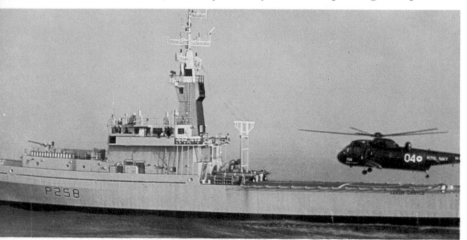

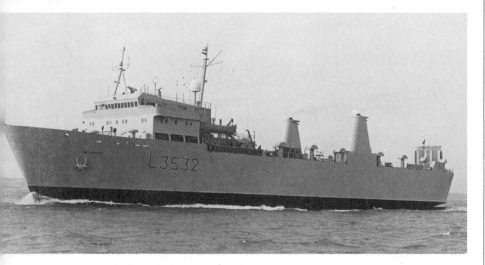

Top: *Leeds Castle*, offshore patrol vessel and 'the Wells Fargo of the South Atlantic'. Above: RFA *Sir Lamorak*, formerly the roll on/roll off vessel *Lake Span Ontario*, which has replaced the ill-fated *Sir Galahad*.

Wizards at work : dockyard magic and the Type 42s

While the programme of repairs was progressing, the dockyard organization also had to cope with the updating of equipment. The refit of HMS *Exeter* has been mentioned, but she was only one of a number of ships which passed through dockyard hands for various additions, not all of them visible to the casual observer. The most common alterations were the additions of twin 30mm guns to all the destroyers, but of course adding a pair of gun mountings is never as simple as it sounds. In the Type 42 guided-missile destroyers it was necessary to remove the port and starboard boats to compensate for the topweight. Then there was the problem of stiffening under the deck to support the extra weight, and a cable run to provide electrical power to the mounting.

Last but not least, some provision had to be made for spare ammunition, as the guns fire some 1000 rounds per minute. Space and weight are not critical for fitting the American Mk36 Super-Rapid Bloom Offboard Chaff system, for it is virtually nothing more than a metal casting fixed to the deck, and occupying no more than a couple of square feet. However a system which has to fire grenades of chaff and infra-red decoys in the path of an incoming Exocet missile must be programmed to fire at exactly the right moment, and that means a control panel and extra wiring to the Operations Room.

Less visible (and highly classified) are the changes to ships' electronic-warfare equipment.

What little has leaked out indicates that a jammer has been added to the standard UAA-1 Abbey Hill EW equipment, and several frigates and destroyers were given additional unspecified equipment. The small antennae on mastheads are only the external part of the equipment, and any major addition to the EW equipment implies additional equipment below decks, in the form of consoles, control panels and yet more wiring.

The worry about PVC coverings to cables, which was blamed for the disastrous amounts of smoke in the four warships lost, led to a major effort to reduce the amount of dangerous insulation. The sheer volume of work (each warship has literally miles of cables inside her) means that recovering takes a long time, nor would it be worthwhile for old ships nearing the end of their useful lives. Another source of worry is furnishings, and wherever possible ships have had to get rid of such unsuitable fittings as formica panels and sponge-rubber cushions and mattresses. Like the problem of cable coverings, it is a gigantic task which has to wait until a ship comes into the dockyard for a routine overhaul.

The publicity given to the sinking of the big container ferry *Atlantic Conveyor* obscured the fact that her sister *Atlantic Causeway* had functioned very effectively as an extemporized helicopter carrier. A little more time was taken over her conversion, and although ambitious plans to give her a ski jump were dropped, she did receive a hangar to accommodate four Sea King helicopters. Experience with her and *Atlantic Conveyor* provided the clinching evidence needed to get the long-deferred 'Arapaho' Project on the move.

'Arapaho' is the codename for a joint Anglo-American plan to test the feasibility of operating helicopters from a large containership hull. Originally it was hoped that the British (the RN) would charter a suitable hull, and the US Navy would provide the helicopters and Naval Reserve pilots. But neither navy could find the funds needed. However, in 1981–82 the US Navy added an aluminium flight deck and prefabricated hangar to a bulk carrier laid up at Newport News, Virginia, to test the feasibility. Then in June 1983 it was announced that the British would be buying this hangar and portable flight deck from the US Navy, and would install it in SS *Astronomer*.

This 27,867 GRT (gross tonnage) container ship had been requisitioned in April 1982, and was given a hangar similar to the one in *Atlantic Causeway*. The walls were made up of containers stacked two deep, on either side forward, and a roof of light sheet steel was laid overhead. In addition the forward end of the container 'walls' were closed off to keep out wind and spray. The ship did not have a proper flight deck, as the container deck simply had obstructions cut or burned away.

Just how *Astronomer* will look after her second

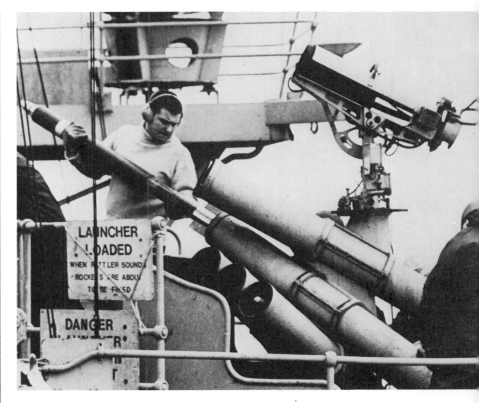

The RN Corvus Chaff launcher, a vital decoy weapon in the deadly cat-and-mouse duel with Exocet.

conversion is not clear, but what is certain is that the chance will not be lost to improve refuelling arrangements and accommodation, and to provide workshops. It is one thing to provide 'spare decks' on board ships operating with a task force, but quite another to ask a containership/carrier to operate independently. During Operation Corporate it was at least in theory possible for a faulty helicopter to be re-routed to one of the carriers or to a warship, whose skilled maintainers might be able to provide the right spares. The purpose of converting *Astronomer* is, however, to provide a 'force multiplier' which could operate independently if needed, and that implies the provision of workshops and a reasonable outfit of spares.

The human factor

Up to now nothing has been said of the human side, the most important of all. The losses in the Falklands fighting came as a great shock to the RN even more than to the public, but as always the real test of morale is how people recover from bad news. In that respect the young sailors serving in the Task Force showed as much resilience as their forebears.

Talking to officers and ratings who served in the Falklands, one can detect an undefined air of 'seniority'. Most will admit that the RN had been getting a bit soft after nearly 40 years of peace, and that the sinking of *Sheffield* provided a much-needed jolt to the Task Force.

This new awareness shows itself in many ways.

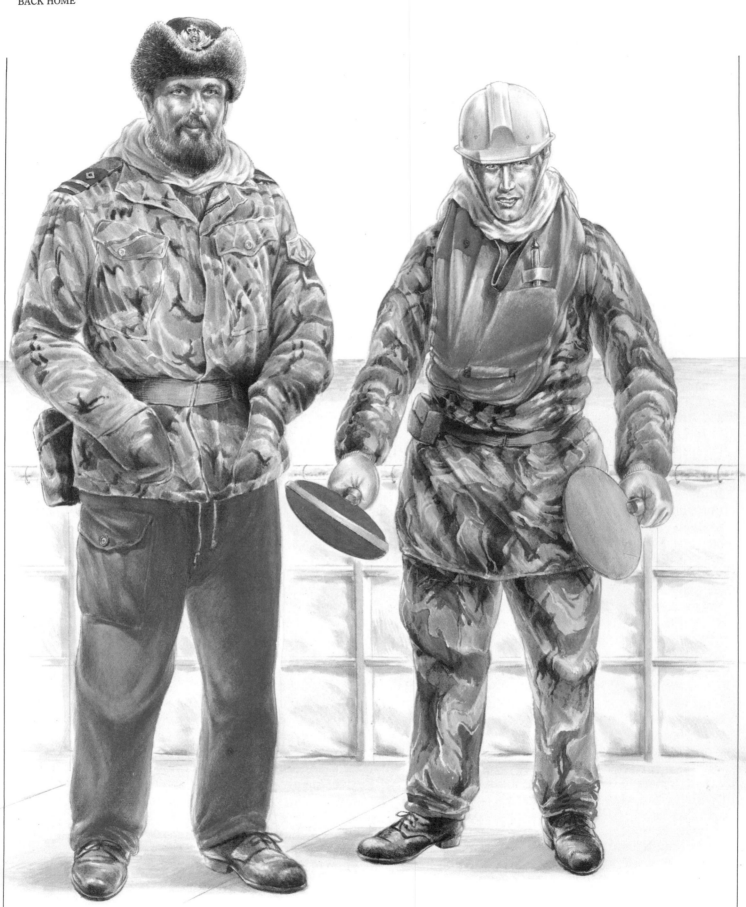

Royal Fleet Auxiliary crew. A so-called Cinderella service, their role in supply replenishment at sea was indispensable. On *Tide-spring*, army gear was worn since there was no time to get Antarctic wear. Note the hats against the cold and the bats for signalling when supplies are passed ship-to-ship.

The new enthusiasm for unrehearsed smoke drills has been mentioned but that is only one type of emergency which is simulated in exercises. The strain of being 'closed up' at Action Stations, or the slightly more relaxed Defence Stations, is now better understood. Old lessons have had to be relearned, such as the World War 2 experience that the human brain cannot concentrate on a radar display for more than 20 minutes.

On the positive side, the RN's approach to training, particularly of its maintainers, has proved to be very good. Not only did the helicopters and Sea Harriers keep flying but the enormously complex equipment in the ships was kept working. Much of it is intended to be repaired 'by replacement', or in other words, not repaired on board. In several instances the maintainers had to develop diagnostic skills at short notice, without drawings or repair manuals, and it is officially admitted that in two different ships a toaster was 'cannibalized' to allow the element to serve as charging choke for a radar set. Stainless-steel wardroom cutlery was also pressed into service when filler rod for welding ran out. The RN takes a lot of trouble to train its maintainers, and such stories prove that the time spent has not been wasted.

The worst jolt to morale was the feeling that the ships of the RN had no counter to the Exocet missile. With one ship sunk and another severely damaged by these deadly weapons it is easy to forget that four out of six Argentine Exocets fired either failed to explode or were decoyed by countermeasures. Nevertheless much of the emphasis in operational training today is to restore confidence in the ability of the Fleet to mount a coordinated defence, not only against anti-ship missiles but the air threat as well. Proving that the RN has a credible defence against Exocet has to be achieved without pretending that Exocet is anything but a very deadly and reliable weapon. The RN itself uses Exocet, and was the first overseas customer for the weapon in the early 1970s.

Today, more than a year after the end of hostilities, the Navy is still learning from the Falklands, from the School of Maritime Operations at HMS *Dryad* down to the ordinary seaman who has to practice irksome fire drills. The electronic battle is on as well, with industry tendering for contracts to design and build two vital pieces of equipment. The surveillance radar which should have been retrofitted to destroyers but was cancelled in 1981, is to be replaced by a new Type 996. The competition for this new radar is nearly settled, as is a similar competition between various manufacturers to produce the new electronic warfare equipment, known as UAF-1, which will replace existing equipment throughout the Fleet.

The next generation of frigates, known as the Type 23 or *Daring* class, were already well advanced on the drawing board before the Falklands, but details of the design have been changed to reduce fire hazards. Four more frigates were ordered last December to replace the destroyers and frigates sunk. Although the Type 42s and Type 21s will not be repeated, two of the Type 22s (*Broadsword* class) ordered will be named *Sheffield* and *Coventry*. Two more will have a 4.5in Mk8 gun on the forecastle and a new long-range guided missile, as well as 'point defence' gun mounting. *Broadsword* and her sister *Brilliant* showed their worth in the South Atlantic, being the only two Sea Wolf-armed ships present, so the addition of four enlarged versions of this magnificent design more than compensates for the losses.

The Falklands experiences have undoubtedly left the RN in better shape than it was before. The losses were bitterly felt, and any overconfidence was rudely shattered by the bravery of the Argentine pilots, but the training and reevaluation which has followed since June last year have put new vigour into the Senior Service. What is equally important is that the RN's battle experience is now being passed to its NATO partners, in the form of revised standards of firefighting and safety, and enhanced air defence, to choose only two examples. Its senior officers have now had experience of command in wartime, something denied to every other NATO force except the US Navy. The sum total of all this is greater efficiency as a fighting force, but the real long-term benefit is that *theories* about the form of naval warfare in the future have been replaced by *experience*.

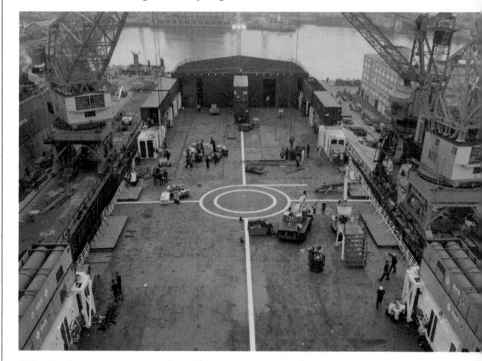

Atlantic Causeway, a container ferry converted at short notice into a helicopter carrier. Her hangar was home to 4 Sea King helicopters and her performance gave new life to plans for operating helicopters in this way.

ONE WHO WAS THERE
Warrant Officer John Phillips

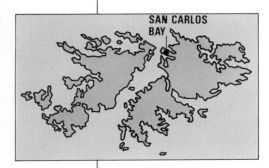

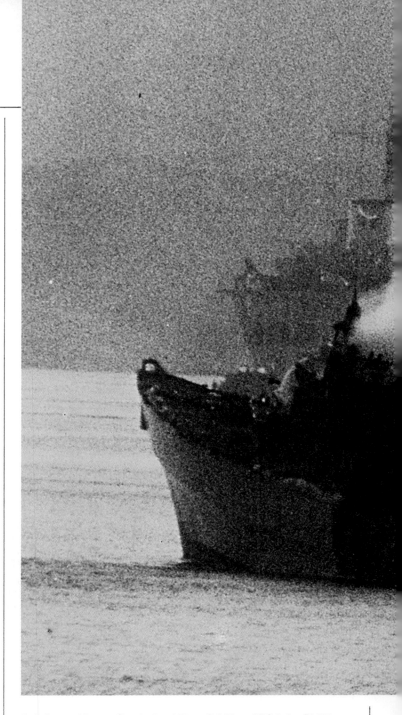

Antelope ablaze after being hit on 24 May. WO John Phillips and Staff Sgt Prescott were called on to render safe the unexploded bombs.

Warrant Officer John Phillips of 49th Explosive Ordnance Disposal Squadron, Royal Engineers, had a short war but a busy one. He arrived at San Carlos Bay aboard RAF *Lancelot* on the night of Thursday, 20 May 1982. His job was to deal with unexploded bombs, mines and shells of all kinds. By the following Tuesday, 25 May, he was aboard the hospital ship *Uganda*. He had lost his left arm, his eardrums were burst, and his friend and fellow bomb-disposal expert, Staff Sergeant James Prescott had been killed at his side by the same bomb-blasted steel door that had mangled WO Phillips' arm beyond repair.

John Phillips has been in the army since he was 15 and has completed 22 years as an adult soldier. As befits an engineer who deals with the delicate and sophisticated mechanisms of deadly weapons, he speaks with great precision; and appears to have an almost photographic memory for details and dates.

Work began the day after *Lancelot* arrived at San Carlos Bay. 'On the Friday night we had warning that HMS *Argonaut* had been hit by two bombs. We were "tasked" on the Friday night, but we never actually got to the job until the Saturday morning, because there was a lot going on. We went to the *Argonaut* with what kit we thought we'd need to deal with the bombs there. They were 1000lb General Purpose bombs, one in the boiler room, and one in the forward magazine. We couldn't deal with the one in the magazine because it was flooded, so we said we'd come back when they'd drained it off. We rendered safe the bomb in the boiler room, which enabled them to make up steam and carry out defensive manoeuvres. Before that they were crippled.'

'We were "tasked" on the Saturday night for HMS *Antelope*. She, again, had been hit twice, both unexploded. We went over on the Sunday, midday. We noticed that there was one bomb in the refrigeration unit, and one forward, in the Petty Officers' mess. We decided to go for the one in the refrigeration unit first because that was easier to get at, and it was identical to the one we'd dealt with the previous day. The process is, you have to remove the firing mechanisms remotely, which entails going up to the bomb, setting up the extraction device — it's called a rocket wrench

— retiring to as safe an area as possible, bearing in mind you're in a confined ship. Firing the mechanism, which is a Catherine-wheel type of thing, causes it to spin round and undoes the firing pistol. The indications were that the bomb was fully armed. However, when it had entered the ship, the pistol, which sticks out of the back, slightly proud, had obviously hit something and was badly damaged. Therefore we couldn't get a good purchase with the wrench. We had four attempts at rendering it safe, all of which failed. It was spinning, but it was spinning so fast it was coming off. It wouldn't extract the pistol.'

'Each time we went as far astern as possible, battening down the doors as we went, to protect ourselves as best we could from the blast. Now they're

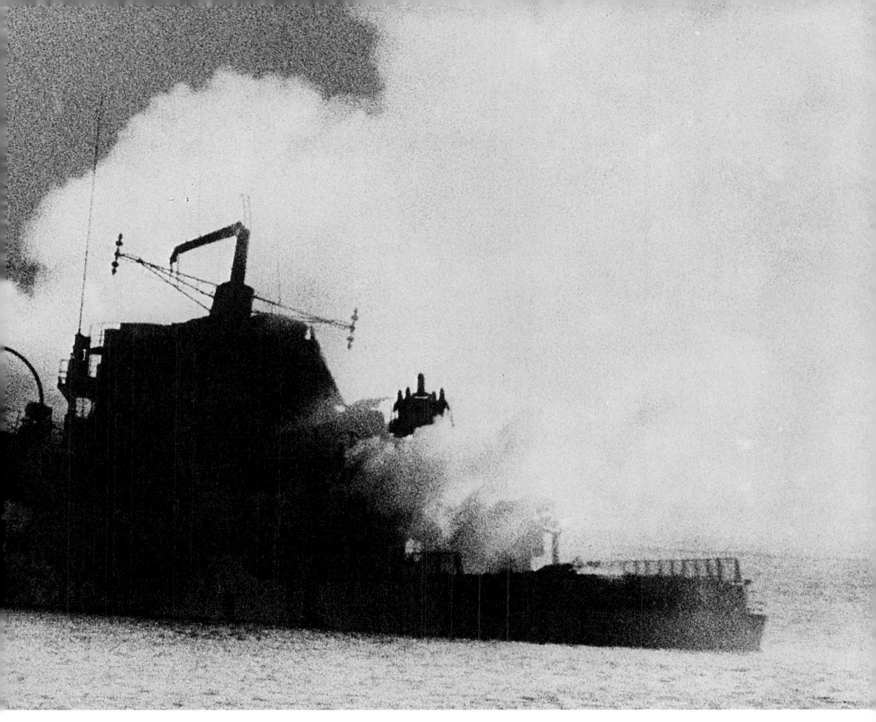

bloody thick doors, and the ship was vented, which is normal procedure anyway for the blast to be vented out. On the fifth attempt it exploded. I remember the build up of pressure, and the next thing I knew I felt this thump in the side, and I was just flying through the air. It seemed in slow motion. Things happen so fast, your brain can't keep up with them.'

'I was something like 30ft away behind two battened-down doors. It was just the pure blast that hit us. And it killed Staff Sergeant Prescott outright. He was right next to me. I was conscious the whole time. I heard the bang. I thought "Jesus! Here we go", and then there was a whoosh, and I was carried through the air the whole length of the flight deck. I remember hitting the wall, and I saw the arm sort of just hanging there. It wasn't completely severed. It was partially severed, so I had a good feel around to see what other injuries there were, hoping that nothing else was serious.'

'Then after a few seconds — though it seemed like minutes — I stood up, expecting to feel pain in my legs, but there was no pain. Then I remember a sailor coming up to me, putting his hand on my shoulder, and saying, "Follow me". I said "What about Jim? Where's my mate?", and he says "Don't worry about him. He's dead." Just like that. There was fire and chaos. I remember walking out past Jim, and the door was bent double in a U-shape. That's quite a thick door, and it obviously hit him and hit me, and took my arm. It was just pure blast and build-up of pressure.'

'We'd told the crew to leave all the stations and go up on the flight deck, so there was no problem there with any injuries on their part. I followed the sailor to the exit, and we went up the hatchway onto the flight deck. They put a tourniquet on, and gave me a morphine jab, and as coincidence would have it the ship's doctor lives no more than a mile away from where I live, so we were talking about Gravesend,

43

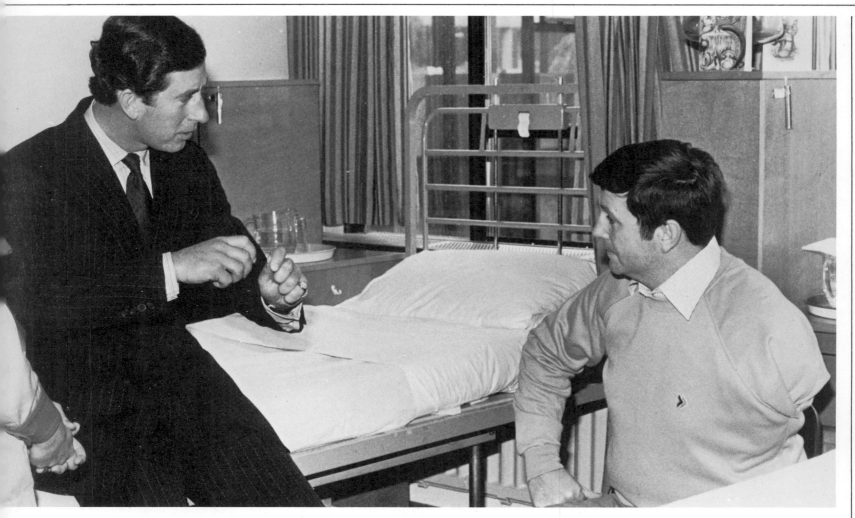

WO John Phillips talks to Prince Charles at the Queen Elizabeth Military Hospital, Woolwich.

where I'm living at the moment. I suppose he was trying to keep me calm, and then after about 30 minutes I abandoned ship with the crew.'

Eventually, as the fire reached the magazines, the *Antelope* blew up, spectacularly. WO Phillips was ferried to an emergency hospital set up in a converted refrigeration unit in Ajax Bay, where they immediately removed his injured arm. Two days later he was helicoptered out to *Uganda*. 'I knew I'd lost it. Because it was in my pullover, and I kept hold of it just in case they could do something, but obviously in those conditions . . . probably back in a proper hospital they might have done something, but in those conditions it was impossible, and there were so many other people coming in anyway. So it had to be done, and that was it. There was no surprise when he woke me up and told me he'd taken it off. No surprise at all. I fully expected it. I was just glad that I was there to listen to him speak.'

He stayed on *Uganda* for two or three weeks, for the wound was infected, and he could not be moved. Eventually he was returned to the UK via Montevideo

and Ascension Island, and was taken to Woolwich hospital. Only two days after arriving on *Uganda* he had started to get out of bed and walk, and deliberately stopped taking most of the pills and tablets being given to him, apart from a simple painkiller. After a week in Woolwich he went home for the weekend. He was in and out of hospital for a short time, then became an outpatient. He had some sick leave, and then, just after the August Bank Holiday, he returned to work. It was less than ten weeks since he had been blown up.

'I was back on duty in September. A discharge wasn't offered at the time, not immediately. All those who were able to return to duty did so. Then the facts were put to them, what their careers were, and what the options were. The decision was left entirely up to myself. The option for me was a medical discharge, with a view to a pension, which I'm entitled to anyway, having completed 22 years. And, obviously, a disability pension and a small lump sum — or soldier on. And I decided to soldier on. I'd reached a position of Warrant Officer 1, which everybody strives for, and

I wanted the chance to be a WO 1. I mean, that's what I've wanted all the way through my army career. And I wasn't going to lose it just for the sake of being ill.'

'So I decided to soldier on, hopefully with the prospect of going on to commissioned rank, and to the age of 55. I'm 40 now. I'm in the army now until July 1985. However, if I'm selected for commissioning, then it will be extended, five years at a time. This is all I know. I left school as a boy soldier at 15. I've never known civvy street. I don't know any other life than the army, and I was given the opportunity, and I took it. After careful consideration. It wasn't an immediate response. I considered it from both sides.'

'Since September I've done normal sergeant major jobs. I returned to the operational roster as well. We have a bomb disposal officer on duty for a week. We're on call-out all the time, you see. Whatever calls come up in that period you go and deal with. We cover the UK. Conventional weapons. World War 2 weapons — general bombs and beach mines.'

What were his feelings on his first call-out after losing his arm? 'Well, I was on the duty roster, and I recall we had a bomb up in a gravel pit near Gravesend. It had been dredged up by a dredger in the Thames, and I don't know whether I'm crackers or what, but I had no fear at all. Because what you're doing, you're carrying out laid-out drills. And all military life is based on laid-out drills. And if you stick to those drills, things go reasonably well. So I had no real fear — I didn't recoil as I approached it or anything like that. We had a job to do. My OC came with me because he obviously had the same worries, and we did it together. That was in October. I did wonder how I'd react. I made a point of, if the call was mine, I went. I didn't let anybody else go instead — probably just to see my own reactions, and they were quite normal. I don't know if I'm a fatalist, or what it is. We did a beach mine as well. The bomb was rendered safe. The mine was exploded.'

John Phillips is up for selection for a commission in January or February, 1984. If selected he would probably finish his two-year tour as WO 1, and then become a full lieutenant. Two years after that he would be made captain. His physical recovery has been remarkably fast. His burst eardrums have healed perfectly, and he fulfils all the fitness requirements of the army medical boards for a man of his age. Understandably, in the beginning, he had fits of depression over the loss of his arm, but says that he received good treatment from his wife, who is a psychiatric nurse. The bouts of depression no longer return. He has had a good adjustable false arm fitted, and can do almost everything necessary for his work without aid. As early as September 1982, he started to drive a car once more, acquiring an automatic with a knob adaptation on the wheel for his false hand to

grip. He often thinks about the Falklands, and wants to return there, as he never did get a chance to see them while he was there. 'I'm arranging a trip in November with the CO. I've dropped enough hints, and he's now taken it up, that we go down for a week, and have a look round, and see what it was all about.'

John Phillips attributes his successful return to duty to his army training. 'I see it as the military background. My military upbringing pushes me on. Everything was lost initially. I thought, "Christ, this is the end," you know, and then after I sat and thought about it for a while, I thought, "Well, why should I give in? Why not continue?" And I've tried to keep everything as normal as possible. If you sit back, and sigh, and say "Well, that's it!" then you're going to permanently sit down. But if you get up and make an effort... It wasn't a conscious decision, I don't think. All this is, I've lost my arm, and that's it. End of story.'

WO Phillips received the Distinguished Service Cross for his work in the Falklands. Staff Sergeant Prescott was awarded the Conspicuous Gallantry Medal posthumously.

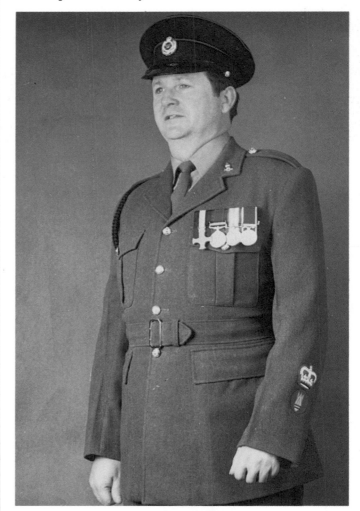

WO John Phillips with the Distinguished Service Cross which he won in the Falklands.

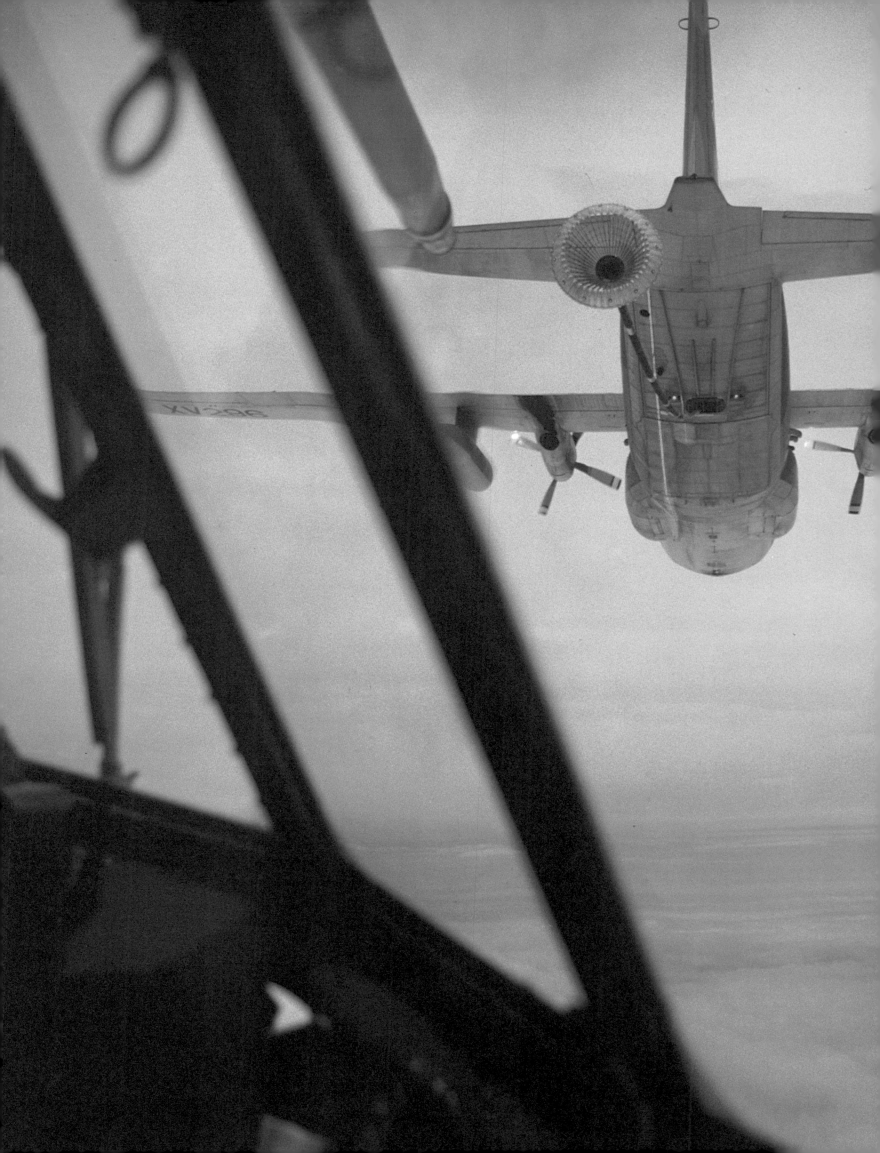

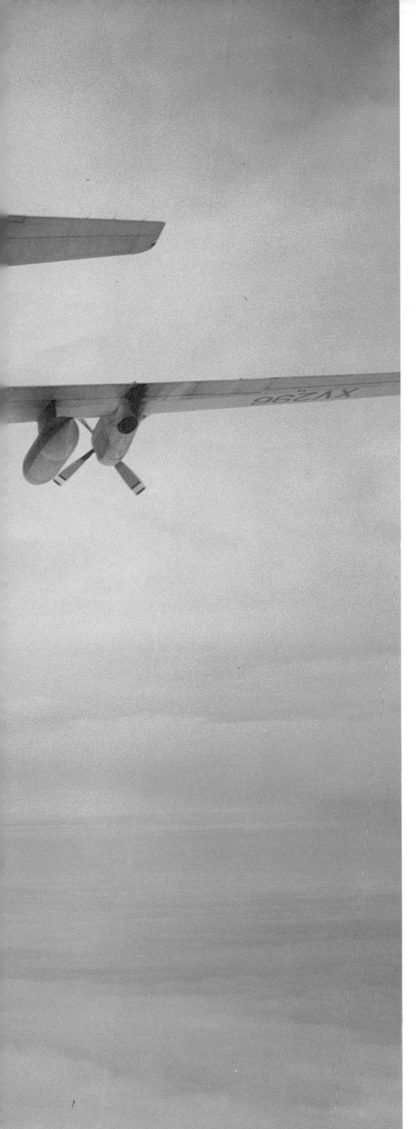

Chapter 3
THE AIR BRIDGE

Britain's vital link with the Falklands is the air bridge which RAF Hercules aircraft maintain by means of complex, expensive inflight refuelling. Now the decision has been taken to build a £220-million strategic airbase on East Falkland. This will allow operations by widebodied TriStar airliners without inflight refuelling, relieving the valiant Hercules of its gruelling workload. For the time being, however, Hercules battles on.

A Lockheed C-130 Hercules tanker refuels its partner on the long flight to Port Stanley.

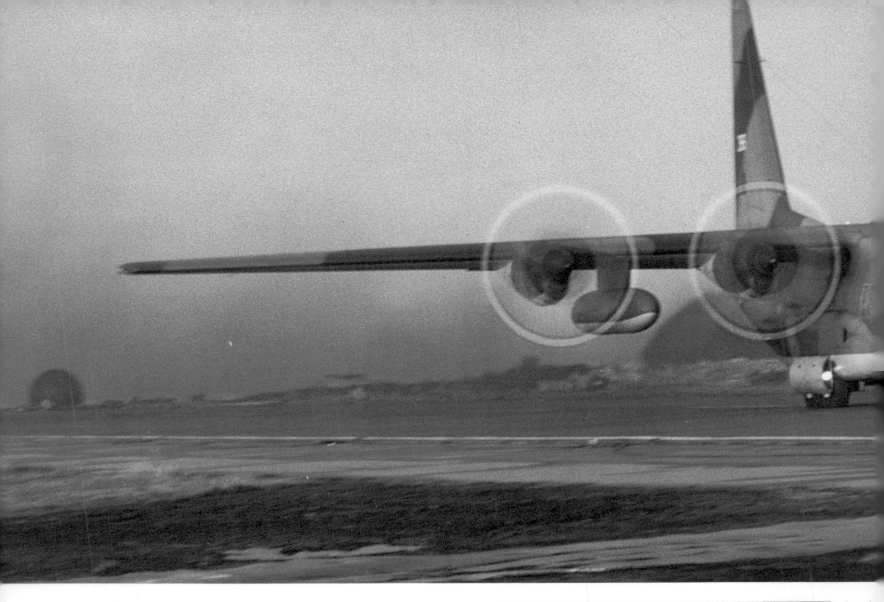

Imagine flying from London to Paris in a ferocious gale aboard a cold, cramped, ear-pounding, bone-shaking Hercules — and making the journey 35 times in a row. Flying to the Falklands has been like that since the war. The islands are almost as far west as New York and over 8000 miles south. RAF planes cannot land routinely in South America, for political reasons, and the weather is a constant threat. In addition Port Stanley airport is inadequate for long-range transport aircraft. Now the decision has been taken to build a major Falklands airbase not far from Stanley. How has the air bridge operated since the Argentine surrender in July 1982, and what is happening at and around RAF Stanley today?

Nature of the air bridge problem

RAF Stanley is at present one of the key airfields in the Western world. Under Station Commander Group Captain Bill Wratten, what in June 1982 had been a battlefield, a year later was an efficient air-logistics terminal and all-weather fighter base (if not a comfortable one). It has been home to almost 1000 people, though during 1983 this number began to decrease as the airfield needed less work and various military personnel dispersed to work in other parts of the islands. Some of the people live in ships, or in buildings in Port Stanley; most are

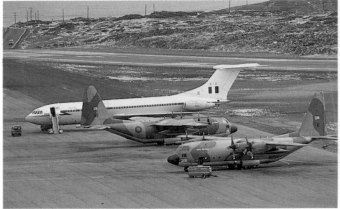

at last in warm Portakabins, and not many have been condemned to a second bitter winter in tents.

Over 100 members of the Tactical Communications Wing provide the full range of air-traffic control and airfield-control staff, met officers, firemen and similar supporting staff. They are in constant contact with ships, with Ascension, and via the Skynet satellite link, with the UK. About 70 serve with the RAF Stanley supply squadron, the air logistics organization. This number may grow. There are also essential maintenance staff, with skilled specialists in the major parts and systems of the Hercules and other aircraft types.

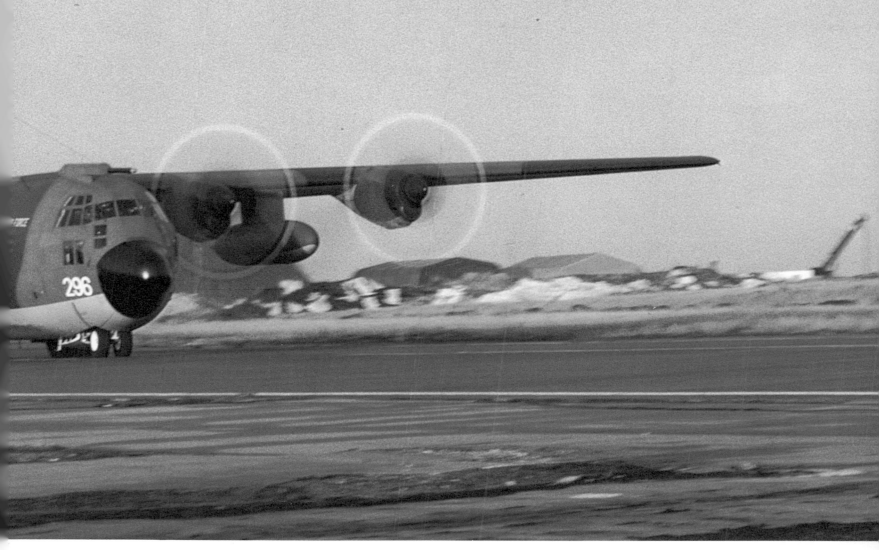

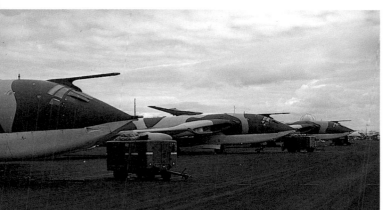

Top: Hercules on the runway at RAF Stanley. Left: One of the RAF's 13 VC10 transports, next to a C-130, Wideawake. Above: Victor K.2 tankers with refuelling probes.

Another important part of the airfield population is the RAF regiment, whose air-defence Rapiers are manned by squadrons on detachment, usually from RAF Germany (63 Squadron Gutersloh provided the first detachment, relieved in September 1982 by 37 Squadron from Brügen.)

If not for Ascension Island and its vital Wide-awake airfield, it would have been totally impossible to bring a single aircraft from Britain to the Falklands apart from helicopters and Harriers. Even with this invaluable staging post at roughly the half-way point the difficulties are enormous. The RAF has no modern long-range military freighter. The only types available are the Lockheed C-130 Hercules, backbone of the British air transport force, and the 13 VC10 C.1 transports operated by 10 Squadron at Brize Norton. The VC10 is reasonably long-ranged but was originally designed as a passenger airliner.

During Operation Corporate (the combined services operation to free the islands) this system was stretched to the utmost. Almost all the RAF aircraft involved were in a matter of days equipped with new weapons, new electronic warfare devices and provisions for inflight refuelling by the standard British probe/drogue method. If ever the technology of refuelling in flight proved worthwhile, Operation Corporate was the occasion. But the distance involved meant that the whole thing became ludicrous. A single round trip from Wideawake to the Total Exclusion Zone (TEZ) meant over 14 hours' nonstop flying (the record was set by a Hercules of 70 Squadron which had headwinds both ways: 28 hrs 4 min) with multiple refuellings. Everything conspired to add to the problems. There were no other options for bases (except possibly Rio de Janeiro) and Brazil was under intense diplomatic pressure from her neighbour Argentina to be at least coldly neutral. The long flight times demanded auxiliary fuel tanks and greatly reduced the available payload. And the tankers which were entailed, Victor K.2s, were designed to refuel fast jets, not slow propeller aircraft.

A short-term, stopgap solution

Although great progress had been made by the time the Argentine forces on the Falklands surrendered on 14 June 1982, it was mere tinkering with a problem that could be permanently solved only by purchasing long-distance aircraft which could fly such distances routinely. In the meantime, stopgap measures were needed. Flight Refuelling Ltd and Marshall of Cambridge (the engineering and support centre for RAF Hercules aircraft) accordingly sought out the required inflight-refuelling probes, designed and proved a probe installation for a Hercules and delivered six probed aircraft to the RAF. Crews had been trained, and a hair-raising downhill refuelling technique called tobogganing had been perfected.

In this technique, a Victor hooks up with a gently diving Hercules so that the latter can hold a speed in excess of 265mph, suitable for the swept-wing jet tanker. A typical refuelling involves such a descent, at 500 to 1000ft/min for about 15 minutes. Then the overweight 'Herc' struggles laboriously back to cruising height at around 23,000ft. The two companies designed and carried out a further modification which converted the Hercules into a tanker.

By chance, the RAF had in storage a number of cylindrical auxiliary fuel tanks originally produced for Andover C.1 aircraft. These are of 825 gal size, holding some 6600lb of fuel, and could easily be fitted inside a Hercules above the floor. Adding two tanks resulted in the LR2 (long-range two-tanks) modification of the Hercules C.1 while for a very few missions the LR4 (with four tanks) was produced. The first examples of each were in use while the fighting was still going on, alongside the final Falklands version, the PLR2 Hercules variant, a probed design with two auxiliary tanks. Another important modification was to install the Omega global navigation aid, a very low frequency (VLF) receiver which dramatically improves track-keeping accuracy, especially in remote regions.

Good navigation is essential in an operation dependent on flight refuelling. In some missions both tanker and receiver flew together in loose formation, but occasionally a rendezvous had to be achieved. None of the Hercules pilots had any experience of air-to-air refuelling (AAR) but they were speedily passed out as qualified and there have been very few major problems. Early in the post-war operations a probe tip was broken — an extremely rare occurrence despite turbulent air at Hercules heights in the South Atlantic — necessitating a diversion to Rio.

Hercules turns tanker

Major internal refitting and a projecting probe turns the Hercules transport into an airborne fuel tanker. Marshall of Cambridge were chosen to complete the conversion at lightning speed. Tanks in the belly of the plane hold the fuel, feeding it out via the hose drum unit (mounted on the cargo ramp) and drogue (bottom right). The receiving aircraft uses a nose probe (below) to make the connection. When the war began, none of the RAF's Hercules pilots had any experience of air-to-air refuelling. The procedure has since become routine. A single trip currently costs £50,000.

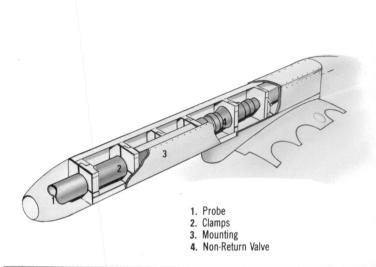

1. Probe
2. Clamps
3. Mounting
4. Non-Return Valve

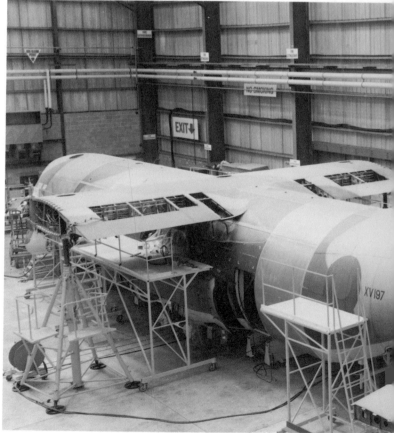

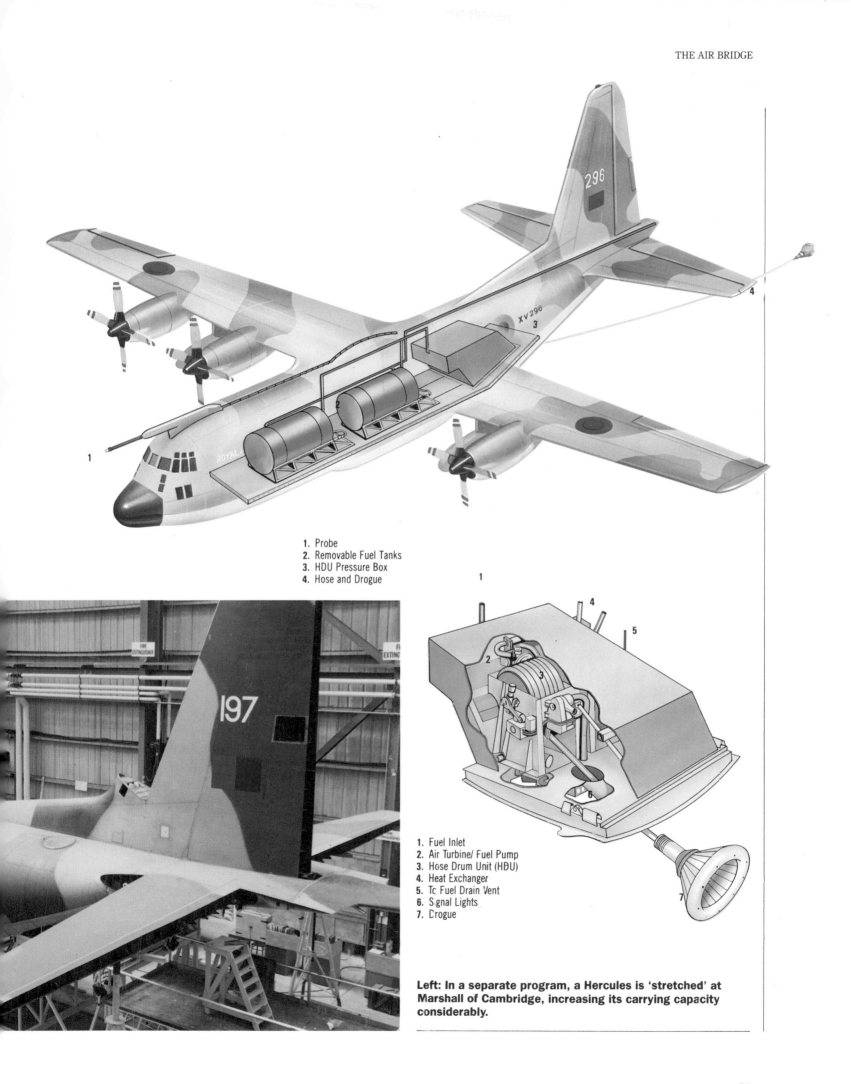

1. Probe
2. Removable Fuel Tanks
3. HDU Pressure Box
4. Hose and Drogue

1. Fuel Inlet
2. Air Turbine/ Fuel Pump
3. Hose Drum Unit (HDU)
4. Heat Exchanger
5. Tc Fuel Drain Vent
6. Signal Lights
7. Drogue

Left: In a separate program, a Hercules is 'stretched' at Marshall of Cambridge, increasing its carrying capacity considerably.

On the whole the vital AAR operation has been a routine affair with the Hercules. On a few occasions, however, sudden unexpected difficulty has been encountered, as when a tanker and Hercules tobogganed into a cloud. When this happened the anti-icing system of the Hercules switched on automatically, drawing hot compressed air from the four T56 turbo-prop engines, and reducing the power transmitted to the propellers by about 15 per cent. The sudden deceleration resulted in a disconnection. There was a potential danger of collision, and the two aircraft gingerly worked their way up into clear air to hook up again.

The airfield on the Falklands is second rate by modern standards, yet from June 1982 it was suddenly the terminus of one of the world's major air routes. Originally called Port Stanley Airport, it became for a time Puerto Argentina and, in late June 1982, RAF Stanley. It was in a terrible state at that time, and even a year later the entire area to the north of the airfield, to the coast of Port William, is dangerous because of numerous mines and the possibility of booby traps. The sheer quantity of explosive devices removed from this site is astonishing. Around the airport was found quite a high proportion of the total 1,477,220 dumped rounds of small-arms ammunition; other abandoned arms, hastily dumped by the fleeing Argentines, included heaps of bombs, mines and napalm.

The weather posed another problem. RAF pilots, especially Hercules captains, are used to bad weather and even landing in poor visibility, and one of the first things done at RAF Stanley was to install not only air-defence radar (completed on June 18) but also air traffic control facilities and an instrument landing system (ILS) to minimize the occasions when aircraft could not land. Crosswinds at Port Stanley are often excessive. The Hercules has a narrow main landing-gear track of 14ft 3in, and if a Force 10 gale is blowing — as in the Falklands winter when the fighting took place — it does not have to be very far off the east-west direction for Hercules landings to be ruled out. Only a highly professional crew can accept such a fact, calmly suffer 25 hours of ear-pounding and discomfort for no purpose, and return to Ascension.

All this work was not in vain. The first Hercules to land at RAF Stanley touched down on 24 June — just 11 days after the last Argentine C-130 had departed — to bring in an air-movements party with the vital equipment needed for loading and unloading aircraft. Most of the aviation-turbine fuel came in by ship. The main purpose of the air bridge was to bring in the endless variety of urgent supplies and specialist personnel and to take out casualties, mail and other loads. Once the air-movements staff had established an operative apron the air bridge quickly built up.

The Black Buck ultra-long-range bombing raids during the war by Vulcans had resulted in just one

Member of RAF ground crew moving into action with a fuel feed. A routine Hercules flight to Port Stanley will involve hundreds of groundcrew from computer operators monitoring loading operations to security guards at Wideawake.

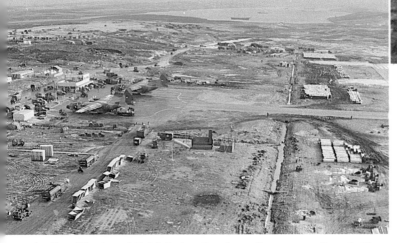

Top: Stanley airfield during the Argentine occupation. In the foreground, in an improvised bay, is a Pucará. On the runway is the temporarily filled crater left by a 1000lb RAF bomb. Above: An aeriel view reveals the formidable task which confronted the Royal Engineers.

large crater from a 1000lb bomb in the middle of the Stanley runway. This served its purpose in closing the runway to Mirages and other high-performance jets, but posed no problem for the Argentine transports, including C-130s, which were airborne long before they reached it on their lightweight takeoffs on return to the mainland. It was a different matter for the RAF Hercules after the Argentine desertion, however, which were so near maximum weight with full tanks that, even into a strong wind, they were still on the ground by the time they met the badly filled crater.

This gave an added urgency to runway improvement, and eventually the decision was taken to close the runway for improvements on 15 August 1982.

A better terminal airport was also needed. Even before the surrender on 14 June the Ministry of Defence in London had begun to discuss the pros and cons of extending Stanley and building a new airport. A decision about this had to await the retaking of the islands and a full survey. The runway issue was more clear cut; it had been apparent from the start that once the islands were restored to British sovereignty it would be essential to improve the Stanley runway, so making life easier for the transports and allowing operations by defending CTOL fighters (conventional takeoff and landing aircraft, as distinct from Harriers). To improve the tattered runway, a quantity of airfield matting (AM-2) made of aluminium was purchased from the US and shipped to the islands to resurface and extend the runway — no easy task, since there were still no proper port facilities, and to lay the matting calls for much heavy plant and equipment. Here again the presence of thousands of explosive devices, a large proportion containing so little metal that they were undetectable by mine detector, greatly hampered the work, which was done in the depth of winter. (The runway could have been extended by conventional means, with concrete, but this would have taken years.)

The air bridge was at once back to 25 or 26-hour round trips, with loads airdropped by various techniques. There was one important addition: a 'snatch' pick-up facility.

Some 30 snatches, for personal mail and official written documents and other loads, were made before the runway improvements allowed Hercules landings to resume on 28 August. The AM-2 matting was not only laid on the original runway, which was tarmac on natural bedrock (very unusual for an airfield), paying special attention to the bomb crater, but it was continued over freshly prepared foundations to extend the runway from 4100ft to a new length of 6000ft. This is adequate, but not overgenerous, for Phantoms to operate with full internal fuel and air-defence weapons such as two pairs of AIM-9L Sidewinders. It solved the length problem for Hercules operations, and made the strip adequate for VC10 operations, but the runway is lacking in strength and width, and so far no VC10 landings have been reported.

As Lt-Colonel PR Ievers wrote in the *Royal Engineers Journal*, repairs to runways do not generally cause problems to a construction squadron trained in airfield repair. On the Falklands, however, many of the important stores and stockpiles were missing. There was no ready crushed rock for crater filling, the main stocks of equipment and spare parts were a 16,000-mile round trip away and finally winds were gusting at 30 knots. There was the added hazard that the aluminium AM2 airfield matting could 'take off' as troops were laying it, and become a dangerous missile.

Runway extension

When it came to laying, eight mixed troops of sappers and infantry worked a three hours-on and six hours-off shift, with two troops at a time on the airfield. The work was completed by 28 August, and the first landing took place a day later.

The runway extension was a demanding task for the plant operators, who before laying a complex sandwich of crushed rock, sand and man-made fibre matting, had to dig out and fill two Vulcan craters.

Rotary Hydraulic Arrester Gear was installed at either end of the runway — three US and two British RHAGs were installed, though it was necessary to prepare six installation points. The high water table, mud, gales, snow, sleet and hail all conspired to make the task a slow and grim one, but by 18 October the men of 3 and 50 Field Squadrons had the satisfaction of seeing the first Phantom take a US RHAG.

A vital part of the whole runway operation was the quarry and rock-crushing work. As demand rose to 1000 tonnes or more per day and the extremely hard Falklands fine-grained quartzite granite began to wear out the drilling and crushing equipment, the quarries became a minor epic in the sapper operation on the Falklands.

A temporary quarry was begun in the winter months of July to provide surface material for roads. On 25 August the old quarry used by the civilian Johnsons contractors who built the airfield was re-opened. It had to be pumped out for three days and then rubbish and ammunition removed. Argentine defensive positions could still be seen above the quarry. The second quarry was taken over by 60 Squadron. Rock production passed from 50 Field Squadron, through Support Squadron to 24 Squadron (who took over from 60 in the summer).

Engineers from Atlas Copco — a rock-drill firm — came out to the Falklands to give expert advice on the Atlas Copco 301 drills. They arrived with two larger 601 drills which they put into use.

More civilian advice came from the firm of Goodwin Barsby whose Goliath rock-crushing equipment was an essential part of the operation.

By early December the quarry teams had produced over 100,000 tonnes of crushed rock for construction projects around the island.

Birth of the new airbase

A larger issue was whether or not to build a new Falklands airfield. Such an undertaking would inevitably mean spending a very large sum in order to construct an infrastructure that could never be taken away and might, in the long term, merely be inherited by Argentina. The decision to mount Operation Corporate in the first place was taken for two reasons: to protect British nationals and to uphold the rule of International Law. But suppose over a long period the environment of what had become a besieged fortress ceased to feel like home to the Falkland Islanders? A giant new airbase would in that case become a major liability.

This kind of consideration weighed in the discussions, and although Cabinet papers will be secret for another 29 years, the 'bottom line' was that there just had to be at least a much better airfield, if not a new one. It is not uncommon for governments to make the wrong decisions because they fear loss of face. Faced with the situation in the summer of 1982, Mrs Thatcher's government could see no alternative to taking the bull by the horns and accepting all the costs and problems of maintaining a major Falklands garrison.

There are good reasons for building the new airbase on a new site. The runway at RAF Stanley could be extended beyond 6000ft only with stupendous effort at great cost. At its present length it is just adequate for Phantoms, and trials at the Aeroplane & Armament Experimental Establishment at Boscombe Down confirmed that it could safely be used by Nimrods, which fly essential long-range patrol, anti-submarine and (in AEW.3 form) high-flying airborne warning and control system missions (Awacs), of the

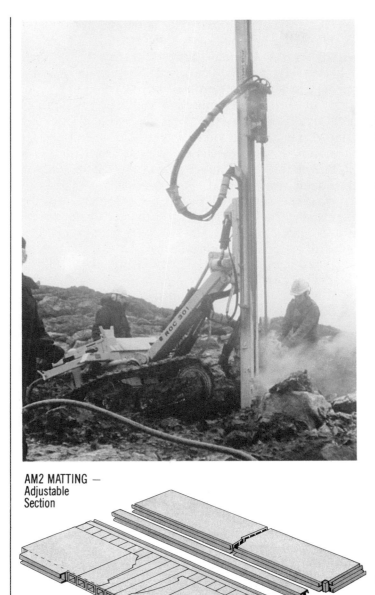

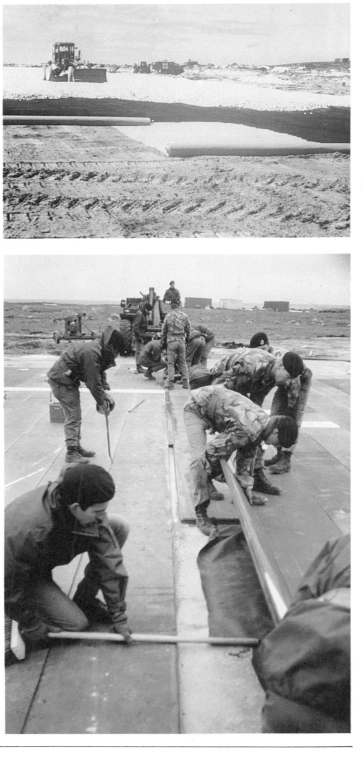

AM2 MATTING —
Adjustable
Section

**Repairing the
tattered runway
required painstaking
preparation. Rock drills extracted vital aggregate (top)
which then formed part of the 4-layer runway 'sandwich'
(top right). The last layer was the AM-2 matting (right and
above). The wind threatened to turn the strips into lethal
frisbees.**

kind lacking during the Operation Corporate.

With severe cross winds the extremely accurate presentation of the Nimrod at the runway threshold places demands on the pilot, flying manually, but safety is not considered to be jeopardized and Nimrod operations might be announced from RAF Stanley before the end of 1983. In addition, a new airbase is needed because more than one runway is called for on a besieged island, and also because (as we have seen) the RAF needs bigger, longer-ranged aircraft for

which the present runway is inadequate.

By July 1983 firm plans had been disclosed. Of two sites surveyed for a possible future Falklands main airbase, the preferred one is called March Ridge near Mount Pleasant, some 20 miles west-south-west of Stanley. Here the terrain is reasonably firm, level and free from waterlogging, and the approaches are quite good (as they are in most parts of the island). The new base will have an 8500ft runway, wider and stronger than that at RAF Stanley, and in view of the

RAF Stanley

In June 1982 Port Stanley Airport was transformed from a sleepy, second rate site into one of the busiest strategic airfields in the Western world. Under the direction of Major Robert C Morgan RE, crucial improvements were made to allow Hercules and Phantom operations. Work was complicated by abandoned explosives. Lack of materials and perilous 30-knot winds made the final achievement still more impressive.

Hangers

Dispersal Area

New 2000′ Runway Extension

Apron

Terminal Building and Control Tower

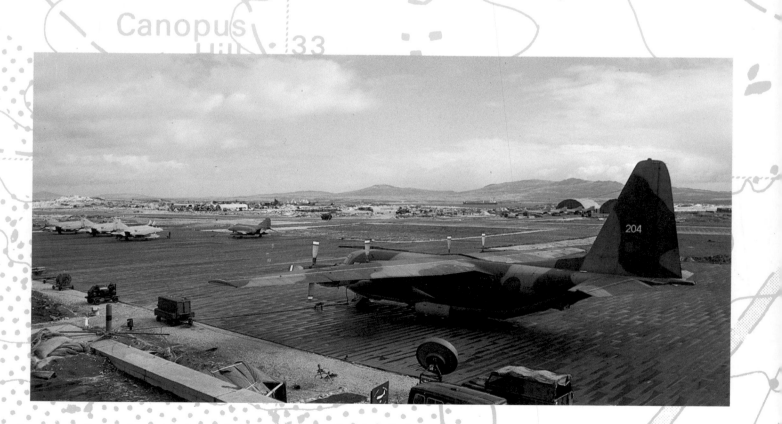

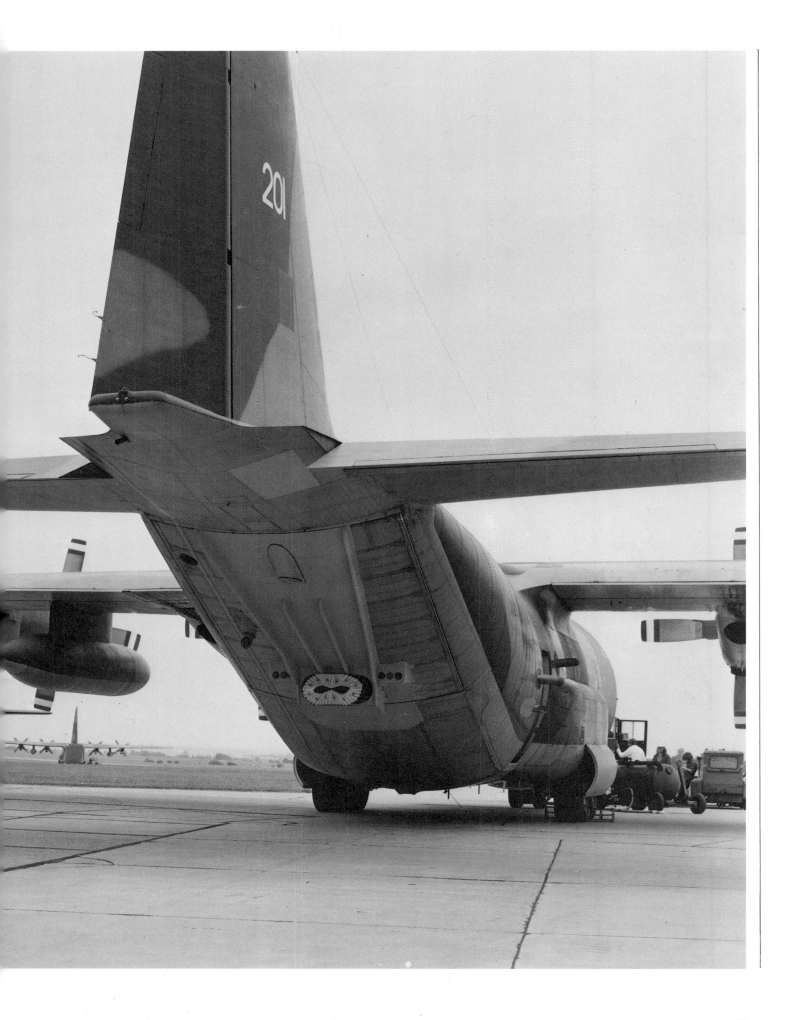

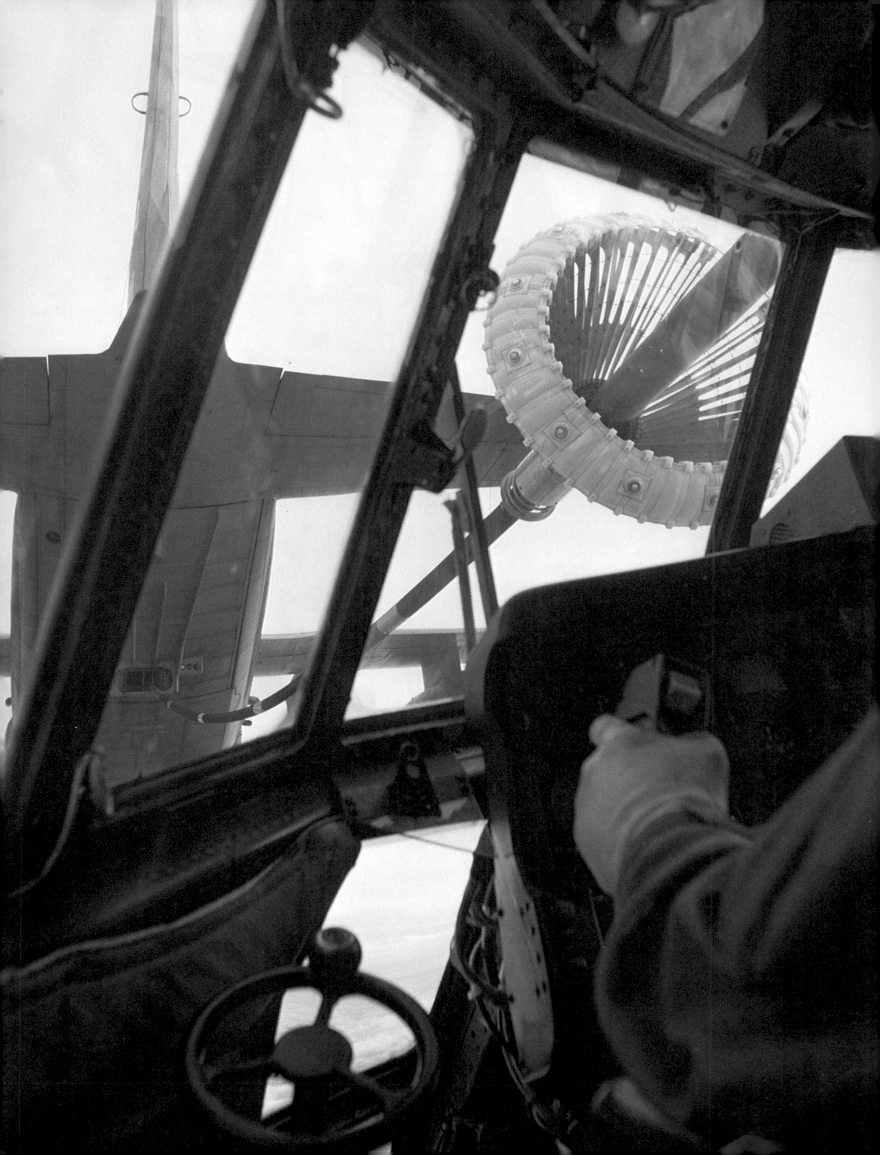